skinnytaste®

high protein

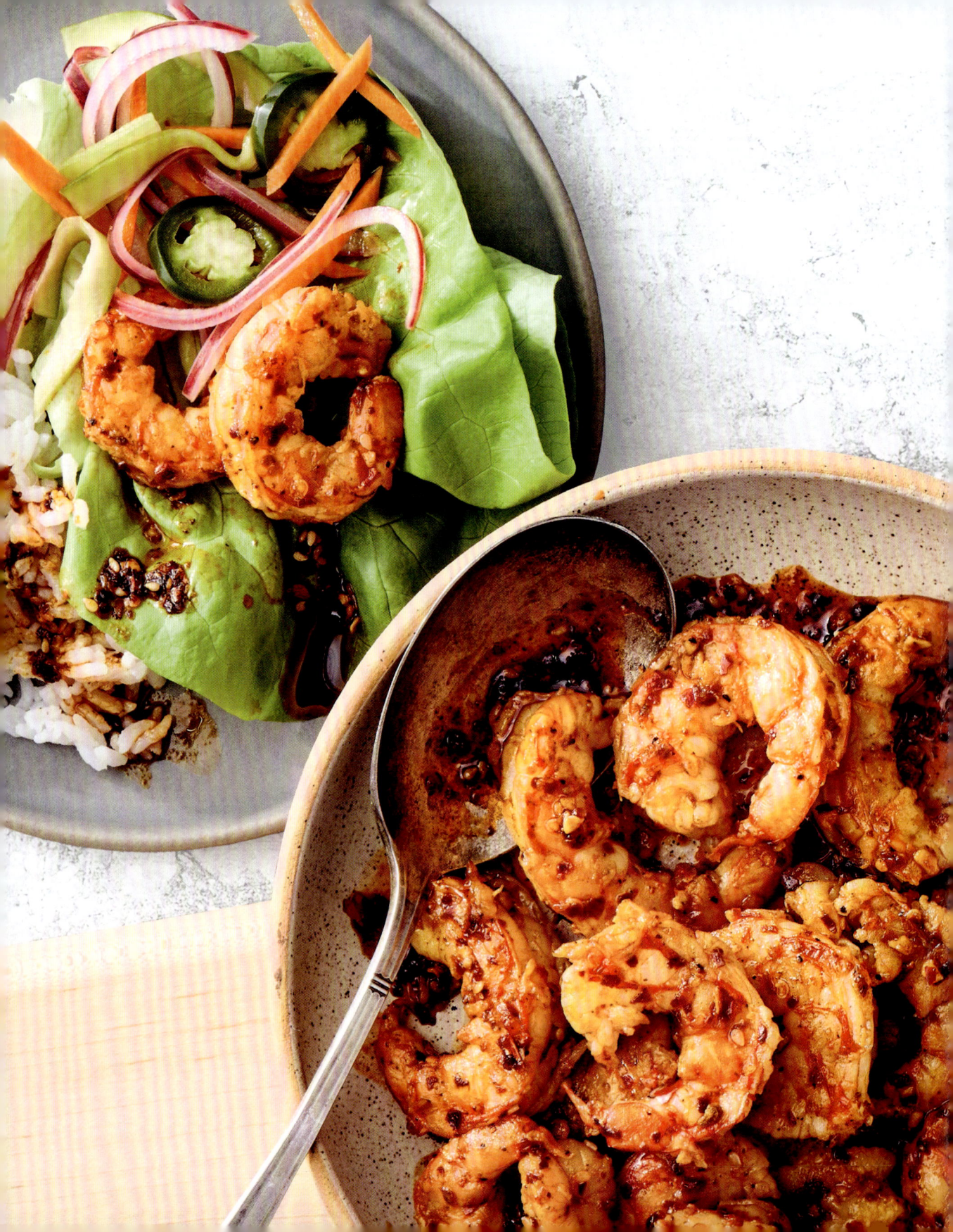

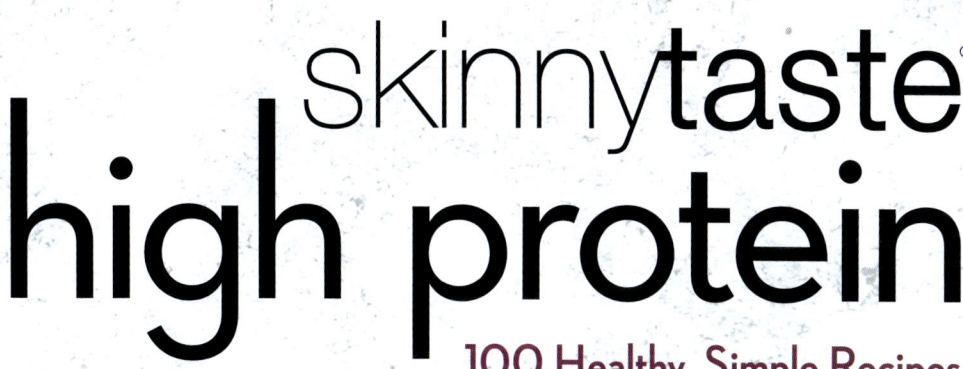

skinnytaste®
high protein

100 Healthy, Simple Recipes
to Fuel Your Day

Gina Homolka
with Heather K. Jones, R.D.

PHOTOGRAPHS BY EVA KOLENKO
LIFESTYLE PHOTOGRAPHS BY VICTORIA JANASHVILI

Clarkson Potter/Publishers
New York

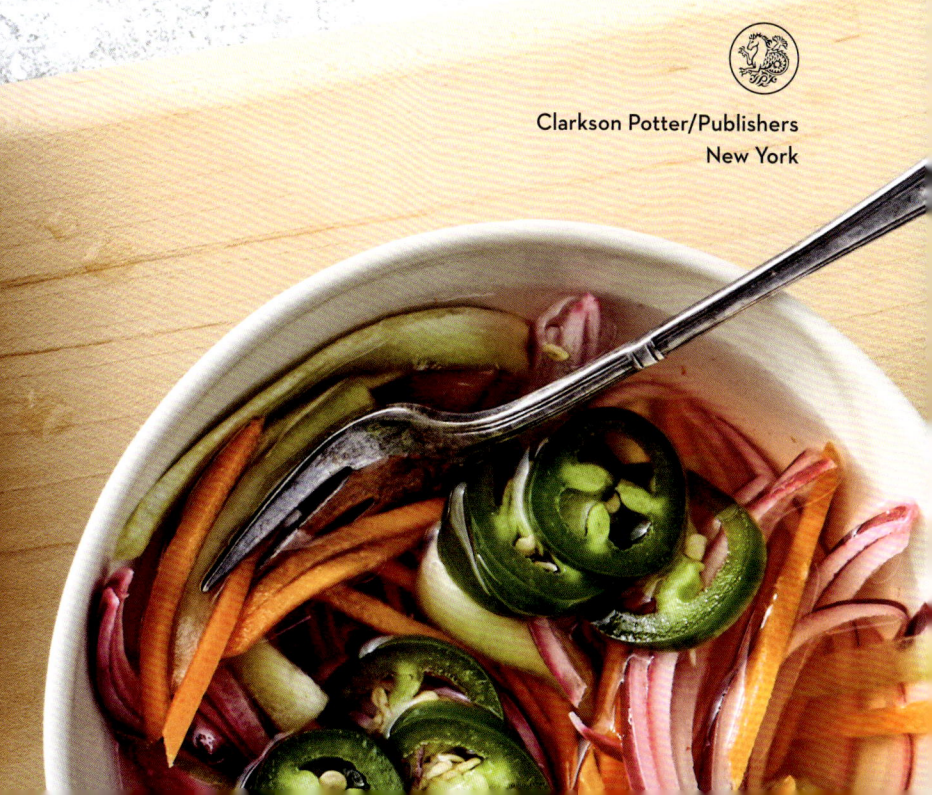

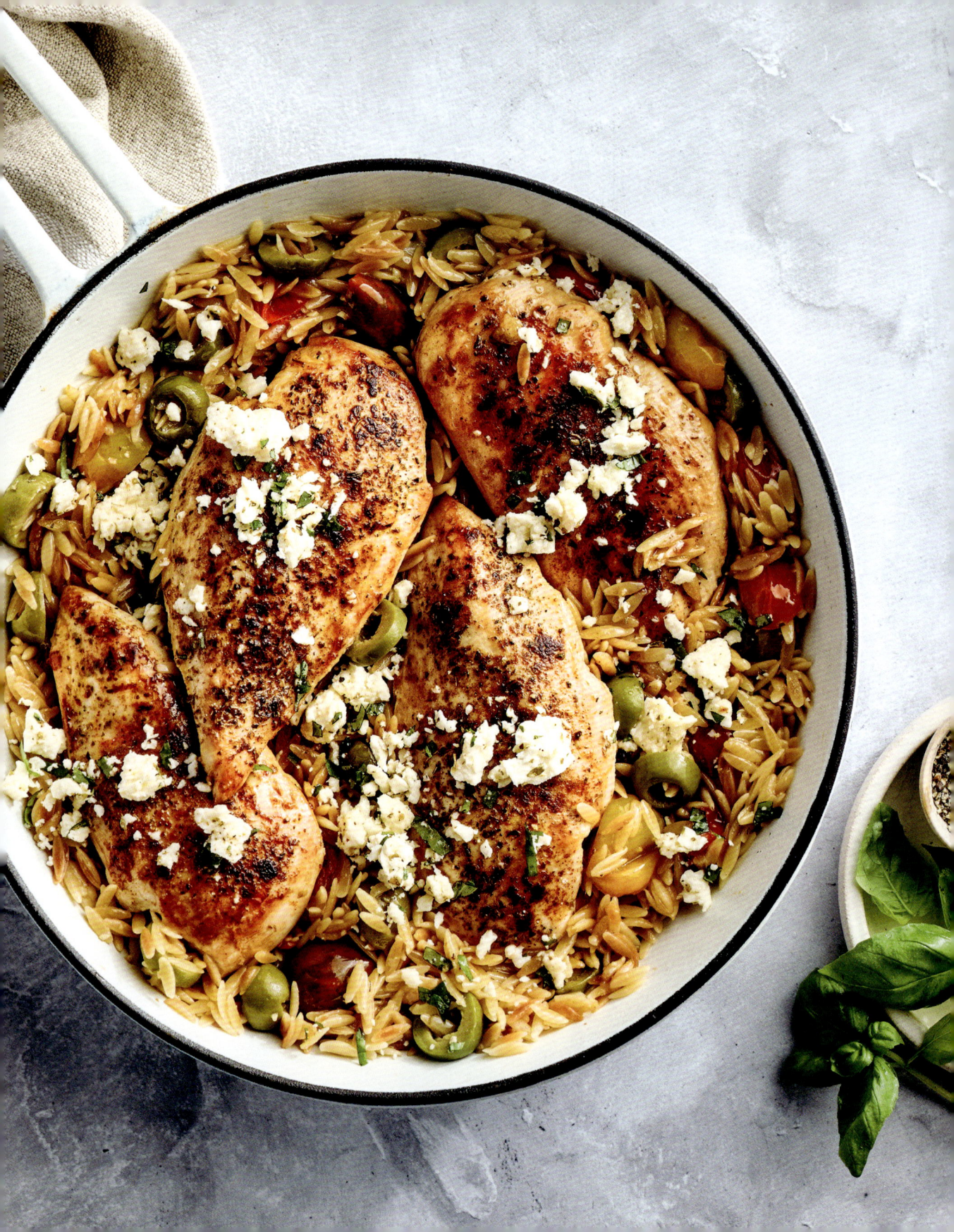

Contents

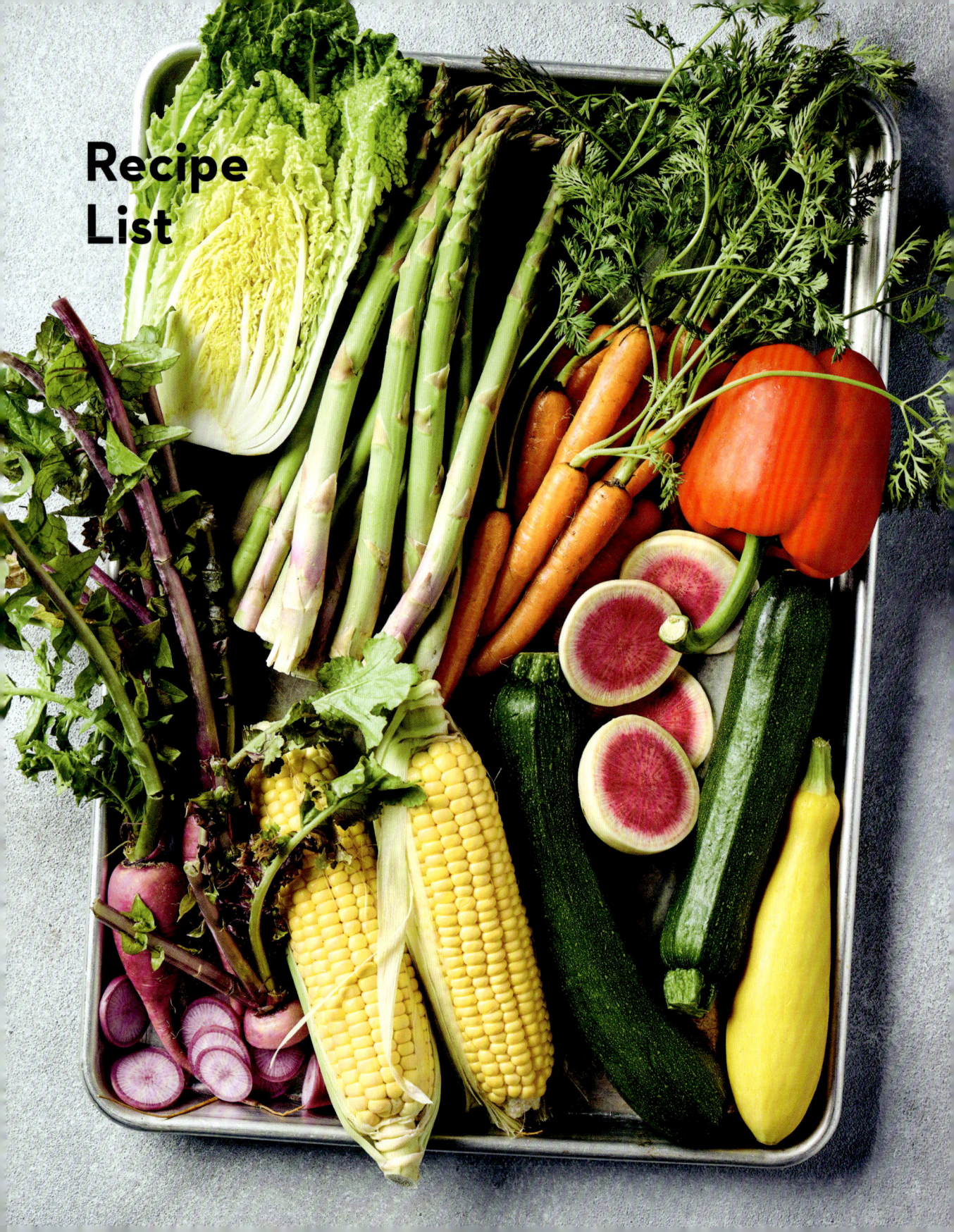

Recipe
List

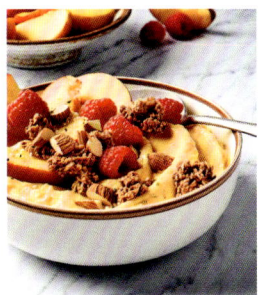

Peaches & Cream Smoothie Bowl, page 33

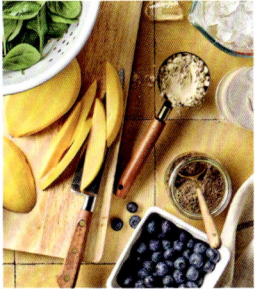

Mango Blueberry Smoothie, page 34

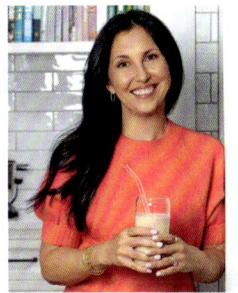

Cinnamon Oatmeal Raisin Smoothie, page 37

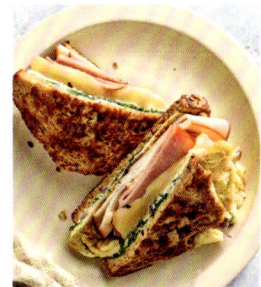

Monte Cristo Omelet Sandwich, page 38

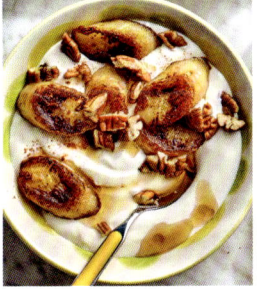

Caramelized Banana Yogurt Bowl with Maple & Pecans, page 41

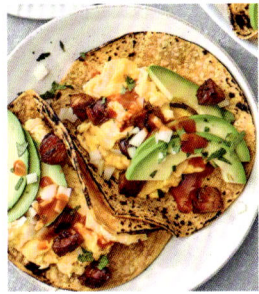

Chicken Chorizo Breakfast Tacos, page 42

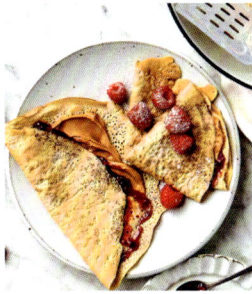

PB&J Crepes, page 45

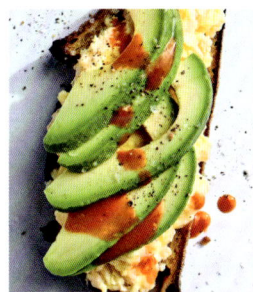

Avocado Toast with Cottage Cheese Eggs, page 46

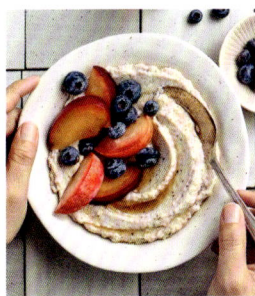

Creamy Protein Oats, page 49

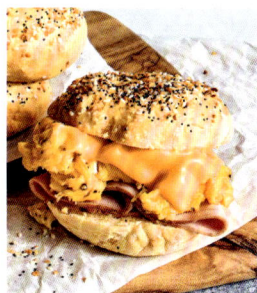

Air Fryer Breakfast Bagel Sandwiches, page 50

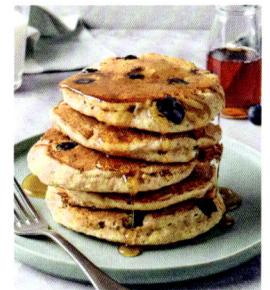

Blueberry-Lemon Cottage Cheese Oat Pancakes, page 53

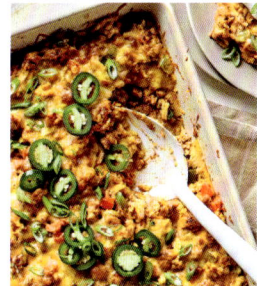

Enchilada Breakfast Casserole, page 54

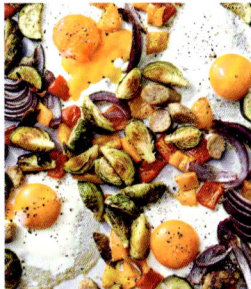

Sheet Pan Breakfast with Veggie Hash, page 57

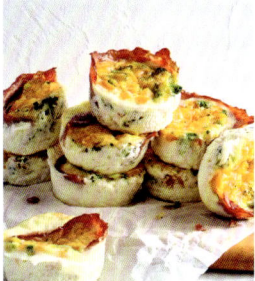

Egg White Cottage Cheese Muffins with Turkey Bacon, page 58

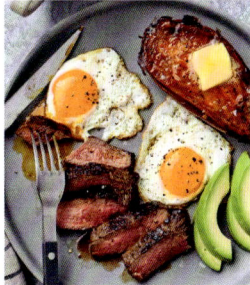

Steak & Eggs, page 61

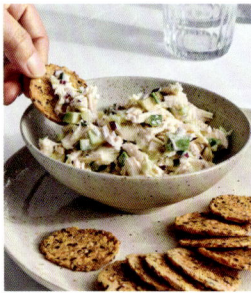

Chicken Avocado Salad
Chip Dip, page 64

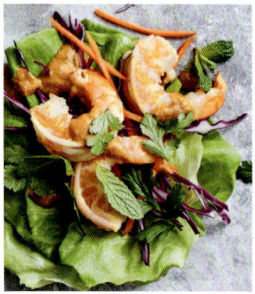

Shrimp Summer Roll
Lettuce Wraps, page 67

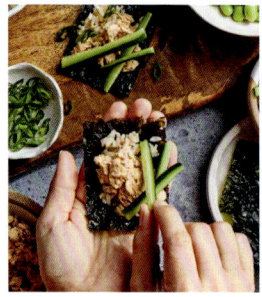

Spicy Salmon Hand
Rolls, page 68

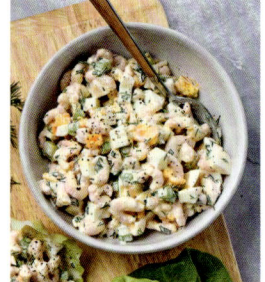

Chilled Shrimp Salad
with Eggs, page 71

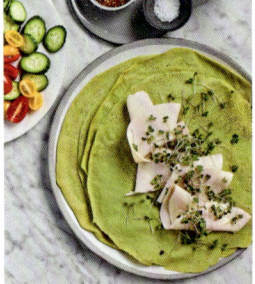

Spinach Egg Wraps,
page 72

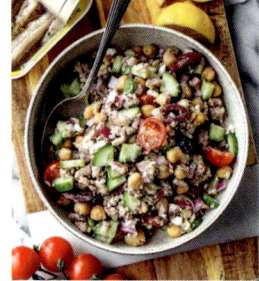

Mediterranean Sardine
Salad, page 75

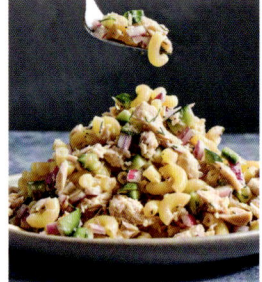

Tuna Macaroni
Salad, page 76

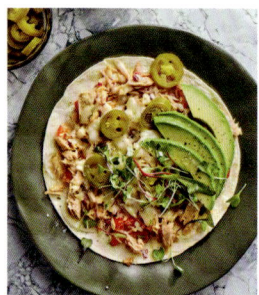

Spicy Tuna Queso
Melt, page 79

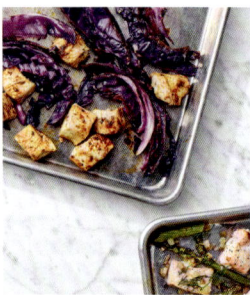

Choose-Your-Adventure
Protein Sheet Pan Bake,
page 80

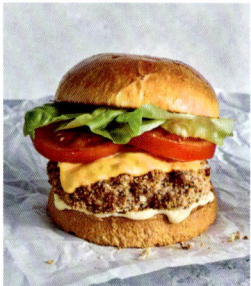

Air Fryer Crispy Chicken
Patty Sandwiches, page 82

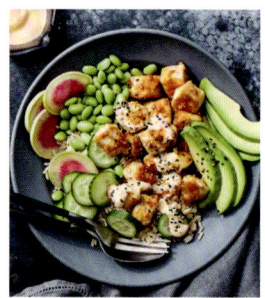

Spicy Chicken Poke Bowl,
page 85

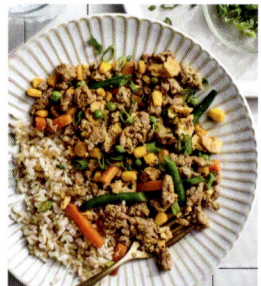

10-Minute Meal Prep
Deconstructed Fried
Rice Bowls, page 86

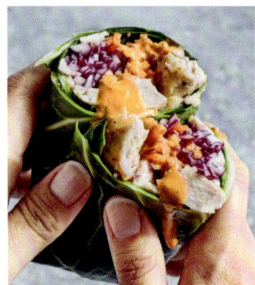

Chicken Collard Wrap
with Peanut Sesame
Dipping Sauce, page 89

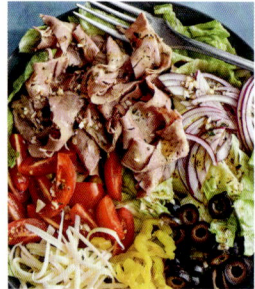

Italian Roast Beef Sub Salad,
page 90

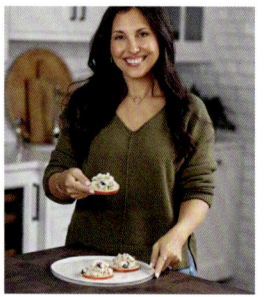

Cranberry Chicken Salad
on Apple Slices, page 93

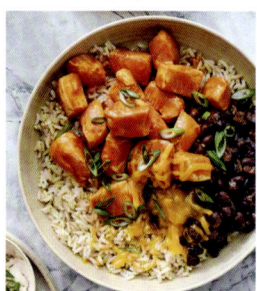

Buffalo Chicken Rice Bowls,
page 94

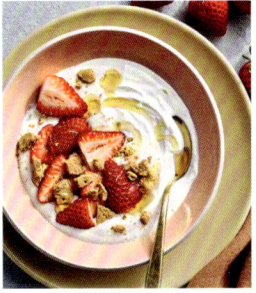

No-Bake Cottage Cheese
Cheesecake Bowl with
Strawberries, page 98

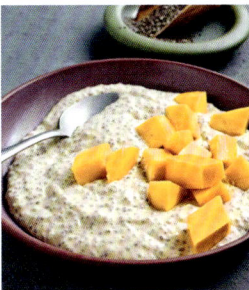

Mango Yogurt Chia
Pudding, page 101

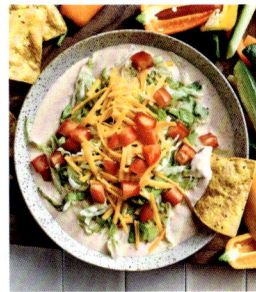

Yogurt Taco Dip,
page 102

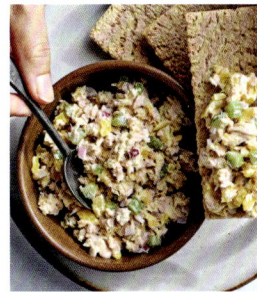

Zesty Banana Pepper
Tuna Salad with
Crackers, page 105

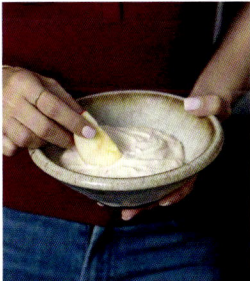

Peanut Butter Yogurt Dip
with Apples, page 106

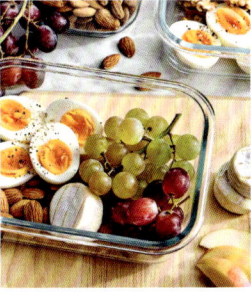

Protein Picnic Boxes,
page 109

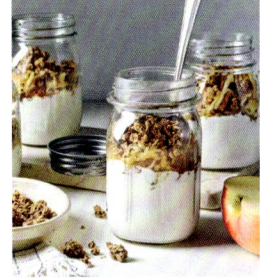

Fall Harvest Jars,
page 110

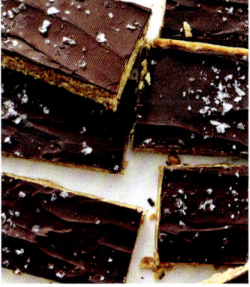

Peanut Butter Chocolate
Protein Bars, page 113

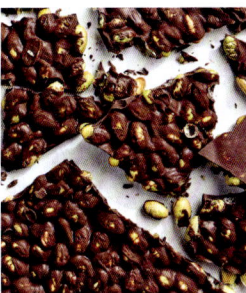

Chocolate Edamame Bark,
page 114

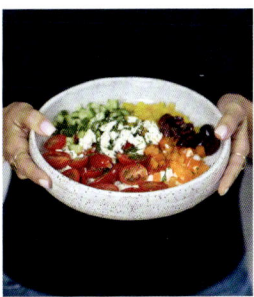

Greek Cottage Cheese
Bowl, page 117

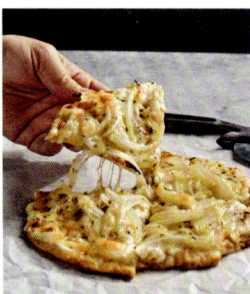

Fugazza (White Onion)
Personal Pizza, page 120

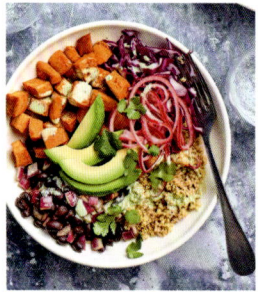

Black Bean Quinoa Bowls,
page 123

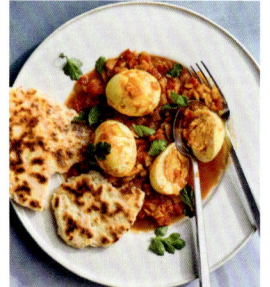

Egg Curry with
Yogurt Naan, page 124

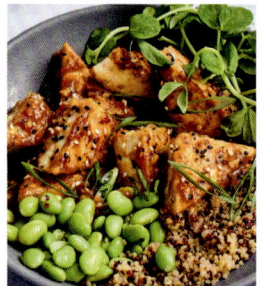

Sticky Glazed Tofu Quinoa
Bowls, page 127

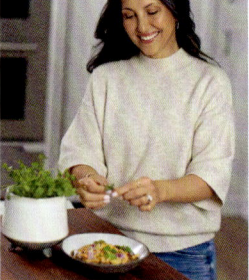

Lentil Chili, page 128

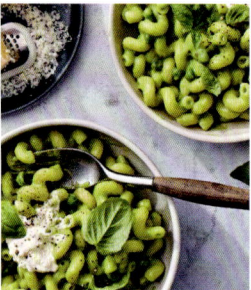

Creamy Parmesan & Peas
Pasta, page 131

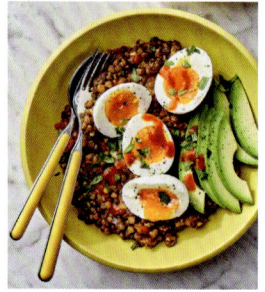

Tomato-Scallion Lentil Bowls
with Jammy Eggs, page 132

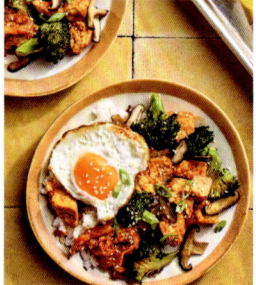

Sheet Pan Gochujang Tofu
with Vegetables, page 135

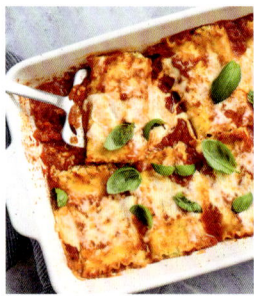

Lasagna Roll-Ups with
Cottage Cheese, page 136

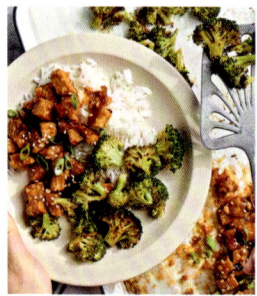

Sheet Pan Tempeh
& Broccoli, page 139

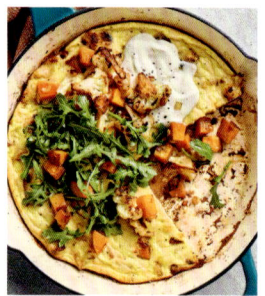

Roasted Autumn Veggie
Frittata, page 140

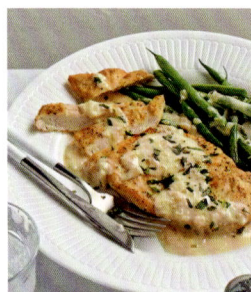

Creamy Mustard
Chicken, page 145

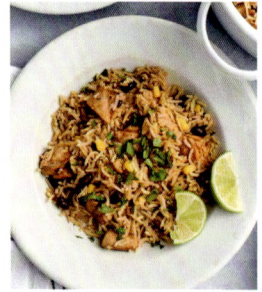

One-Pot Fiesta Chicken
& Rice, page 146

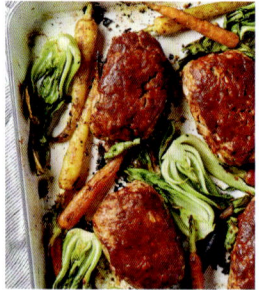

Sheet Pan Soy-Glazed
Meatloaf & Veggies,
page 149

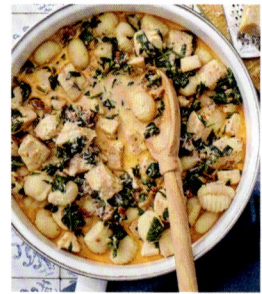

Marry Me Chicken
& Gnocchi, page 150

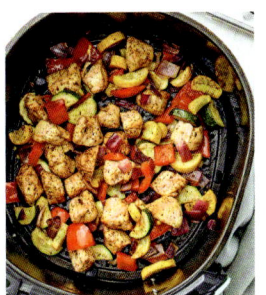

Air Fryer Cajun Chicken & Veggies, page 153

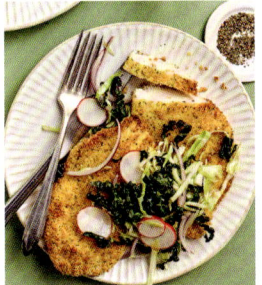

Air Fryer Chicken Schnitzel with Cabbage-Kale Slaw, page 154

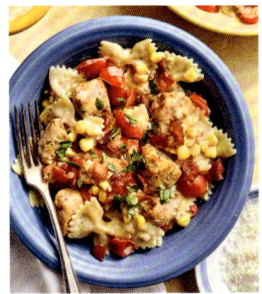

One-Pot Summer Pasta with Chicken, Corn & Bacon, page 157

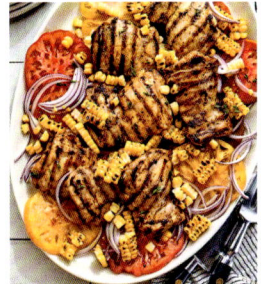

Grilled Chicken Thighs & Charred Corn Summer Salad, page 158

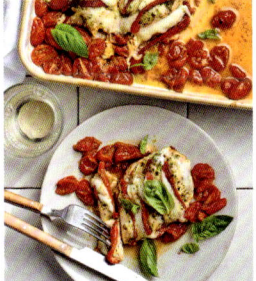

Pesto Pizza Chicken Bake, page 161

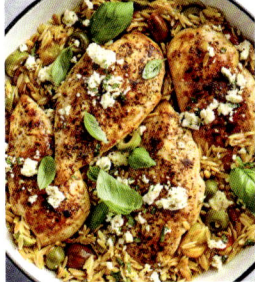

One-Pot Chicken Orzo Caprese, page 162

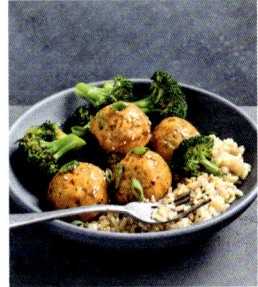

Baked Teriyaki Chicken Meatballs, page 165

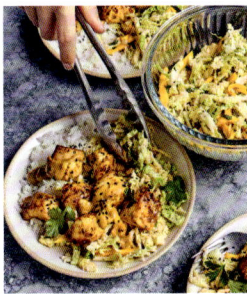

Air Fryer Chicken Satay Bowls with Spicy Peanut Sauce & Mango Slaw, page 166

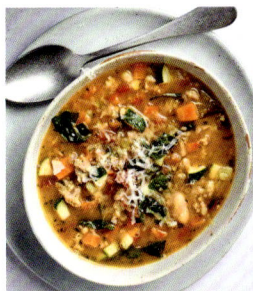

Shortcut Turkey Meatball Minestrone, page 169

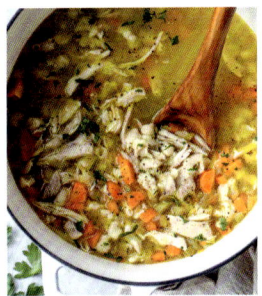

Chicken Spaetzle Soup, page 172

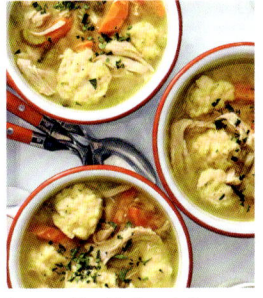

Instant Pot Turkey & Sage Dumpling Soup, page 175

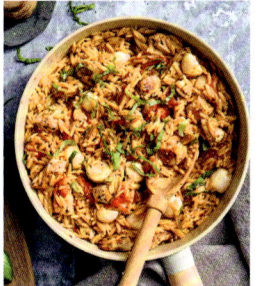

One-Pot Lemony Orzo with Chicken & Feta, page 176

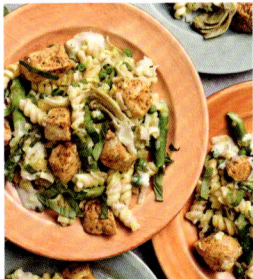

One-Pot Chicken Pasta Primavera, page 179

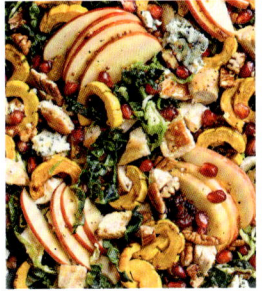

Hearty Autumn Salad with Chicken & Maple-Dijon Dressing, page 180

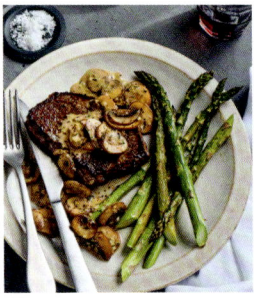

Seared Steaks with Dijon-Mushroom Sauce & Roasted Asparagus, page 185

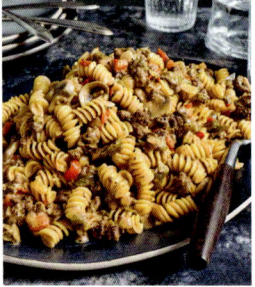

One-Pot Philly Cheesesteak Pasta, page 186

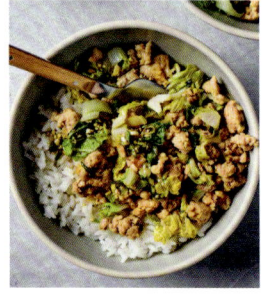

Potsticker Rice Bowls, page 189

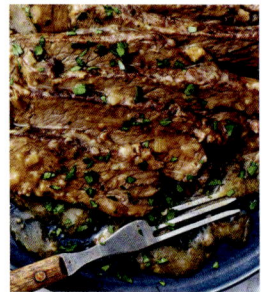

Sunday Pot Roast with Gravy, page 190

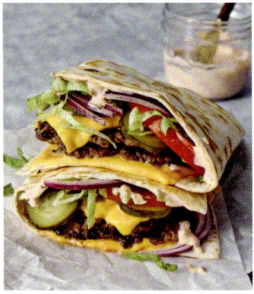

Smash Burgerdilla, page 193

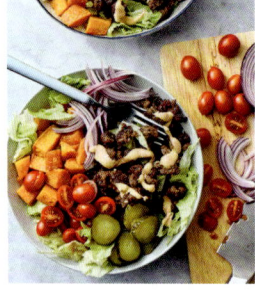

Sweet Potato Burger Bowls with Special Sauce, page 194

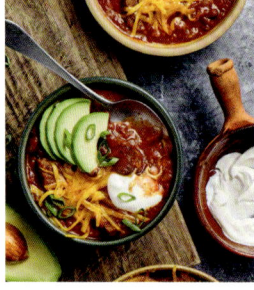

Slow Cooker Chili con Carne, page 197

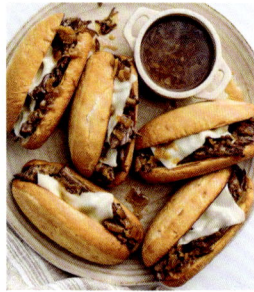

Instant Pot French Dip au Jus, page 199

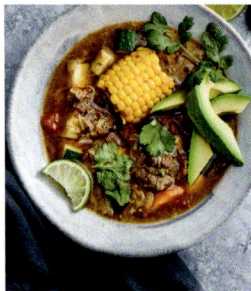

Instant Pot Caldo de Res (Mexican Beef Soup), page 203

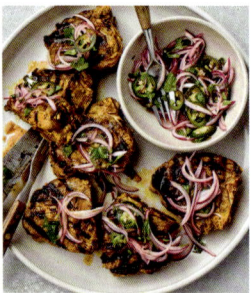

Spiced Yogurt-Marinated Lamb Chops, page 204

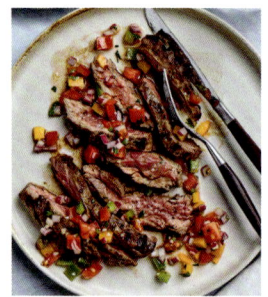

Churrasco with Salsa Criolla, page 207

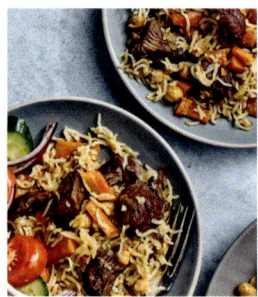

Instant Pot Uzbek Plov, page 208

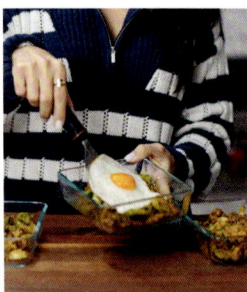

Spicy Pork Brussels Bowls, page 211

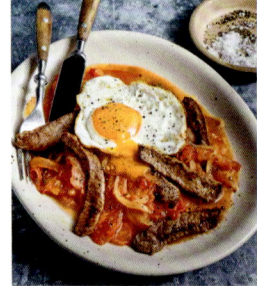

Carne Bistec a Caballo (Colombian Thin-Cut Steaks with Fried Egg), page 212

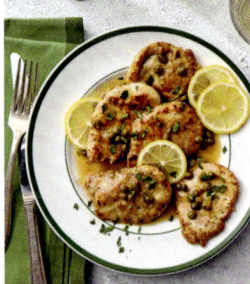

Pork Tenderloin Piccata, page 215

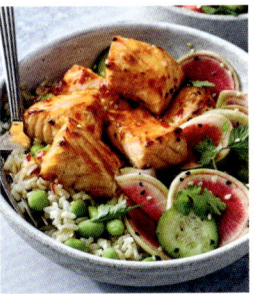

Sweet & Spicy Salmon Bowls with Edamame Rice, page 219

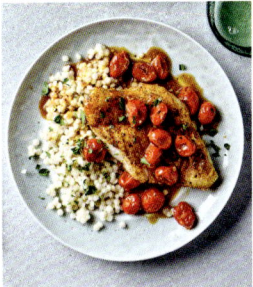

Seared Cod with Roasted Cherry Tomato Sauce, page 220

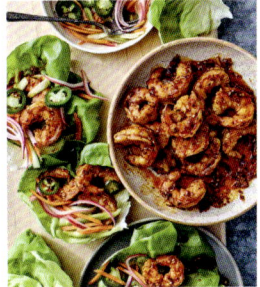

Chili Crisp Shrimp Lettuce Wraps with Pickled Veggies, page 223

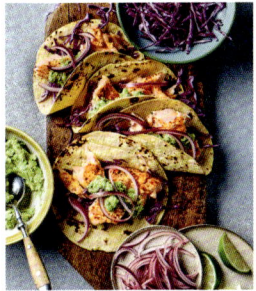

Sheet Pan Tajín Salmon Tacos, page 224

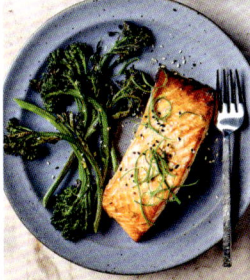

Sheet Pan Miso-Soy Steelhead Trout with Charred Broccolini, page 227

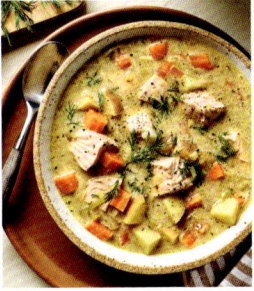

Salmon & Potato Leek Soup, page 228

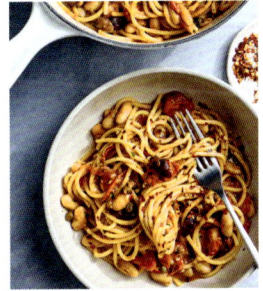

One-Pot White Bean Pasta Puttanesca, page 231

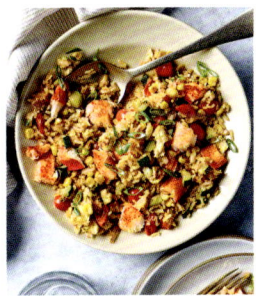

Summer Farmers' Market Lobster Fried Rice, page 232

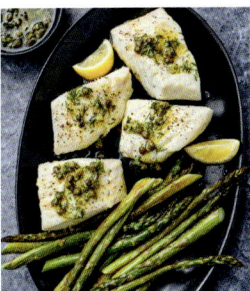

Broiled Fish with Lemony-Dill Sauce, page 235

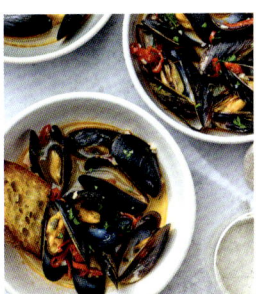

Calabrian Chili Mussels with Garlic Toast, page 236

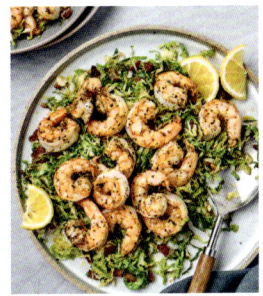

Sautéed Shrimp with Shredded Brussels & Bacon, page 239

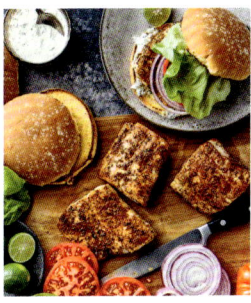

Air Fryer Blackened Mahimahi Sandwiches, page 240

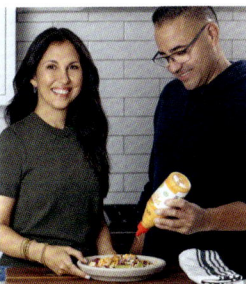

Air Fryer Fish Taco Bowls, page 243

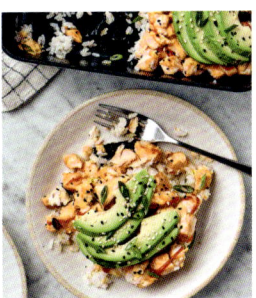

Spicy Salmon Sushi Bake, page 244

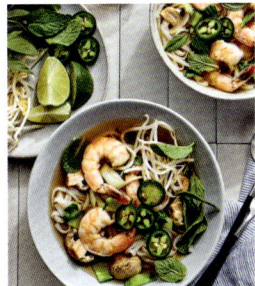

Pho the Love of Shrimp, page 247

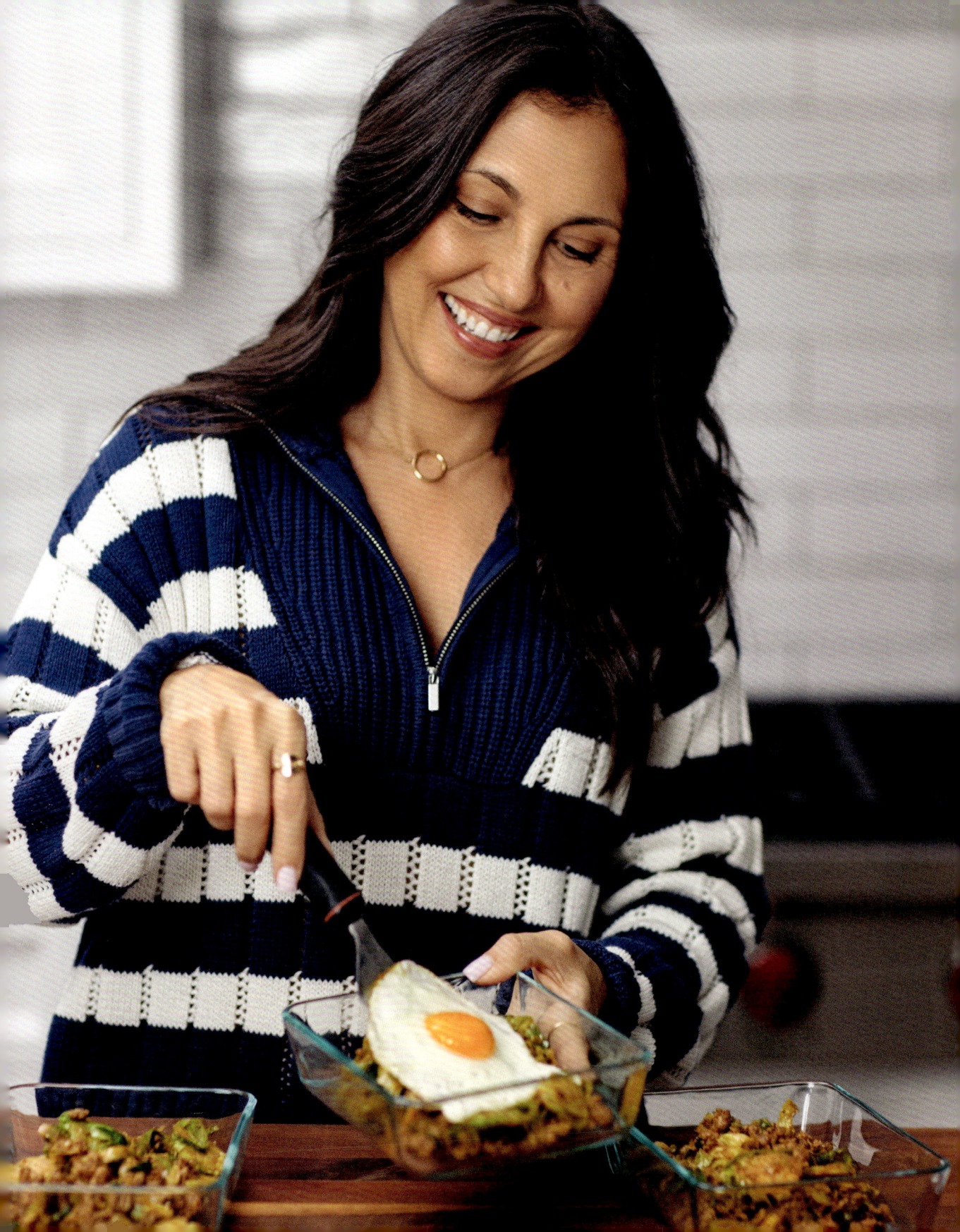

Finding Balance Through High-Protein Cooking

While this is a high-protein cookbook, it's also a personal reflection of my own health journey that began in 2020.

Like many, 2020 turned my world upside down. With gyms closed, social outings on pause, and the uncertainty of the year, I found comfort in baking and indulging in nostalgic foods to cope with the chaos. With all of this, combined with the onset of my menopause journey, I found myself not only gaining some weight but also feeling out of sync with my body. My energy levels were low, my body felt sluggish, my memory wasn't as sharp, and I struggled to stay motivated throughout the day. On top of that, I began noticing a loss of muscle mass, even though I was sticking to my usual workout routine.

But I wasn't too worried. I thought, when things return to normal, I'll just get back to my usual healthy cooking and exercise routine. However, when life finally did settle down, I found myself still struggling, and despite doing everything "right"—eating balanced meals and moving more—I just wasn't seeing the progress I'd expected.

That's when I discovered the power of a high-protein diet, and it was truly a game changer for me. I learned how much protein was right for my body (see calculators on page 21) and made significant changes to my daily intake. I started tracking how many grams of protein I was eating during each meal and snack to ensure I was meeting my goals. To keep things balanced, I included at least 1 cup of produce with my meals and aimed for 25 grams of fiber each day. Skipping breakfast had been a habit of mine, but my new routine included a protein-packed morning meal that set the tone for my day.

Beyond just focusing on protein, I made it a priority to stay hydrated, aiming for 80 to 100 ounces of water daily—a change that significantly reduced the frequency of my headaches. Sleep also became a critical focus. By establishing a consistent nighttime routine, going to bed at the same time each night, reducing my alcohol consumption, and experimenting with supplements and teas to improve sleep quality, I began to get seven to eight hours of rest regularly—a shift that had a profound impact on how I felt each day.

Stress management was another key factor in my journey. I committed to walking daily in addition to my weight training, which drastically improved both my mood and energy levels. Walking became a nonnegotiable part of my routine, helping me manage stress while supporting my physical and mental well-being.

It's been a journey, but I'm so happy to finally be at a place where I feel like myself again. I've regained my energy, feel stronger than ever, and, most important, have found a sustainable way to nourish my body without feeling deprived. At this stage in my life, my focus isn't on the number on the scale—it's on feeling good in my body, reducing stress, maintaining muscle, and living a long, active, and healthy life!

This cookbook is the culmination of that journey to find balance—a collection of high-protein recipes designed to fuel your body, support your nutritional goals, and make mealtime enjoyable. Whether you're looking to incorporate more protein into your diet, manage your weight, gain muscle, or simply eat delicious food that keeps you feeling satisfied, these recipes are here to help.

Many of you have shared with me on social media that you're struggling to get enough protein in your diet, and that's also why I wrote this book—to provide you with a variety of delicious, high-protein recipes that will reignite your excitement for cooking. In the recipe chapters, you'll discover everything from hearty breakfasts like Creamy Protein Oats (page 49) to lazy girl lunches like Tuna Macaroni Salad (page 76), quick one-pot meals like One-Pot Lemony Orzo with Chicken & Feta (page 176), flavorful meatless options such as Lentil Chili (page 128), and even satisfying snacks like my Peanut Butter Chocolate Protein Bars (page 113).

With this book, I hope to help you simplify the process of eating more protein, while enjoying every bite! It's a collection of my absolute favorite high-protein recipes for breakfast, lunch, and dinner, each with 30 grams of protein or more (snacks with 10 grams or more).

These aren't just recipes I've perfected through countless tests—they're the ones I turn to time and again in my own home. They're quick, easy, and packed with flavor, striking the perfect balance between healthy and delicious—so much so that even the pickiest eaters in my family can't get enough of them.

You'll discover meals for every kind of cook and schedule. There are recipes that come together quickly with just a little prep, like Air Fryer Cajun

Chicken & Veggies (page 153), others that are made entirely in one pot for easy cleanup, like Spicy Salmon Sushi Bake (page 244), and plenty that are perfect for meal-prepping ahead of a busy week—Sweet Potato Burger Bowls (page 194) and 10-Minute Meal Prep Deconstructed Fried Rice Bowls (page 86). I've included a hearty meatless section for vegetarians, along with chapters dedicated to poultry, seafood, and meats for every craving. You'll also find many recipes that are gluten-free and dairy-free, ensuring that those with dietary restrictions can enjoy these protein-packed meals, too. Plus, I've included a few high-protein snack ideas for those in-between moments or post-dinner bites.

In my personal life, I also incorporate at least 1 cup of vegetables or fruit into every meal to ensure I get plenty of fiber and overall nutritional balance. And while this is a high-protein cookbook, many recipes in this book reflect this approach; and for those that don't, I offer suggestions for perfect pairings to help you complete your plate with vibrant, nutrient-rich produce.

You'll find protein calculators and the many benefits of eating a high-protein diet from Heather K. Jones, our longtime Skinnytaste dietitian, on page 19, but for me, the easiest way to hit my daily protein goal is to divide it across three meals and a snack. I aim for around 30 grams of protein per meal and 10 to 15 grams per snack.

To help you even more, I've included a 4-week meal plan (see page 26) to make sticking to your goals easier than ever. A handy Protein Cheat Sheet on page 22 is a quick guide to the highest-protein foods, so you can confidently create your own balanced meals.

This cookbook isn't just about fueling your body—it's about enjoying the process, eating foods you love, and discovering how easy it can be to prioritize protein in your everyday life, no matter your dietary needs. I hope you love this high-protein cookbook as much as I do!

Recipe Key

Look for these helpful icons throughout the book:

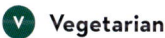 **Quick**
(ready in 30 minutes or less)

V **Vegetarian**

GF **Gluten-Free**

DF **Dairy-Free**

FF **Freezer-Friendly**

Weight Watchers Points

For those of you on WW, I've linked all my recipes to the WW recipe builder, which will give you your points when logged into the WW app, conveniently located on my website under the cookbook tab:

www.skinnytaste.com/cookbook-index/

A Note About Salt

Different brands and different types of salt vary not only in the amount of sodium per measured amount, but also for taste. For consistency in my recipes—both for flavor and for the sodium values listed with the recipes—I use Diamond Crystal kosher salt. If you use another type of salt or a different brand of kosher salt, just remember to taste as you go.

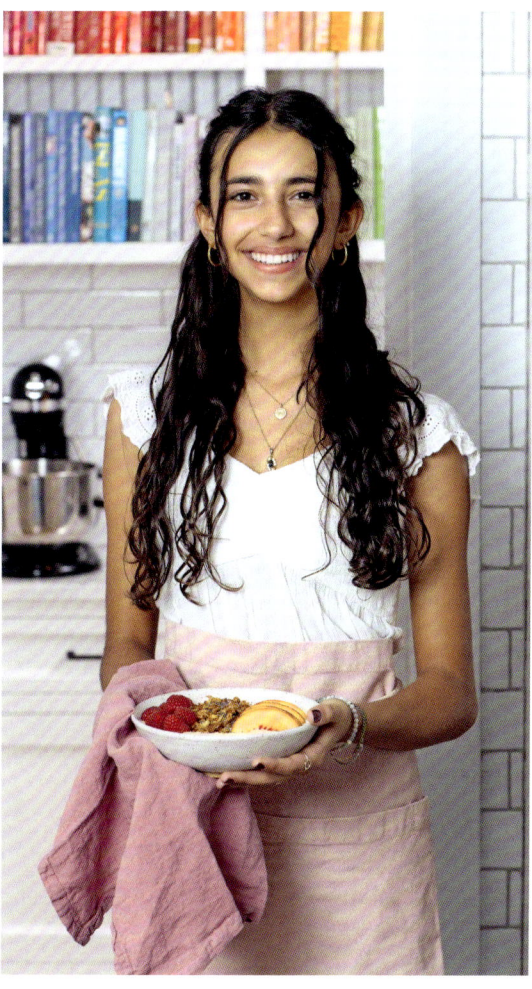

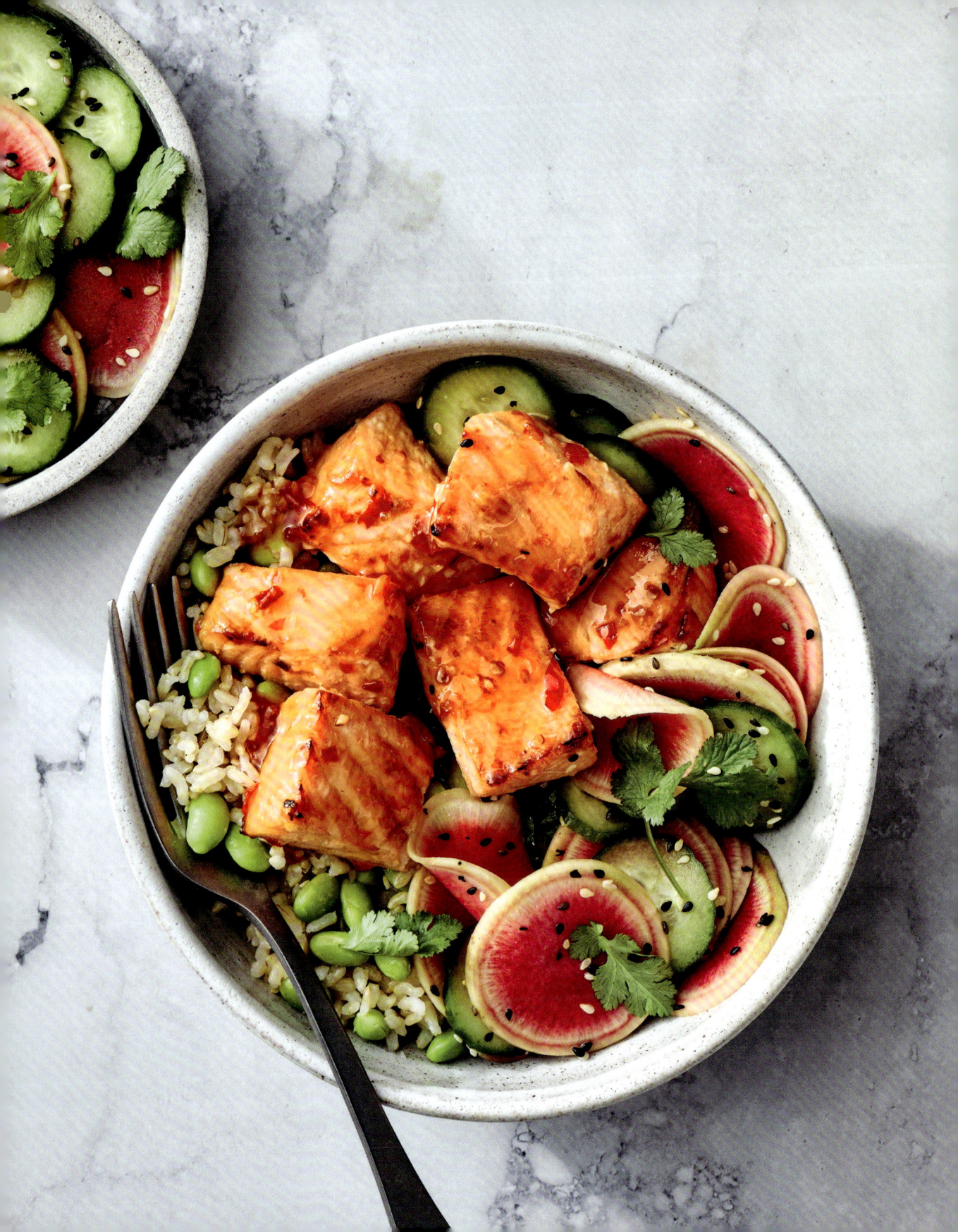

Protein 101

HEATHER K. JONES, RD

Protein isn't just important: It's essential for life! As one of the three macronutrients—along with carbohydrates and fats—fueling your body with sufficient amounts of protein is one of the best things you can do to support your health today and in the future.

Where things get confusing is knowing how much protein is sufficient. This is because there's a difference between the amount of protein *required* to support your body's basic nutritional needs, and the amount considered *optimal* for your unique physiology. Still, a growing body of research suggests that higher protein intakes may be best for our muscles, bones, and metabolic and mental health, especially as we age.

Here are the top 10 reasons to eat more protein:

Regulate Food Intake

According to the eye-opening protein leverage hypothesis, the body's primary appetite is for protein. So, if we don't eat enough protein throughout the day—especially in the morning—we might eat excess calories to compensate for the deficit. Enter a high-protein diet! A good baseline is consuming 30 grams of protein per meal, but you could benefit from more (or less) protein depending on your health goals, age, activity levels, and total caloric intake (see protein calculators on page 21).

Reduce Snacking + Cravings

If we begin each day with a high-protein breakfast we may be less likely to snack on chips and other nutrient-empty foods—particularly in the evening. Research suggests that consuming at least 30 grams of protein in the morning reduces hunger and increases satiety throughout the day, which may help control urges to snack (and as a result, promote a healthy weight!). Which brings me to my next point . . .

Control Hunger + Appetite

Protein helps control hunger signals in the brain, leading to increased feelings of fullness. Why? Protein is highly satiating, helping us feel more satisfied between meals—even when fewer calories are consumed with meals and snacks.

Build + Maintain Muscle Mass

When protein intake is evenly distributed over three meals daily—rather than packed into one meal—it may increase our 24-hour muscle protein synthesis by as much as 25 percent! This can help us build and maintain muscle mass, which is super important as we age. Protein also helps reduce the loss of lean body and muscle mass during weight loss.

Improve Metabolic Health + Support Weight Loss

Some studies have reported reductions in blood pressure, waist circumference, and triglycerides with higher-protein diets. Consuming more calories from quality protein sources may also increase insulin sensitivity, improve cholesterol levels, and may promote healthy eating behaviors to better support your weight loss goals.

Improve Sleep

Adequate protein intake—especially at breakfast—plays a role in stabilizing our circadian rhythm. Our circadian rhythm not only regulates the body's 24-hour internal schedule—affecting sleep and wake times, sleep quality, and overall health—but also helps regulate our metabolism and weight.

Stimulate Inner Stability

Protein is a critical building block for your nervous system, and without enough protein you can't produce enough of the neurotransmitters needed for emotional and mental regulation. Boosting protein consumption, on the other hand, promotes better mood regulation and increases serotonin—a key factor in overall mental health.

Promote Healthy Bones in Menopause

Although we generally need fewer calories overall as we age, we require more calories from protein in order to maintain our muscle mass and bone density. This is especially important during menopause when estrogen levels decline and our risk for osteopenia, osteoporosis, and sarcopenia increases. To reduce your risk of bone fractures after menopause, make sure you're getting plenty of calcium and vitamin D, too. Calcium, vitamin D, and protein are all needed for optimal bone health as we age.

Create Healthier Skin + Hair

Eating more protein ensures that your body has the necessary building blocks to create keratin (a fibrous protein that is essential for stronger and healthier hair, nails, and skin) and collagen (a key protein that contributes to skin elasticity and smoothness).

Prevent Cognitive Decline

As another benefit of increasing our protein intake, protein sufficiency may reduce our risk of cognitive decline and dementia. Higher protein intakes also seem to improve episodic memory and overall cognition among those with dementia, making protein a particularly important macronutrient for brain health.

How Much Protein Do You *Really* Need?

Ready to hop on the high-protein bandwagon, Skinnytaste-style? Your first step is figuring out how much protein is optimal for *you*.

While there's no magic number for optimum protein intake, there are guidelines you can follow to ensure you're getting the right amount of protein to support your health goals. Aiming for 30 grams of protein per meal and 10 to 15 grams per snack is a good baseline, but you could benefit from more or less in some cases.

Your RDA for Protein

Your RDA (recommended daily allowance) for protein refers to the minimum—not the optimum—amount of protein required daily for your body to meet its basic nutritional requirements.

Here's how to calculate your minimum RDA for protein:

Calculating Your Minimum RDA for Protein

Divide your body weight in pounds by 2.2 to get your weight in kilograms

(your weight in kg) × (0.8 grams of protein) = your protein needs

Example:
140 pounds / 2.2 = 64 kg × 0.8 = 51 grams protein

The minimum RDA for protein provides enough protein to prevent a deficiency, but this amount may not be sufficient to maintain muscle strength, bone mass, or weight loss. Rather, your **optimal protein intake** may be more than double your minimum RDA, especially as you age.

These are the rough guidelines I typically recommend for clients, but if you're overweight, your weight will need to be adjusted to your ideal weight before calculating your protein needs.

If you're changing up your diet in a significant way, always remember to consult a dietitian or physician as well. There are also certain health conditions (such as gout, liver disease, and kidney disease) that do not work with a high-protein diet, so again, make sure to consult your doctor first.

Calculating Your Optimum Daily Protein Intake

If You Are Lightly Active

Divide your ideal body weight in pounds by 2.2 to get your weight in kilograms

(your weight in kg) × (1.2 grams of protein) = your protein needs

Example:
140 pounds / 2.2 = 64 kg × 1.2 = 77 grams protein

If You Are Moderately Active

Divide your ideal body weight in pounds by 2.2 to get your weight in kilograms

(your weight in kg) × (1.6 grams of protein) = your protein needs

Example:
140 pounds / 2.2 = 64 kg × 1.6 = 102 grams protein

If You're Very Active and Lifting Weights Two to Four Times per Week

Divide your ideal body weight in pounds by 2.2 to get your weight in kilograms

(your weight in kg) × (2.2 grams of protein) = your protein needs

Example:
140 pounds / 2.2 = 64 kg × 2.2 = 141 grams protein

What if You're in Menopause?

Women going through menopause will have higher minimum protein needs due to the increased risk of muscle loss during this time. Increased needs can range from 1.2 to 2.2 grams per weight in kilograms, depending on activity level.

Protein Cheat Sheet

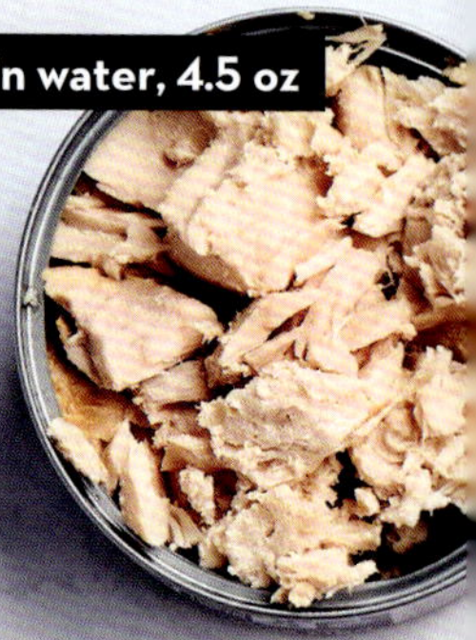

While the right amount of protein for you depends on factors such as your age, caloric intake, activity level, and health goals, aiming for 30 grams of protein per meal is a good baseline. Of course, if your daily target is closer to 100 or 120 grams, you could aim for around 40 grams of protein per meal or enjoy a couple of high-protein snacks throughout the day.

I like dividing my protein goals across three meals and two or three snacks. I aim for 30 grams of protein with meals and 10 to 20 grams per snack. What does 30 grams of protein look like? Here's a cheat sheet to help you reach your daily target.

Each of these servings of food contains around 30 grams of protein.

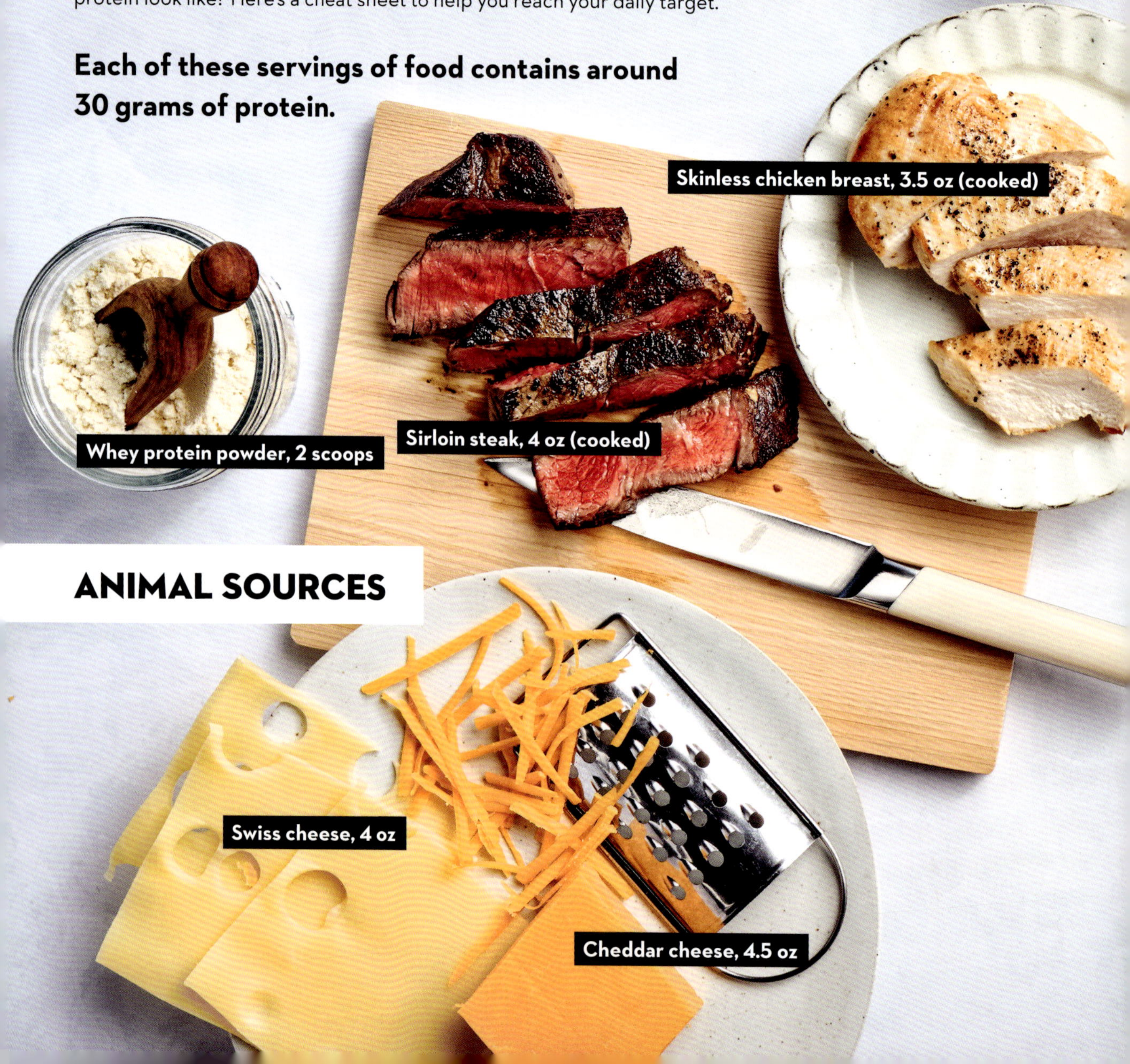

Canned tuna in water, 4.5 oz

Skinless chicken breast, 3.5 oz (cooked)

Sirloin steak, 4 oz (cooked)

Whey protein powder, 2 scoops

ANIMAL SOURCES

Swiss cheese, 4 oz

Cheddar cheese, 4.5 oz

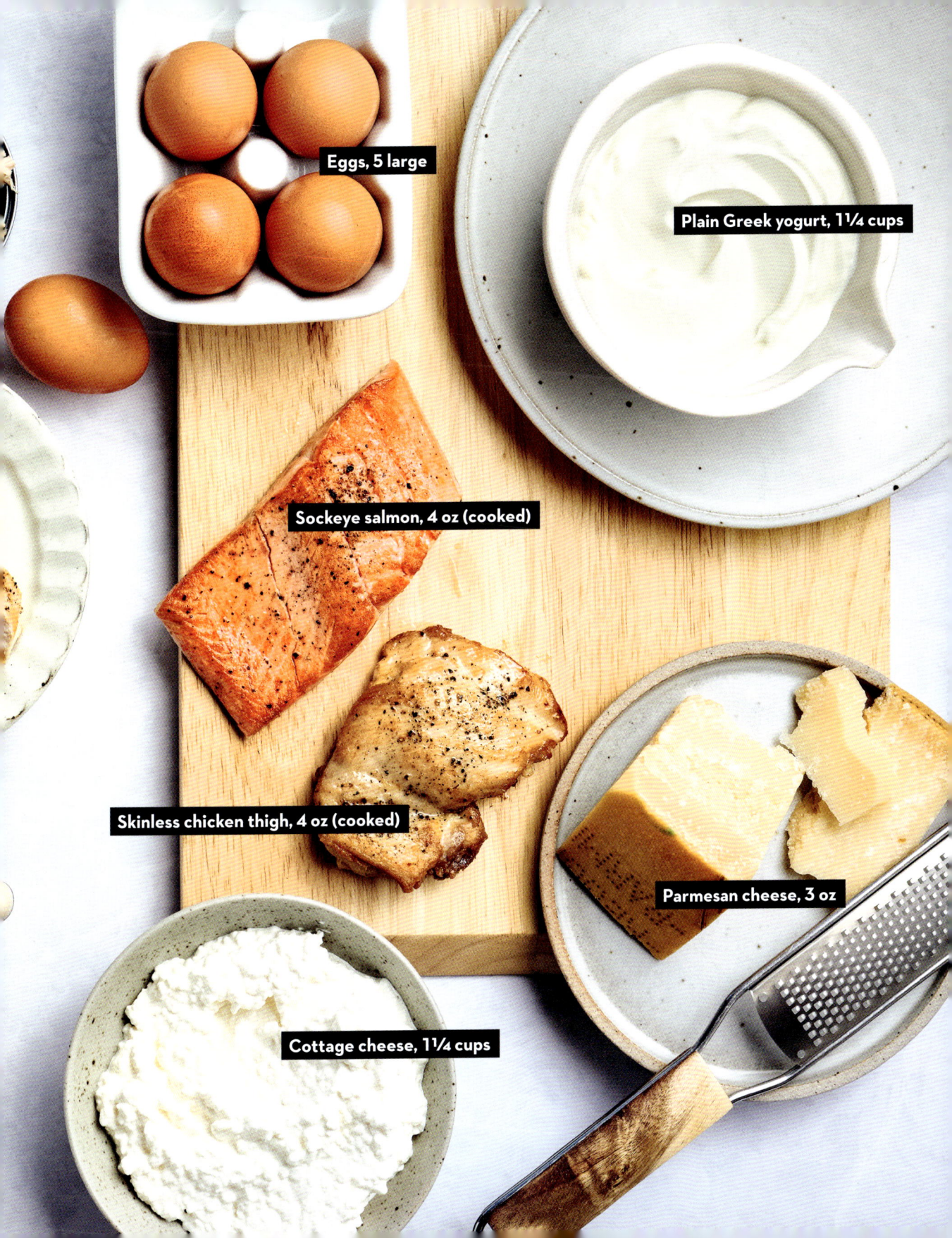

Eggs, 5 large

Plain Greek yogurt, 1¼ cups

Sockeye salmon, 4 oz (cooked)

Skinless chicken thigh, 4 oz (cooked)

Parmesan cheese, 3 oz

Cottage cheese, 1¼ cups

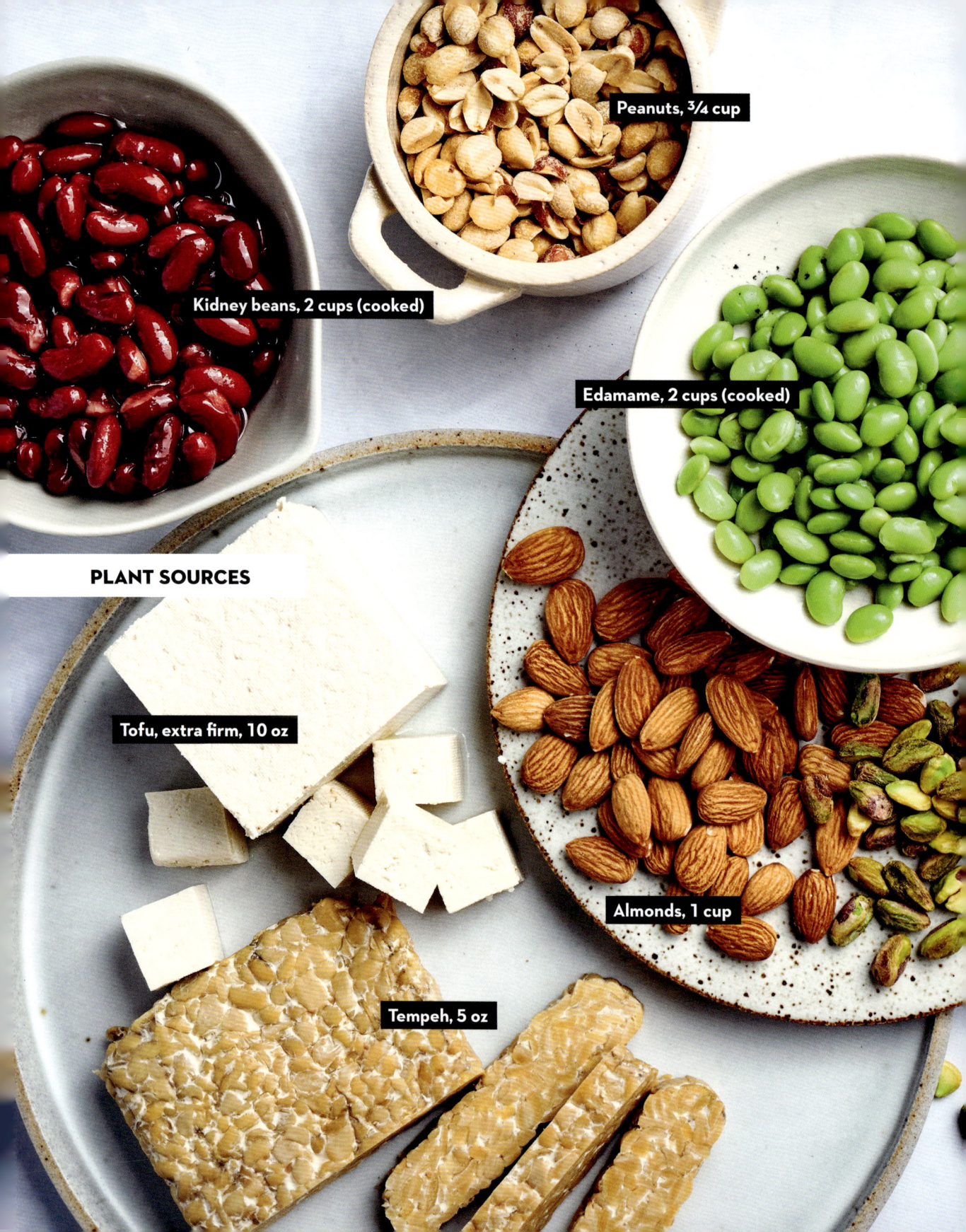

Peanuts, ¾ cup

Kidney beans, 2 cups (cooked)

Edamame, 2 cups (cooked)

PLANT SOURCES

Tofu, extra firm, 10 oz

Almonds, 1 cup

Tempeh, 5 oz

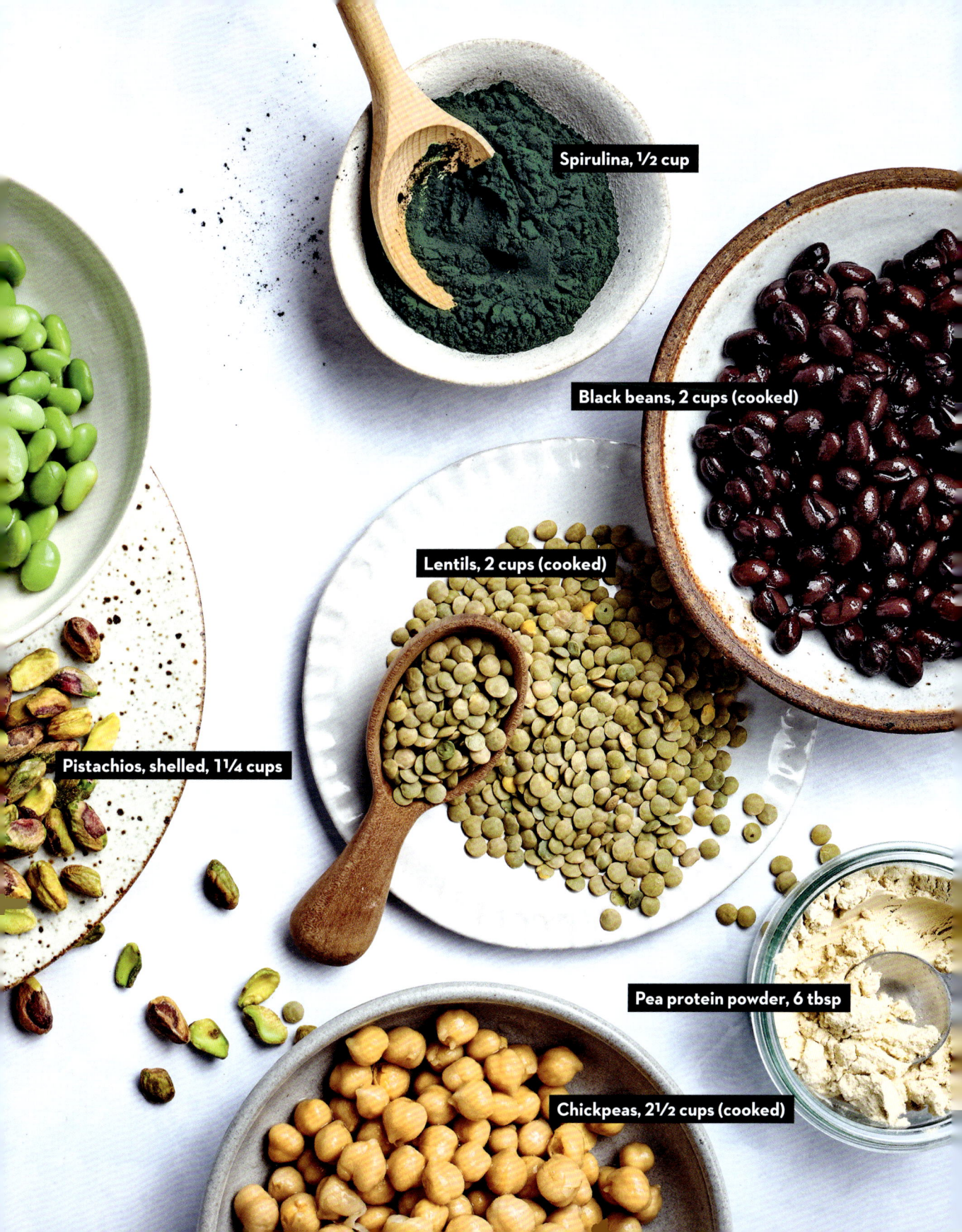

Spirulina, ½ cup

Black beans, 2 cups (cooked)

Lentils, 2 cups (cooked)

Pistachios, shelled, 1¼ cups

Pea protein powder, 6 tbsp

Chickpeas, 2½ cups (cooked)

4-Week High-Protein Meal Plan

	Sunday CALS: 1,503 PRO: 120 G	Monday CALS: 1,457 PRO: 125 G	Tuesday CALS: 1,493 PRO: 126 G	Wednesday CALS: 1,515 PRO: 122 G	Thursday CALS: 1,512 PRO: 137 G	Friday CALS: 1,436 PRO: 118 G	Saturday CALS: 1,062 PRO: 70 G
BREAKFAST	Sheet Pan Breakfast with Veggie Hash (p. 57) Cals: 358 Pro: 30 g Carbs: 18 g Fat: 20 g	Egg White Cottage Cheese Muffins with Turkey Bacon (p. 58) Cals: 201 Pro: 30 g Carbs: 8 g Fat: 8 g	Egg White Cottage Cheese Muffins with Turkey Bacon (p. 58) Cals: 201 Pro: 30 g Carbs: 8 g Fat: 8 g	Egg White Cottage Cheese Muffins with Turkey Bacon (p. 58) Cals: 201 Pro: 30 g Carbs: 8 g Fat: 8 g	Egg White Cottage Cheese Muffins with Turkey Bacon (p. 58) Cals: 201 Pro: 30 g Carbs: 8 g Fat: 8 g	Peaches & Cream Smoothie Bowl (p. 33) Cals: 406 Pro: 32 g Carbs: 43 g Fat: 13 g	Peaches & Cream Smoothie Bowl* (p. 33) Cals: 406 Pro: 32 g Carbs: 43 g Fat: 13 g
LUNCH	Chicken Avocado Salad Chip Dip* (p. 64) Cals: 446 Pro: 33 g Carbs: 19 g Fat: 27 g	Leftover Sunday Pot Roast with Gravy (p. 190) + 1 cup steamed green beans Cals: 533 Pro: 47 g Carbs: 18 g Fat: 31 g	Leftover Sunday Pot Roast with Gravy (p. 190) + 1 cup steamed green beans Cals: 533 Pro: 47 g Carbs: 18 g Fat: 31 g	Leftover Lentil Chili (p. 128) Cals: 503 Pro: 35 g Carbs: 67 g Fat: 13 g	Leftover Lentil Chili (p. 128) Cals: 503 Pro: 35 g Carbs: 67 g Fat: 13 g	Chicken Collard Wrap with Peanut Sesame Dipping Sauce (p. 89) + an apple Cals: 409 Pro: 36 g Carbs: 49 g Fat: 10 g	Chilled Shrimp Salad with Eggs† (p. 71) Cals: 392 Pro: 31 g Carbs: 3 g Fat: 29 g
SNACK	Chocolate Edamame Bark (p. 114) Cals: 166 Pro: 10 g Carbs: 17 g Fat: 10 g	1 string cheese + ¼ cup raw almonds Cals: 220 Pro: 13 g Carbs: 6 g Fat: 18 g	1 string cheese + ¼ cup raw almonds Cals: 220 Pro: 13 g Carbs: 6 g Fat: 18 g	Zesty Banana Pepper Tuna Salad with Crackers (p. 105) + 1 cup grapes Cals: 361 Pro: 27 g Carbs: 41 g Fat: 11 g	Zesty Banana Pepper Tuna Salad with Crackers (p. 105) + 1 cup grapes Cals: 361 Pro: 27 g Carbs: 41 g Fat: 11 g	1 string cheese + ¼ cup raw almonds + an orange Cals: 282 Pro: 14 g Carbs: 21 g Fat: 18 g	¼ cup raw almonds + 1 cup grapes Cals: 264 Pro: 7 g Carbs: 33 g Fat: 14 g
DINNER	Sunday Pot Roast with Gravy (p. 190) + 1 cup steamed green beans Cals: 533 Pro: 47 g Carbs: 18 g Fat: 31 g	Lentil Chili (p. 128) Cals: 503 Pro: 35 g Carbs: 67 g Fat: 13 g	One-Pot Fiesta Chicken & Rice (p. 146) + 2 ounces avocado Cals: 539 Pro: 36 g Carbs: 63 g Fat: 16 g	Baked Teriyaki Chicken Meatballs (p. 165) Cals: 450 Pro: 30 g Carbs: 51 g Fat: 14 g	Spiced Yogurt-Marinated Lamb Chops (p. 204) Cals: 447 Pro: 45 g Carbs: 39 g Fat: 11 g	Sautéed Shrimp with Shredded Brussels & Bacon (p. 239) Cals: 339 Pro: 36 g Carbs: 12 g Fat: 16 g	**Dinner Out!**

*Quadruple the recipe.

†Double the recipe.

NOTE FOR ALL 4 WEEKS: Breakfast and lunch Monday–Friday are designed to serve 1, while dinners and all meals on Saturday and Sunday are designed to serve a family of 4. Some recipes make enough leftovers for two nights or lunch the next day.

WEEK 2

	Sunday	Monday	Tuesday	Wednesday	Thursday	Friday	Saturday
	CALS: 1,447 **PRO: 127 G**	**CALS: 1,568** **PRO: 121 G**	**CALS: 1,527** **PRO: 129 G**	**CALS: 1,471** **PRO: 121 G**	**CALS: 1,481** **PRO: 126 G**	**CALS: 1,454** **PRO: 118 G**	**CALS: 1,072** **PRO: 79 G**
BREAKFAST	Roasted Autumn Veggie Frittata (p. 140) Cals: 489 Pro: 36 g Carbs: 29 g Fat: 27 g	Caramelized Banana Yogurt Bowl with Maple & Pecans (p. 41) Cals: 377 Pro: 31 g Carbs: 36 g Fat: 14 g	Caramelized Banana Yogurt Bowl with Maple & Pecans (p. 41) Cals: 377 Pro: 31 g Carbs: 36 g Fat: 14 g	Caramelized Banana Yogurt Bowl with Maple & Pecans (p. 41) Cals: 377 Pro: 31 g Carbs: 36 g Fat: 14 g	Cinnamon Oatmeal Raisin Smoothie (p. 37) Cals: 396 Pro: 34 g Carbs: 56 g Fat: 4 g	Cinnamon Oatmeal Raisin Smoothie (p. 37) Cals: 396 Pro: 34 g Carbs: 56 g Fat: 4 g	PB&J Crepes (p. 45) Cals: 562 Pro: 36 g Carbs: 34 g Fat: 35 g
LUNCH	Spicy Tuna Queso Melt* (p. 79) + 1 cup sliced cucumbers Cals: 357 Pro: 37 g Carbs: 30 g Fat: 16 g	Leftover Caldo de Res (p. 203) Cals: 354 Pro: 40 g Carbs: 26 g Fat: 11 g	Leftover Caldo de Res (p. 203) Cals: 354 Pro: 40 g Carbs: 26 g Fat: 11 g	Mediterranean Sardine Salad (p. 75) Cals: 410 Pro: 31 g Carbs: 29 g Fat: 22 g	Leftover Shortcut Turkey Meatball Minestrone (p. 169) Cals: 378 Pro: 40 g Carbs: 31 g Fat: 12 g	Leftover Shortcut Turkey Meatball Minestrone (p. 169) Cals: 378 Pro: 40 g Carbs: 31 g Fat: 12 g	Italian Roast Beef Sub Salad* (p. 90) Cals: 448 Pro: 42 Carbs: 11 g Fat: 26 g
SNACK	Peanut Butter Chocolate Protein Bars (p. 113) Cals: 247 Pro: 14 g Carbs: 20 g Fat: 15 g	2 hard-boiled eggs + 1 string cheese Cals: 203 Pro: 20 g Carbs: 1 g Fat: 13 g	Protein Picnic Boxes† (p. 109) Cals: 306 Pro: 19 g Carbs: 13 g Fat: 21 g	Protein Picnic Boxes (p. 109) Cals: 306 Pro: 19 g Carbs: 13 g Fat: 21 g	2 hard-boiled eggs + 1 string cheese Cals: 203 Pro: 20 g Carbs: 1 g Fat: 13 g	Peanut Butter Chocolate Protein Bars (p. 113) Cals: 247 Pro: 14 g Carbs: 20 g Fat: 15 g	1 medium orange Cals: 62 Pro: 1 g Carbs: 16 g Fat: 0 g
DINNER	Instant Pot Caldo de Res (p. 203) Cals: 354 Pro: 40 g Carbs: 26 g Fat: 11 g	Black Bean Quinoa Bowls (p. 123) Cals: 634 Pro: 30 g Carbs: 106 g Fat: 11 g	Sheet Pan Tajín Salmon Tacos (p. 224) Cals: 490 Pro: 39 g Carbs: 42 g Fat: 19 g	Shortcut Turkey Meatball Minestrone (p. 169) Cals: 378 Pro: 40 g Carbs: 31 g Fat: 12 g	Potsticker Rice Bowls (p. 189) Cals: 504 Pro: 32 g Carbs: 41 g Fat: 23 g	Summer Farmers' Market Lobster Fried Rice (p. 232) Cals: 433 Pro: 30 g Carbs: 55 g Fat: 10 g	**Dinner Out!**

*Quadruple the recipe.

†Make half the recipe.

	Sunday	Monday	Tuesday	Wednesday	Thursday	Friday	Saturday
	CALS: 1,573 **PRO: 128 G**	**CALS: 1,466** **PRO: 137 G**	**CALS: 1,450** **PRO: 134 G**	**CALS: 1,621** **PRO: 134 G**	**CALS: 1,507** **PRO: 121 G**	**CALS: 1,502** **PRO: 125 G**	**CALS: 892** **PRO: 82 G**
BREAKFAST	Enchilada Breakfast Casserole (p. 54) Cals: 407 Pro: 43 g Carbs: 26 g Fat: 16 g	Leftover Enchilada Breakfast Casserole (p. 54) Cals: 407 Pro: 43 g Carbs: 26 g Fat: 16 g	Leftover Enchilada Breakfast Casserole (p. 54) Cals: 407 Pro: 43 g Carbs: 26 g Fat: 16 g	Creamy Protein Oats (p. 49) Cals: 383 Pro: 31 g Carbs: 54 g Fat: 6 g	Creamy Protein Oats (p. 49) Cals: 383 Pro: 31 g Carbs: 54 g Fat: 6 g	Creamy Protein Oats (p. 49) Cals: 383 Pro: 31 g Carbs: 54 g Fat: 6 g	Monte Cristo Omelet Sandwich* (p. 38) + an orange Cals: 518 Pro: 50 g Carbs: 49 g Fat: 16 g
LUNCH	Spicy Chicken Poke Bowl* (p. 85) Cals: 546 Pro: 48 g Carbs: 45 g Fat: 19 g	Spinach Egg Wraps (p. 72) + 3 ounces deli turkey + ½ cup arugula + 2 teaspoons mustard + an apple Cals: 305 Pro: 37 g Carbs: 30 g Fat: 5 g	Spinach Egg Wraps (p. 72) + 3 ounces deli turkey + ½ cup arugula + 2 teaspoons mustard + an apple Cals: 305 Pro: 37 g Carbs: 30 g Fat: 5 g	Spinach Egg Wraps (p. 72) + 3 ounces deli turkey + ½ cup arugula + 2 teaspoons mustard + an apple Cals: 305 Pro: 37 g Carbs: 30 g Fat: 5 g	Leftover Instant Pot Uzbek Plov (p. 208) Cals: 467 Pro: 31 g Carbs: 71 g Fat: 6 g	Leftover Instant Pot Uzbek Plov (p. 208) Cals: 467 Pro: 31 g Carbs: 71 g Fat: 6 g	Shrimp Summer Roll Lettuce Wraps* (p. 67) Cals: 312 Pro: 31 g Carbs: 26 g Fat: 11 g
SNACK	1 medium orange Cals: 62 Pro: 1 g Carbs: 16 g Fat: 0 g	½ cup dry roasted edamame Cals: 195 Pro: 21 g Carbs: 14 g Fat: 8 g	½ cup dry roasted edamame + an orange Cals: 257 Pro: 22 g Carbs: 30 g Fat: 8 g	Mango Blueberry Smoothie (p. 34) Cals: 396 Pro: 32 g Carbs: 60 g Fat: 6 g	Greek Cottage Cheese Bowl (p. 117) Cals: 205 Pro: 23 g Carbs: 10 g Fat: 10 g	Greek Cottage Cheese Bowl (p. 117) Cals: 205 Pro: 23 g Carbs: 10 g Fat: 10 g	1 medium orange Cals: 62 Pro: 1 g Carbs: 16 g Fat: 0 g
DINNER	Instant Pot French Dip au Jus (p. 199) + ½ sliced red bell pepper Cals: 558 Pro: 36 g Carbs: 58 g Fat: 20 g	Leftover Instant Pot French Dip au Jus (p. 199) + 1 cup sliced cucumbers Cals: 559 Pro: 36 g Carbs: 58 g Fat: 20 g	Creamy Parmesan & Peas Pasta (p. 131) Cals: 521 Pro: 32 g Carbs: 75 g Fat: 13 g	Instant Pot Uzbek Plov (p. 208) + a green salad† Cals: 537 Pro: 34 g Carbs: 82 g Fat: 8 g	One-Pot Chicken Orzo Caprese (p. 162) Cals: 452 Pro: 37 g Carbs: 44 g Fat: 13 g	Chili Crisp Shrimp Lettuce Wraps with Pickled Veggies (p. 223) Cals: 447 Pro: 40 g Carbs: 41 g Fat: 11 g	**Dinner Out!**

*Quadruple the recipe.

†Green salad per serving includes 2 cups romaine, ½ tomato (sliced), 6 cucumber slices, 3 red onion rings, and 1 tablespoon light vinaigrette.

	Sunday	Monday	Tuesday	Wednesday	Thursday	Friday	Saturday
	CALS: 1,509 **PRO: 125 G**	**CALS: 1,641** **PRO: 125 G**	**CALS: 1,682** **PRO: 129 G**	**CALS: 1,538** **PRO: 128 G**	**CALS: 1,509** **PRO: 137 G**	**CALS: 1,543** **PRO: 133 G**	**CALS: 1,162** **PRO: 79 G**
BREAKFAST	Sheet Pan Breakfast with Veggie Hash (p. 57) Calories: 358￼ Protein: 30 g Carbs: 18 g Fat: 20 g	Air Fryer Breakfast Bagel Sandwiches (p. 50) + an orange Cals: 507 Pro: 33 g Carbs: 31 g Fat: 21 g	Air Fryer Breakfast Bagel Sandwiches (p. 50) + an orange Cals: 507 Pro: 33 g Carbs: 31 g Fat: 21 g	Avocado Toast with Cottage Cheese Eggs (p. 46) Cals: 328 Pro: 30 g Carbs: 27 g Fat: 12 g	Avocado Toast with Cottage Cheese Eggs (p. 46) Cals: 328 Pro: 30 g Carbs: 27 g Fat: 12 g	Mango Blueberry Smoothie (p. 34) Cals: 396 Pro: 32 g Carbs: 60 g Fat: 6 g	Chicken Chorizo Breakfast Tacos (p. 42) Cals: 412 Pro: 32 g Carbs: 27 g Fat: 20 g
LUNCH	Hearty Autumn Salad with Chicken & Maple-Dijon Dressing (p. 180) Cals: 529 Pro: 40 g Carbs: 37 g Fat: 27 g	Cranberry Chicken Salad on Apple Slices (p. 93) Cals: 452 Pro: 36 g Carbs: 21 g Fat: 20	Cranberry Chicken Salad on Apple Slices (p. 93) Cals: 452 Pro: 36 g Carbs: 21 g Fat: 20	Tuna Macaroni Salad (p. 76) over 2 cups baby spinach Cals: 441 Pro: 37 g Carbs: 45 g Fat: 15 g	Tuna Macaroni Salad (p. 76) over 2 cups baby spinach Cals: 441 Pro: 37 g Carbs: 45 g Fat: 15 g	Leftover Instant Pot Turkey & Sage Dumpling Soup (p. 175) + 2 ounces multigrain baguette Cals: 407 Pro: 37 g Carbs: 52 g Fat: 5 g	Spicy Salmon Hand Rolls* (p. 68) Cals: 452 Pro: 41 g Carbs: 34 g Fat: 17 g
SNACK	1 cup 0% Greek yogurt + ½ cup sliced strawberries Cals: 143 Pro: 24 g Carbs: 12 g Fat: 0 g	1 cup 0% Greek yogurt + ½ cup sliced strawberries Cals: 143 Pro: 24 g Carbs: 12 g Fat: 0 g	2 ounces turkey jerky Cals: 133 Pro: 23 g Carbs: 9 g Fat: 2 g	2 ounces turkey jerky + 1 cup strawberries Cals: 179 Pro: 24 g Carbs: 20 g Fat: 2 g	Fall Harvest Jars† (p. 110) Cals: 333 Pro: 33 g Carbs: 39 g Fat: 6 g	Fall Harvest Jars (p. 110) Cals: 333 Pro: 33 g Carbs: 39 g Fat: 6 g	¼ cup mixed nuts + an apple Cals: 298 Pro: 6 g Carbs: 34 g Fat: 18 g
DINNER	One-Pot White Bean Pasta Puttanesca (p. 231) Cals: 479 Pro: 31 g Carbs: 78 g Fat: 7 g	Egg Curry with Yogurt Naan (p. 124) Cals: 539 Pro: 32 g Carbs: 51 g Fat: 23 g	Slow Cooker Chili con Carne (p. 197) + ¾ cup brown rice + 1 ounce avocado Cals: 590 Pro: 37 g Carbs: 65 g Fat: 22 g	Leftover Slow Cooker Chili con Carne (p. 197) + ¾ cup brown rice + 1 ounce avocado Cals: 590 Pro: 37 g Carbs: 65 g Fat: 22 g	Instant Pot Turkey & Sage Dumpling Soup (p. 175) + 2 ounces multigrain baguette Cals: 407 Pro: 37 g Carbs: 52 g Fat: 5 g	Sweet & Spicy Salmon Bowls with Edamame Rice‡ (p. 219) Cals: 407 Pro: 31 g Carbs: 41 g Fat: 13 g	**Dinner Out!**

*Quadruple the recipe.

†Make half the recipe.

‡Double the recipe.

NOURISHING MORNINGS

I was never a big breakfast person. For years, I would either skip breakfast altogether, or grab something quick and light, assuming I didn't really need a morning meal to get me through the day. But when I started eating a high-protein diet, I quickly realized that I could never meet my protein goals without eating a proper breakfast. I'd often find myself scrambling to catch up by the end of the day, eating snacks after dinner to make up for what I missed earlier.

That's when I began to rethink how I approached breakfast. I wanted meals that weren't just high in protein but also satisfying, energizing, and—most important—something I'd actually look forward to eating. Starting my day with a protein-packed breakfast not only helped me hit my daily targets, but also kept me full and focused all morning.

This chapter is filled with high-protein breakfast meals that are both practical and delicious, from quick grab-and-go options to recipes you can make ahead for busy weekdays. Whether you're an early riser looking for a way to fuel your day, or if, like me, you're someone who has been resisting making breakfast a priority, these recipes will show you just how easy getting at least 30 grams of protein in the morning can be to start your day strong.

With protein-packed smoothies like the Mango-Blueberry Smoothie (page 34), savory egg dishes like Sheet Pan Breakfast with Veggie Hash (page 57), and even sweet options like PB&J Crepes (page 45) that won't leave you crashing midmorning, you'll find something to suit every mood and schedule.

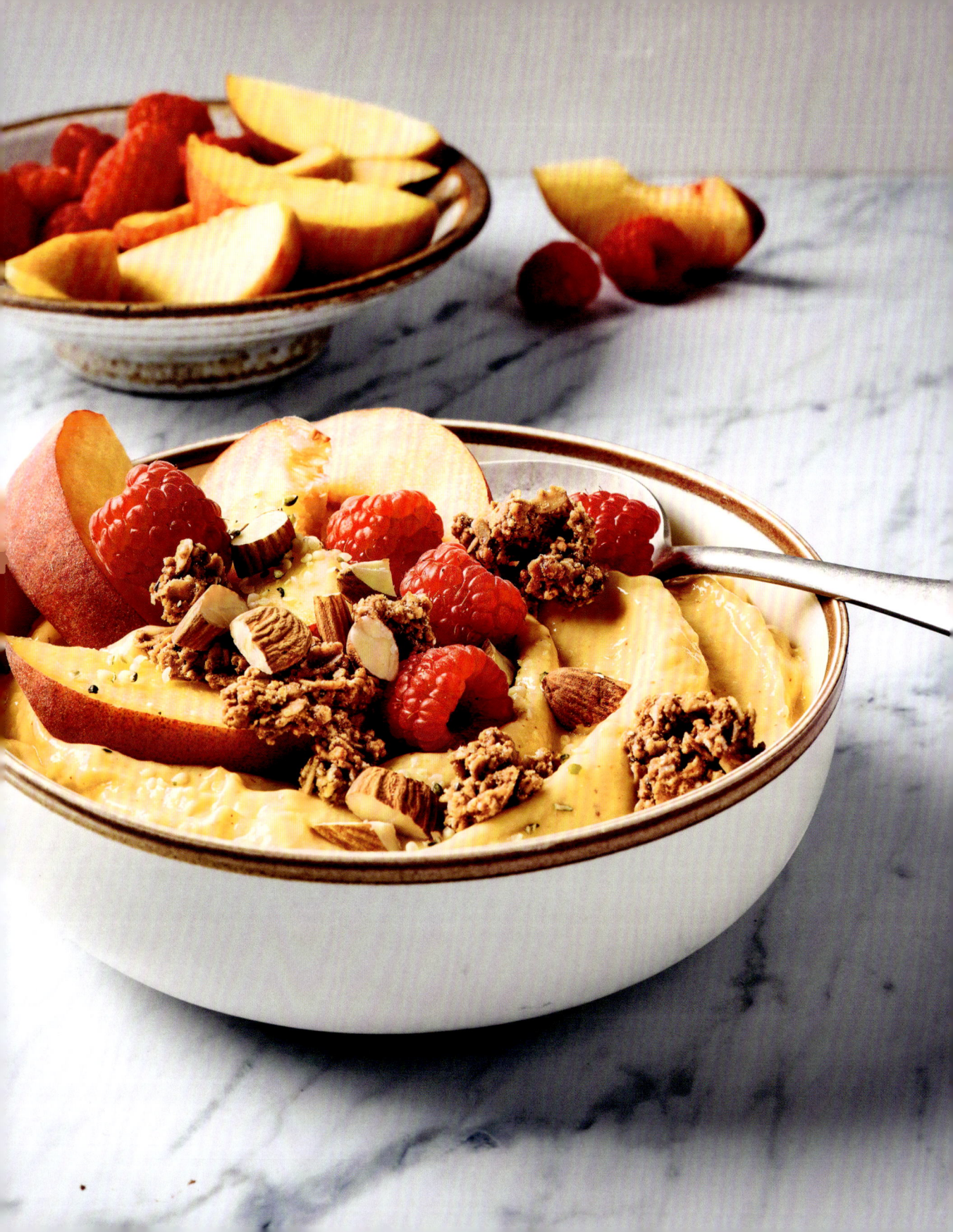

PEACHES & CREAM SMOOTHIE BOWL

In the summer when peaches are at their sweetest, I can't get enough of this creamy and healthy peach smoothie bowl. It's not only high in protein, but it also has more than 6 grams of fiber per serving. If peaches aren't in season, frozen peaches or mango would also work. For toppings, use whatever fruit, nuts, and seeds you like to make it your own. Strawberries, blueberries, and shredded coconut are personal faves in addition to this combination here. It's so flexible, too—you can serve it as a snack, breakfast, or dessert!

Freeze the peach slices in a small container or zip-top plastic bag until solid, 4 hours or overnight. (If you want to use store-bought frozen peaches instead, it's about 1 cup.)

In a blender, combine the frozen peaches, milk, yogurt, and collagen and blend on high speed until smooth, 15 to 20 seconds.

TO SERVE: Scoop into a bowl and top with sliced fresh peaches, raspberries, granola, hemp seeds, and almonds.

SERVES 1

1 peach, sliced

¼ cup fat-free milk or milk of choice

1 (5.3-ounce) container vanilla yogurt, such as Oikos Pro or Ratio

1 teaspoon unflavored collagen peptide or vegetarian collagen peptide powder

FOR SERVING

½ peach, sliced

4 raspberries

2 tablespoons gluten-free granola, such as Purely Elizabeth Ancient Grain

1 teaspoon hemp or chia seeds

2 tablespoons chopped raw almonds

Per Serving | Calories 406 | **Protein 32 g** | Carbohydrate 43 g | Fiber 6.5 g | Sugars 29 g | Fat 13 g | Saturated Fat 2.5 g | Cholesterol 19 mg | Sodium 137 mg

MANGO BLUEBERRY SMOOTHIE

Don't be turned off by the brown color of this smoothie—this refreshing drink is perfect for a post-workout pick-me-up or a healthy breakfast on the go! It's packed with protein and fiber, making this a great way to start the day. Plus, mangoes are rich in vitamins C and A, while blueberries are loaded with antioxidants. Need even more reasons to love this super smoothie? Coconut water provides electrolytes like potassium and magnesium, and spinach adds a boost of folate, and vitamins A and K.

In a blender, combine the coconut water, mango, blueberries, spinach, flaxseeds, pea protein, and ice and blend until smooth.

TIP: Double the recipe. Drink one today, then portion out the ingredients for the second one (minus the ice and coconut water) and store in the fridge, ready to blend tomorrow.

SERVES 1

¾ cup coconut water

¾ cup fresh or frozen mango slices

¾ cup blueberries, fresh or frozen

¾ cup baby spinach

2 tablespoons ground flaxseeds

¼ cup unflavored pea protein (or a scoop of your favorite protein powder)

1 cup ice

Per Serving | Calories 396 | **Protein 32 g** | Carbohydrate 60 g | Fiber 8.5 g | Sugars 44 g | Fat 6 g | Saturated Fat 0 g | Cholesterol 0 mg | Sodium 223 mg

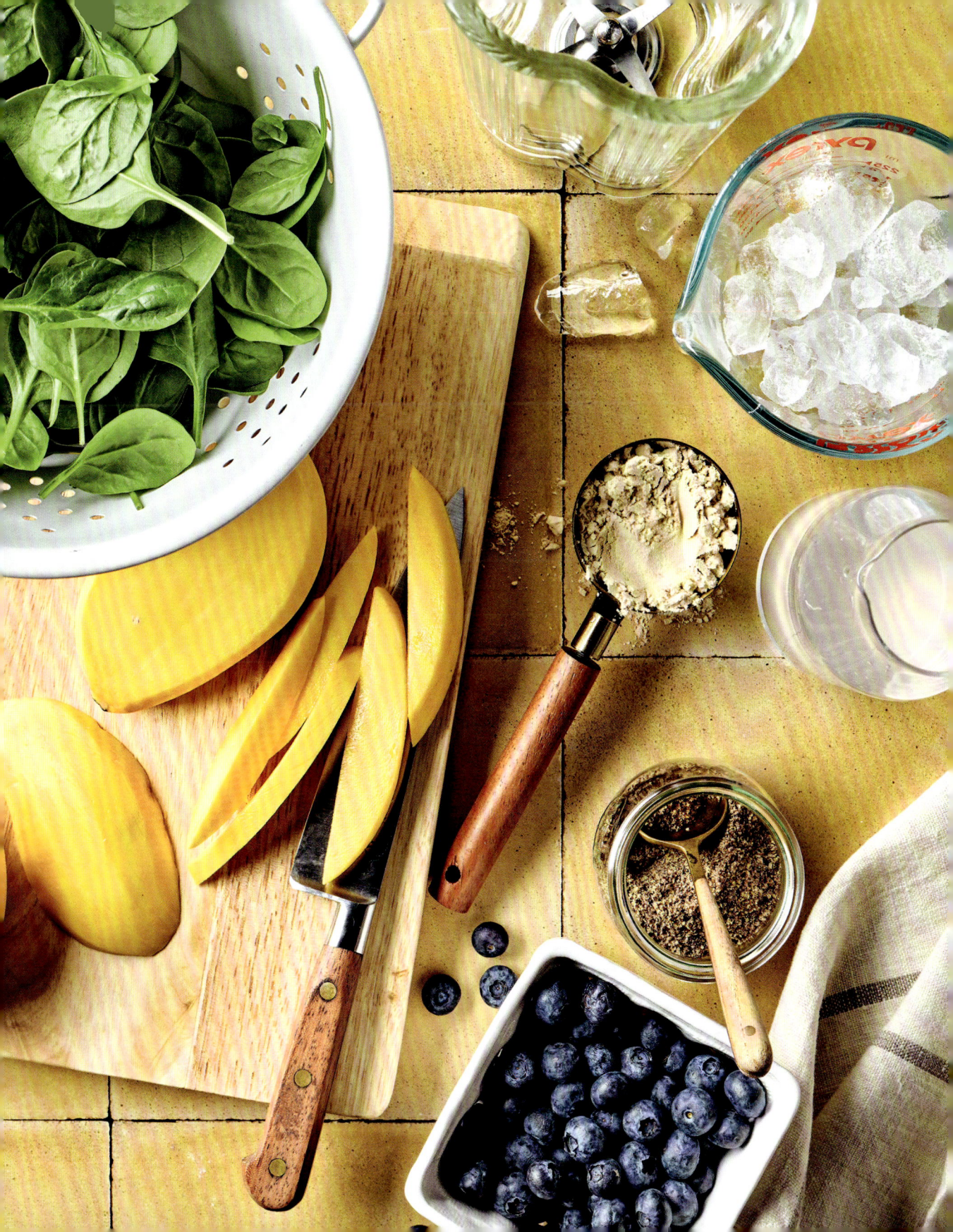

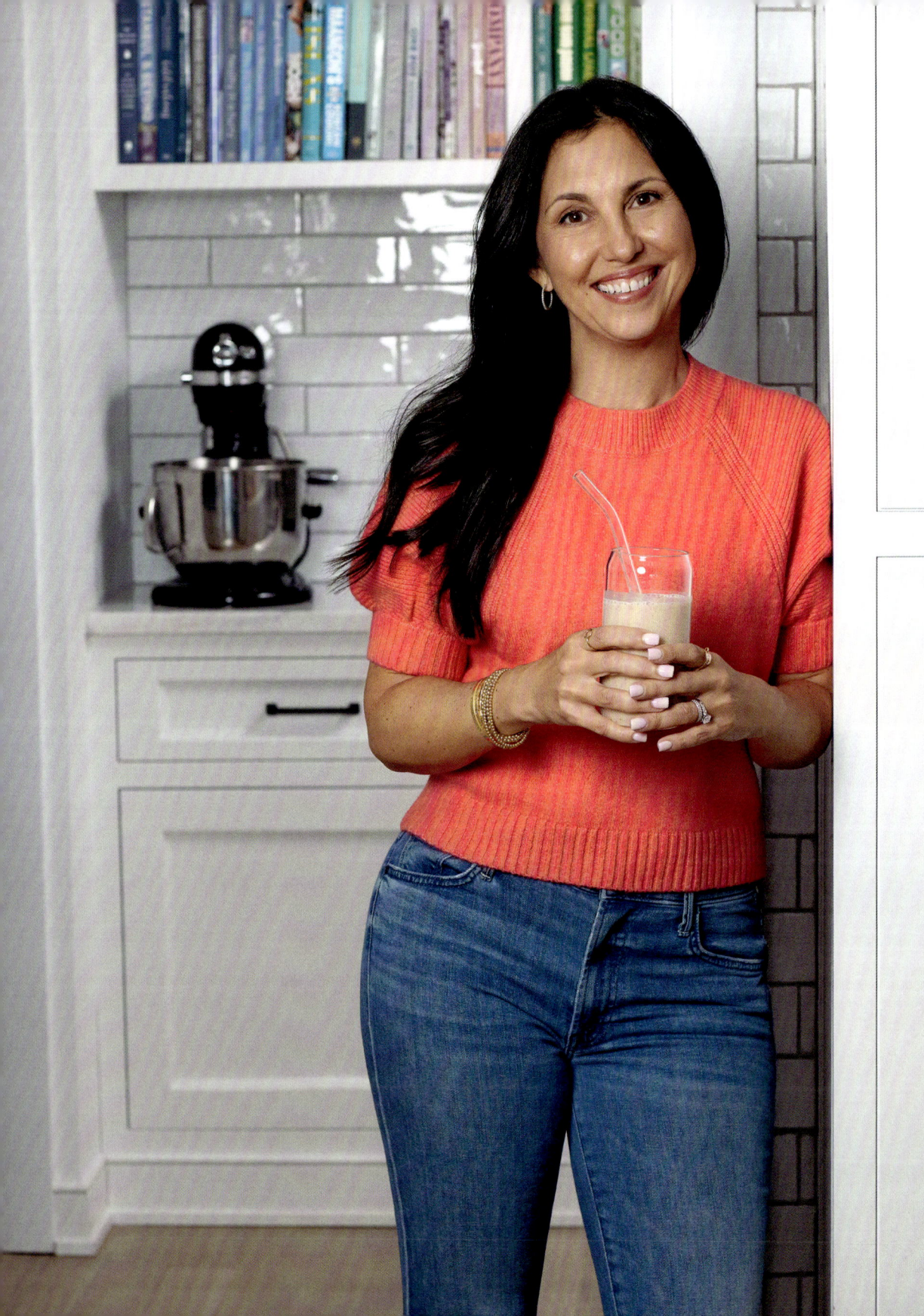

CINNAMON OATMEAL RAISIN SMOOTHIE

I love adding oatmeal to my smoothies—it boosts the fiber, thickens the texture, and provides long-lasting energy for a more satisfying and nutritious drink. I enjoy cinnamon and raisins in my hot oatmeal, so I thought why not also include them in my oatmeal smoothie? This tasty smoothie is naturally sweetened with a banana, and a dash of turmeric provides an extra boost of flavor and health benefits!

In a blender, combine the milk, oats, and raisins and let them sit for a few minutes to soften, if desired.

Add the banana, protein powder, cinnamon, turmeric, and ice and blend until smooth. Serve immediately.

TIP: Add spinach, chia seeds, flaxseeds, or collagen for an extra boost of nutrition.

SERVES 1

1 cup fat-free milk
or nondairy milk

¼ cup quick-cooking oats*

1 tablespoon raisins

1 medium banana

¼ cup pea protein powder or
protein powder of your choice

¾ teaspoon ground cinnamon

½ teaspoon ground turmeric

1 cup ice

*Read the label to be sure this product is gluten-free.

Per Serving | Calories 421 | **Protein 35 g** | Carbohydrate 62 g | Fiber 7 g |
Sugars 32 g | Fat 4 g | Saturated Fat 0.5 g | Cholesterol 5 mg | Sodium 135 mg

MONTE CRISTO OMELET SANDWICH

Is it a sandwich or an omelet? Well, it's a little bit of both! I love a Monte Cristo sandwich—it reminds me of my younger years hanging out with my mom at her luncheonette. This special sandwich is typically made with ham, turkey, and Swiss cheese, and then dipped in beaten egg and pan-fried, similar to the way you prepare French toast. Some people like it with a little berry jam on the side. My healthier version includes spinach, and it actually cooks in the omelet (so you get extra protein from the egg), and then it folds back into a sandwich. It's delicious!

In a small bowl, beat the whole egg and egg whites. Add the spinach, onion, salt, and pepper to taste.

Heat a nonstick skillet (large enough to fit 2 slices of bread side by side) over low heat and spray with oil. When hot, pour the eggs into the skillet. Quickly place the bread on the eggs and then flip the bread over so both sides are wet and coated with the egg. Cover and cook until the eggs are set, 4 to 5 minutes, then uncover and flip the omelet with a spatula.

Place the ham, turkey, and cheese directly over where the bread is and cover the skillet until the cheese melts and the bottom of the omelet is browned, 2 to 3 minutes. Once browned, fold the omelet in half to form a sandwich and transfer to a plate. Cut in half and enjoy!

SERVES 1

1 large egg

½ cup egg whites

¼ cup chopped baby spinach

2 tablespoons chopped red onion

⅛ teaspoon kosher salt

Freshly ground black pepper

Olive oil spray

2 slices thin-sliced whole-grain bread, such as Dave's Killer Bread Good Seed, or your favorite gluten-free bread

2 ounces sliced reduced-sodium ham

1 ounce sliced reduced-sodium turkey breast

1 ounce (2 slices) light Swiss cheese (I like Finlandia Light Swiss)

Per Serving | Calories 456 | **Protein 49 g** | Carbohydrate 34 g | Fiber 10.5 g | Sugars 9 g | Fat 15 g | Saturated Fat 5.5 g | Cholesterol 236 mg | Sodium 1,284 mg

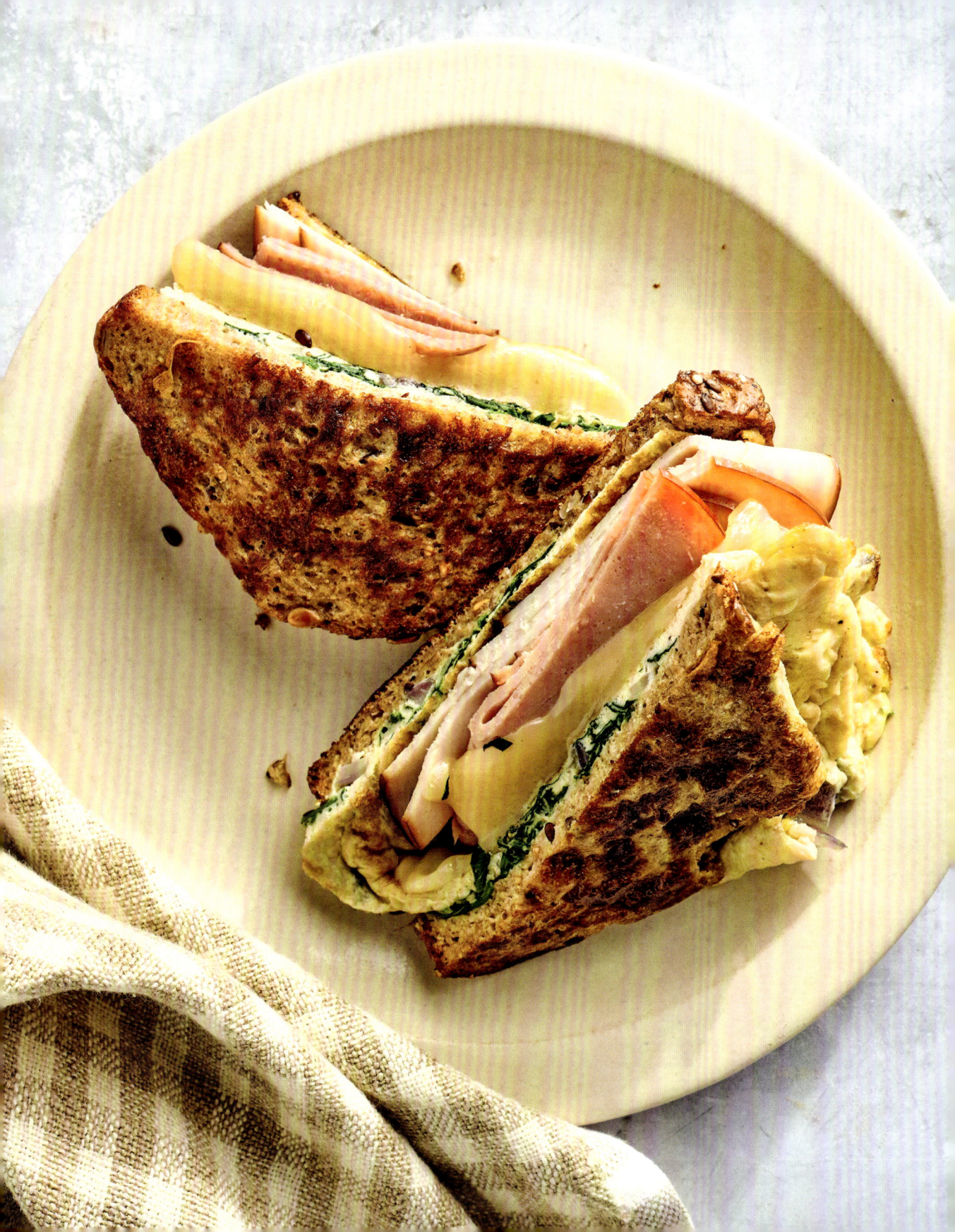

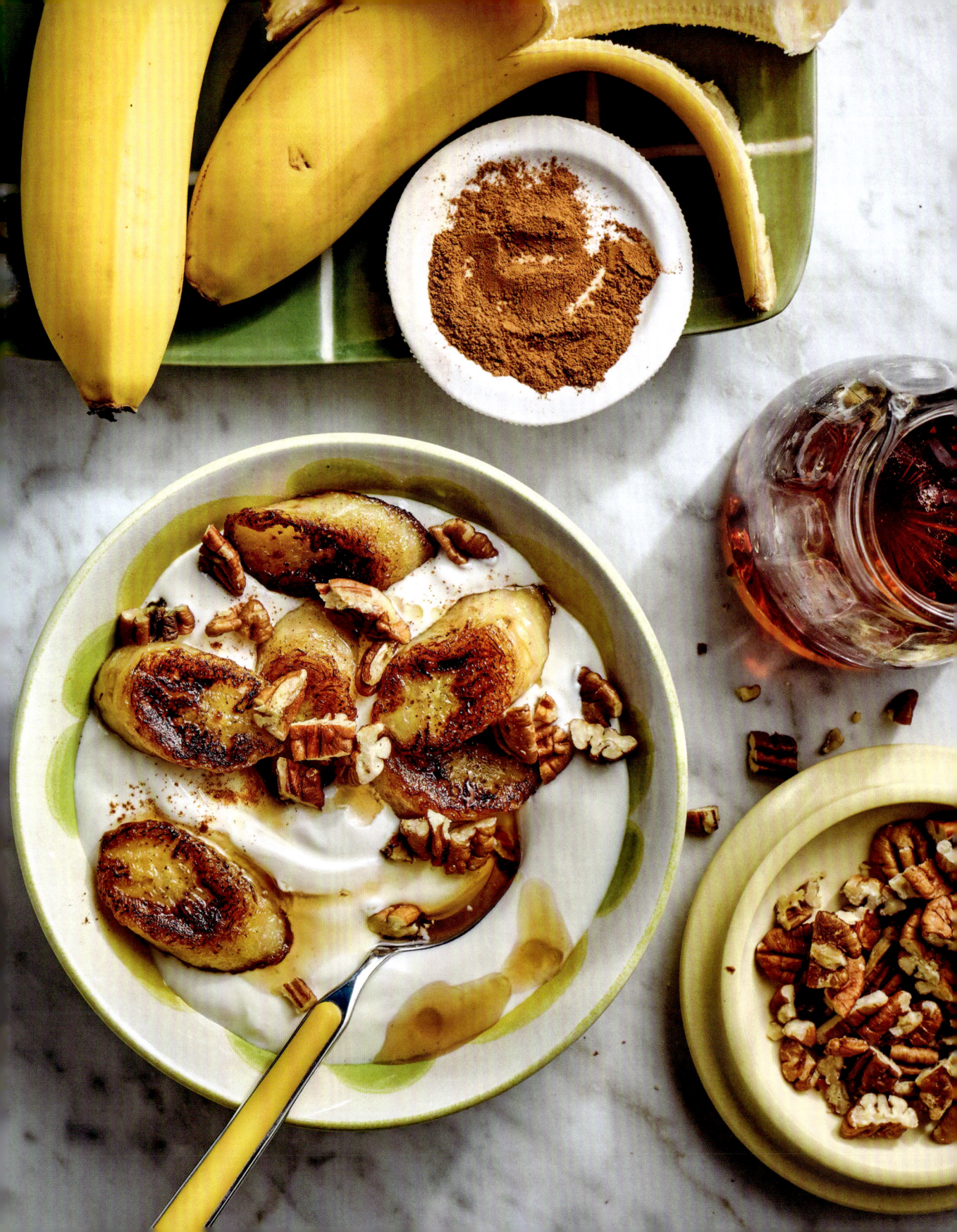

CARAMELIZED BANANA YOGURT BOWL

with Maple & Pecans

This 10-minute yogurt bowl with caramelized bananas and pecans tastes like you're having dessert for breakfast! It's also great as a midday snack or as an actual dessert. The natural sugars in bananas help them caramelize without needing to add any butter or sugar. I experimented with mixing a tablespoon of unflavored collagen in with the yogurt to increase the protein, and it blended seamlessly. A little pure maple syrup goes a long way to sweeten the yogurt, but you can also use sugar-free syrup, if you prefer.

Spray a nonstick medium pan with coconut oil and heat over medium-low heat. Place the banana slices in the pan and sprinkle with cinnamon. Cover and cook for 3 minutes on each side until they are caramelized and turn golden brown.

In a shallow serving bowl, thoroughly stir together the yogurt and the collagen, then smooth it with the back of a spoon. Drizzle the top with the maple syrup. Arrange the caramelized bananas on top, sprinkle with the chopped pecans, and serve.

SERVES 1

Coconut oil spray

1 small banana (about 6 inches long), sliced

Pinch of ground cinnamon

1 cup 2% Greek yogurt (I love Fage)

1 tablespoon unflavored collagen peptide powder or vegetarian collagen peptide powder

1 teaspoon pure maple syrup

2 tablespoons raw pecans, roughly chopped

Per Serving | Calories 377 | **Protein 31 g** | Carbohydrate 36 g | Fiber 4 g | Sugars 24 g | Fat 14 g | Saturated Fat 4 g | Cholesterol 27 mg | Sodium 112 mg

CHICKEN CHORIZO BREAKFAST TACOS

On mornings when I'm famished, I love to whip up tacos for breakfast. They're easy, filling, and you can make them so many different ways. To increase the protein without increasing the fat, I usually do a mix of whole egg and egg whites, but feel free to use 12 whole eggs instead, if you prefer. If you can't find chicken chorizo, chicken breakfast sausage works just as well. If you want to keep these vegetarian, use vegan chorizo crumbles.

Heat a large nonstick skillet over medium heat and spray with oil. Add the chorizo and cook until browned, 2 to 3 minutes. Remove the chorizo from the skillet and set aside. Spray the skillet with more oil and add the whole eggs and egg whites. Season with the salt and cook, stirring, until just done, 2 to 3 minutes. Remove from the heat and fold in the cheddar and sausage.

While the egg cooks, char the tortillas for 30 seconds on each side over a flame on the stove. To assemble the tacos, place 2 tortillas on each plate and divide the eggs and avocado evenly among the tortillas. Finish the tacos with cilantro, diced onion, and your hot sauce of choice (if using).

TIP: I always keep a carton of egg whites in my refrigerator for a lean protein source to add to eggs, oatmeal, and more.

SERVES 4

Olive oil spray

1 (3-ounce) link fully cooked chicken chorizo, such as Boar's Head or Aidells, chopped

4 large eggs, beaten

2 cups egg whites

¼ teaspoon kosher salt

¾ cup shredded reduced-fat cheddar cheese (3 ounces) or nondairy cheddar, such as Violife

8 corn tortillas

4 ounces sliced avocado (about 1 small Hass)

¼ cup chopped fresh cilantro

½ small yellow onion, finely diced

Salsa roja or Cholula hot sauce (optional), for serving

Per Serving (2 tacos) | Calories 412 | **Protein 32 g** | Carbohydrate 27 g | Fiber 5 g | Sugars 2 g | Fat 20 g | Saturated Fat 7 g | Cholesterol 227 mg | Sodium 676 mg

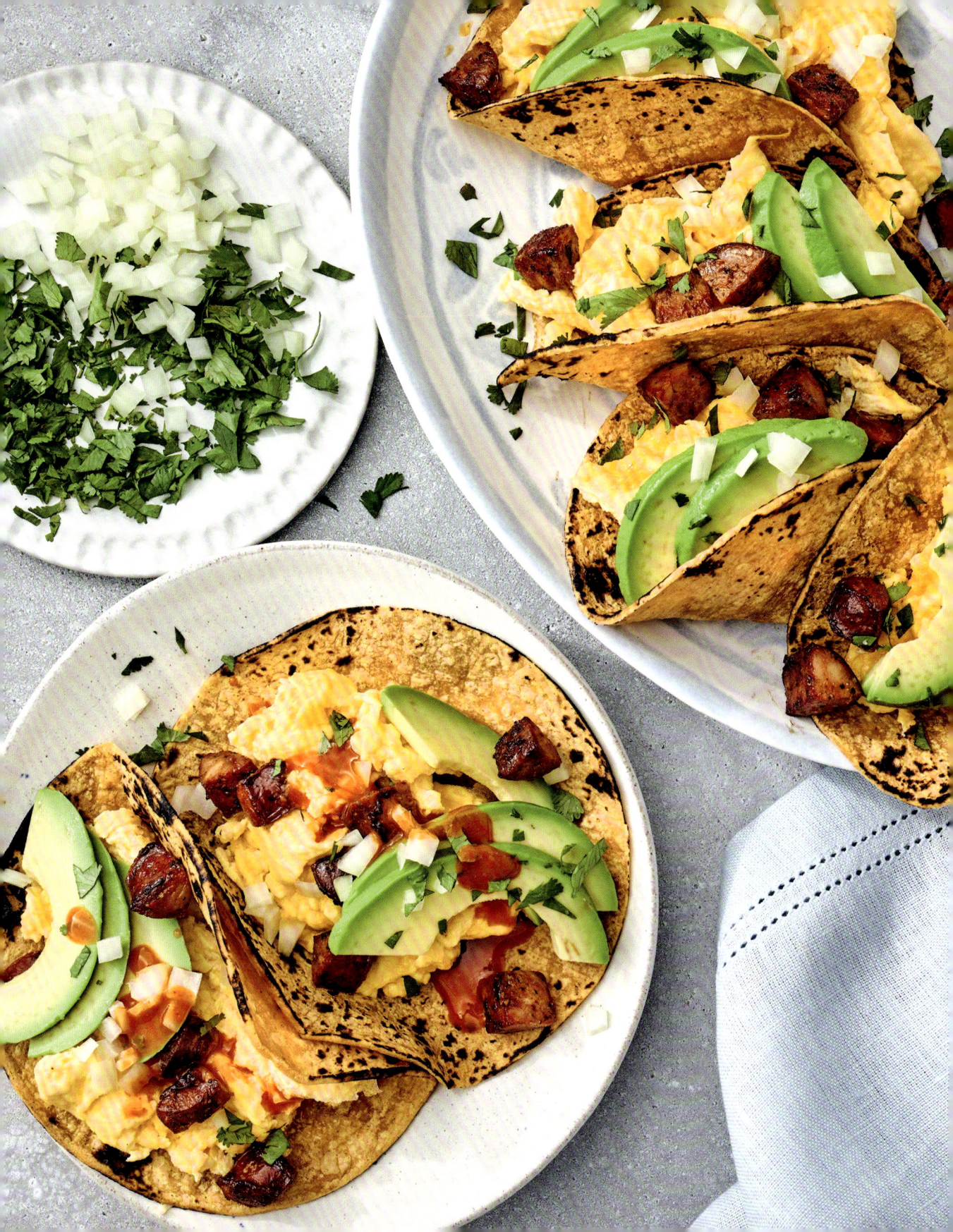

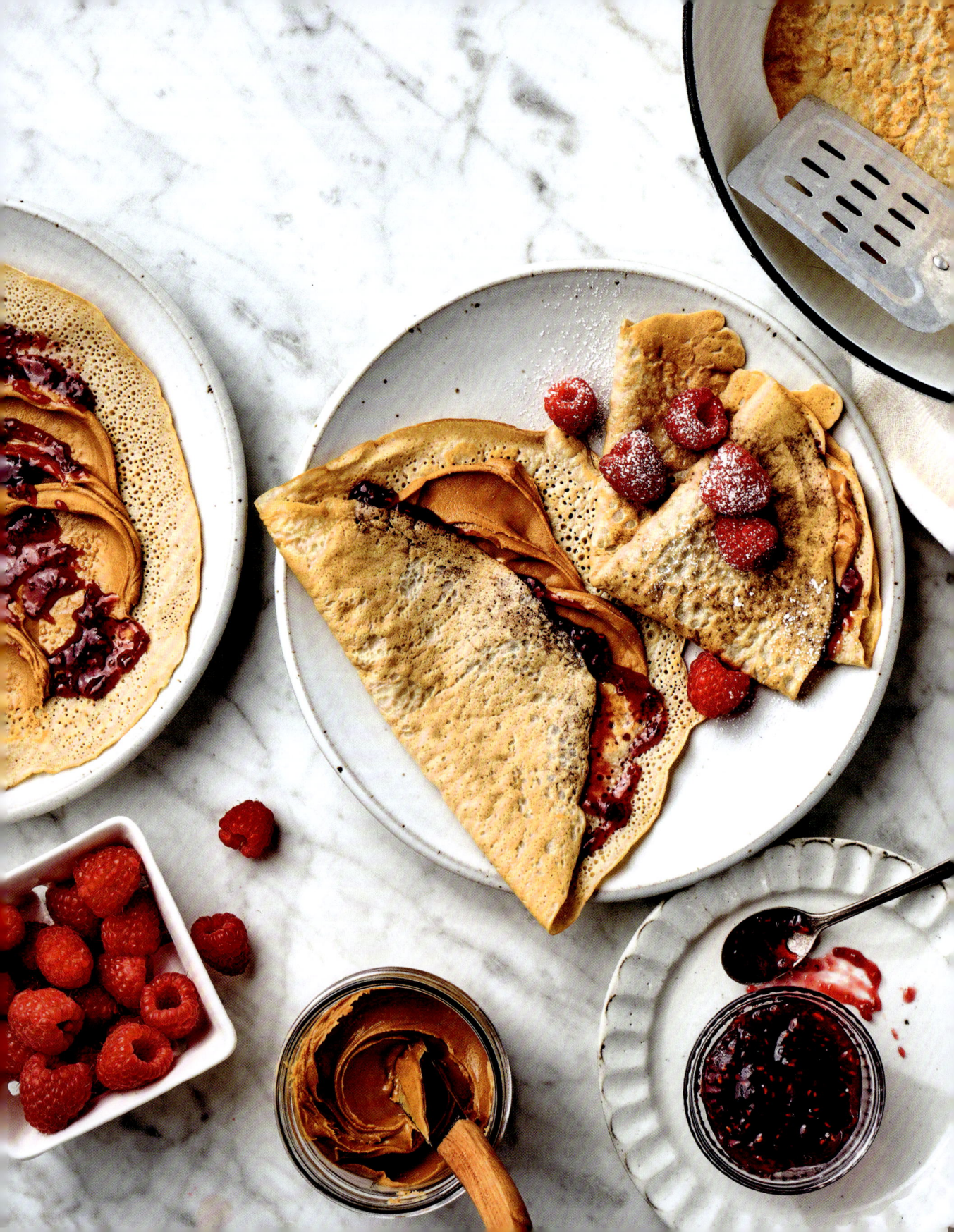

PB&J CREPES

Fun fact: Crepes were the very first recipe my mom taught me to cook as a kid! I grew up eating crepes practically every week, and these high-protein blender crepes taste just like the ones I had as a child but are made with a lot more protein and no flour. You can top or fill them with even more protein like yogurt, cottage cheese, nut butters, ricotta, eggs, or whatever you can think of! Here, I went with peanut butter and jam, one of my favorite sandwich combinations that's just as delicious rolled in a crepe. With all the extra protein, these crepes will keep you and your kids feeling satisfied longer.

SERVES 4

8 High-Protein Crepes (recipe follows)

½ cup creamy peanut butter or your favorite nut butter

¼ cup sugar-free raspberry preserves, such as Polaner Sugar Free

2 cups fresh raspberries

Powdered sugar (optional), for topping

Prepare the crepes as instructed in the recipe that follows.

In a small microwave-safe bowl, melt the peanut butter in the microwave for 30 to 60 seconds, until it's easy to spread. Spread 1½ teaspoons of preserves on the bottom half of each crepe, followed by 1 tablespoon peanut butter. Fold in half, then in quarters, and top with raspberries. Sprinkle with powdered sugar, if desired.

Per Serving (2 crepes) | Calories 562 | **Protein 36 g** | Carbohydrate 34 g | Fiber 13 g | Sugars 9 g | Fat 35 g | Saturated Fat 6.5 g | Cholesterol 2 mg | Sodium 348 mg

HIGH-PROTEIN CREPES

In a blender, combine the egg whites, milk, protein powder, oat flour, vanilla, and sweetener, if desired. Pulse for 10 seconds until the batter is smooth and blended.

Heat a 10-inch nonstick skillet over medium-low heat. Once hot, lightly coat the skillet with cooking spray.

Pour about ¼ cup of the batter into the skillet, tilting it to spread the batter evenly into a thin layer. Cook until the bottom is lightly browned, about 1 minute. Carefully flip the crepe with a spatula and cook the other side. Avoid flipping too soon to prevent the crepe from breaking apart. Transfer the crepe to a plate and repeat with the remaining batter.

Per Serving (2 crepes) | Calories 140 | **Protein 20 g** | Carbohydrate 8 g | Fiber 1 g | Sugars 2 g | Fat 2 g | Saturated Fat 0.5 g | Cholesterol 2 mg | Sodium 127 mg

MAKES 8 CREPES

1 cup egg whites

½ cup 2% milk or nondairy protein milk, such as Ripple

½ cup unflavored pumpkin seed protein, pea protein powder, or vanilla protein powder of your choice

¼ cup oat flour*

1 teaspoon vanilla extract

1 tablespoon monk fruit sweetener (optional)

Cooking oil spray

*Read the label to be sure this product is gluten-free.

AVOCADO TOAST
with Cottage Cheese Eggs

Avocado toast on its own is delicious, but it's definitely lacking in protein. Adding eggs is an easy fix, and because I like to get 30 grams of protein with my breakfast, I do a combo of eggs, egg whites, and cottage cheese. Adding cottage cheese to your eggs not only ups the protein but also makes them super creamy, just like cheesy eggs. I usually top this toast with sriracha because I like it spicy, but that's totally optional.

Toast the bread. Meanwhile, heat a small nonstick skillet over medium heat. Spray with oil and add the whole egg, egg whites, and cottage cheese. Scramble right in the skillet, stirring to break up the eggs and combine with the cottage cheese. Add the salt and cook, stirring, until the liquid from the cottage cheese evaporates, 4 to 5 minutes.

Spread the eggs over the toast and top with avocado slices. Finish with another pinch of salt and Sriracha, hot sauce, or pepper flakes, if desired.

TIP: To make this dairy-free while keeping the protein high, swap the cottage cheese for ⅓ cup more egg whites.

SERVES 1

1 (1½-ounce) slice sourdough bread or gluten-free bread

Cooking oil spray

1 large egg

⅓ cup egg whites

⅓ cup low-fat (2%) cottage cheese (I love Good Culture)

Pinch of kosher salt, plus more for topping

1 ounce sliced avocado (about ¼ small Hass)

Sriracha, hot sauce, or crushed red pepper flakes (optional), for topping

Per Serving | Calories 328 | **Protein 30 g** | Carbohydrate 27 g | Fiber 3 g | Sugars 5 g | Fat 12 g | Saturated Fat 3.5 g | Cholesterol 196 mg | Sodium 830 mg

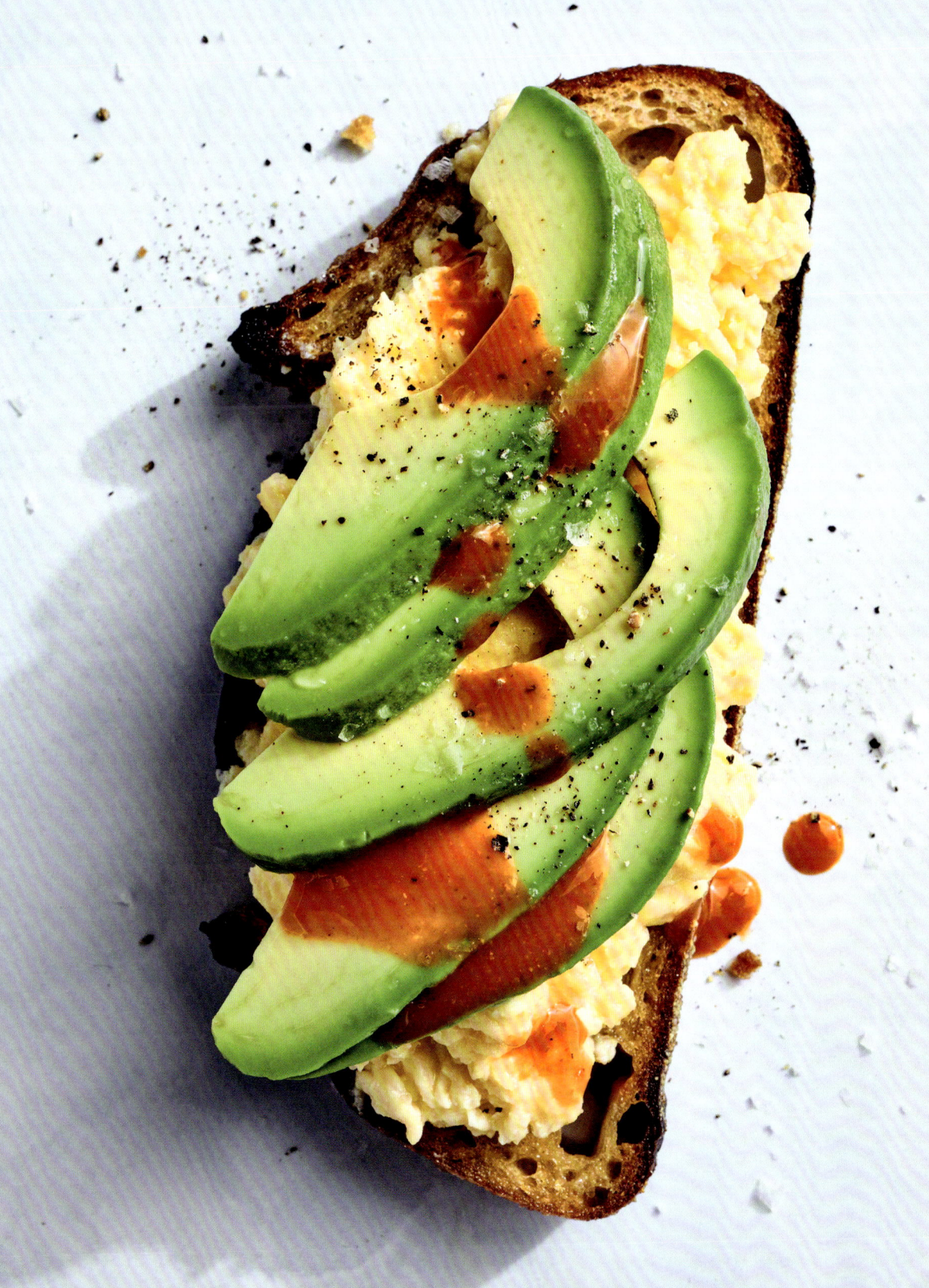

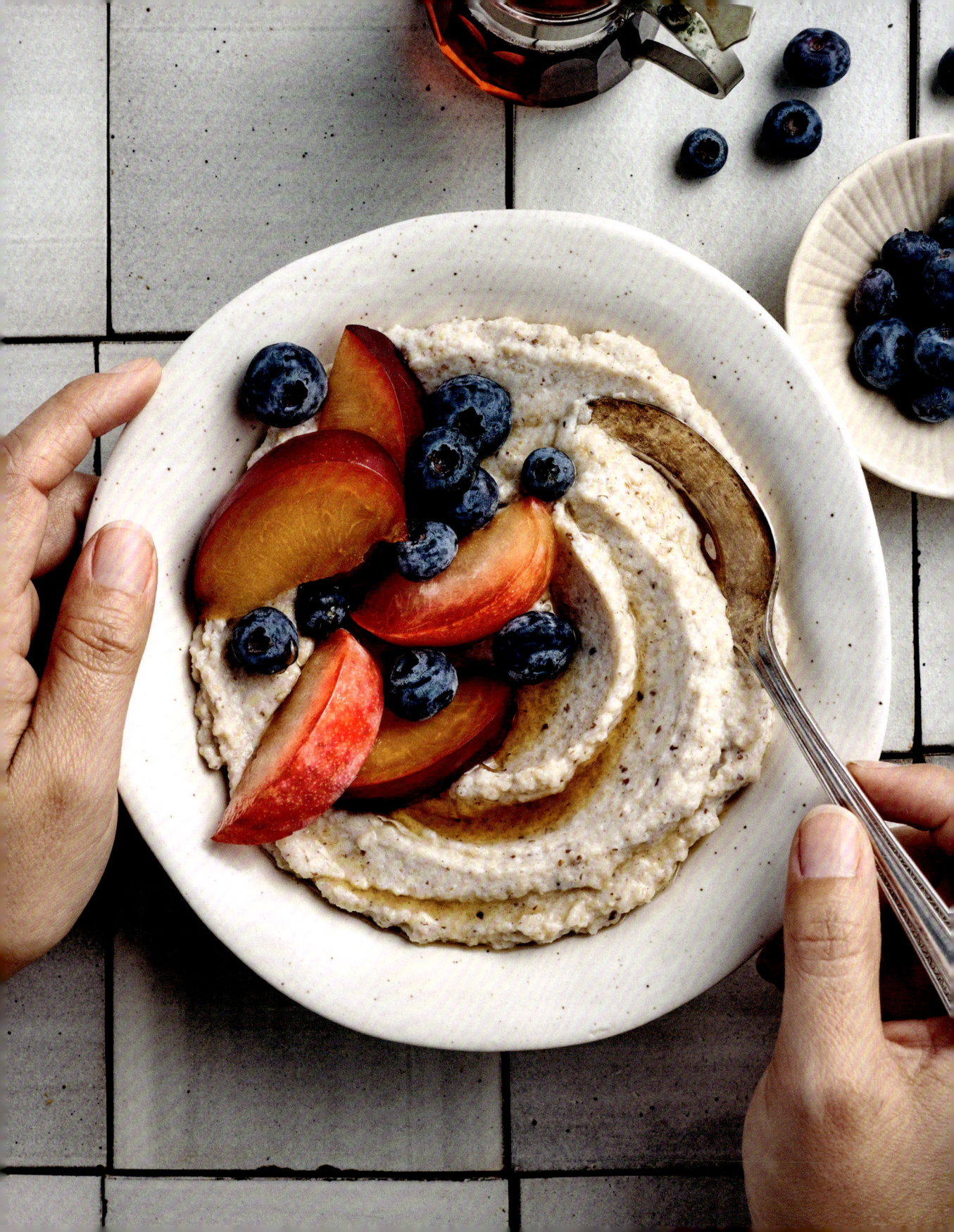

CREAMY PROTEIN OATS

When I was a kid, my mom always made me and my brother hot cereals like oatmeal, cream of wheat, and farina with milk, sugar, and cinnamon for breakfast. It was such a comforting way to start the day. I recently discovered oat bran cereal, which is the outer layer of the oat groat—it's high in fiber, vitamins, minerals, and antioxidants, and it's creamy when cooked, just like oatmeal. I've been including hot oat bran in my breakfast rotation, and to make it high protein, I add milk, egg whites, and a little whey protein. Since I'm always aiming to get at least 25 grams of fiber in my day, I even add flaxmeal for a boost of nutrients. Topped with cinnamon and seasonal fruit, this makes the creamiest, most comforting hot breakfast that reminds me of my mom's.

In a small saucepan, combine 1 cup of the milk, ½ cup water, the oat bran, egg whites, protein powder, flaxmeal, cinnamon, and sweetener of your choice and whisk well until no lumps remain. Bring to a boil over medium-low heat, stirring. Once boiling, reduce the heat to low and simmer, stirring constantly so the milk doesn't scorch, until thick and creamy, about 3 minutes.

Pour into a bowl and stir in the remaining ¼ cup milk to loosen and another pinch of cinnamon. Top with fruit and enjoy immediately.

SERVES 1

1¼ cups fat-free milk or dairy-free protein milk

⅓ cup oat bran hot cereal or protein oats,* such as Bob's Red Mill

3 tablespoons egg whites

2 tablespoons unflavored whey or pea protein powder

1 tablespoon ground flaxseeds

⅛ teaspoon ground cinnamon, plus more for topping

1 tablespoon sweetener of choice, or to taste (I use monk fruit)

½ cup seasonal fruit for topping, such as blueberries, or sliced peaches or nectarines

*Read the label to be sure this product is gluten-free.

Per Serving | Calories 383 | **Protein 31 g** | Carbohydrate 54 g | Fiber 7 g | Sugars 23 g | Fat 6 g | Saturated Fat 0.5 g | Cholesterol 27 mg | Sodium 220 mg

AIR FRYER BREAKFAST BAGEL SANDWICHES

Ham, egg, and cheese is my go-to breakfast sandwich, but I've never seen one pack this much protein! To make this high protein, I use my homemade Greek yogurt egg bagels—they're light, fluffy, and the perfect base for a protein-packed start to the day (just make sure your baking powder is not expired or the dough won't rise). You can make the bagels in the air fryer or in the oven, and they're also ideal for meal prep (see tip). Serve this with a cup of fruit to make it a meal and feel free to swap the toppings, such as Canadian bacon or turkey/chicken breakfast sausage in place of the ham.

MAKE THE YOGURT EGG BAGELS: In a medium bowl, combine the flour, baking powder, and salt and whisk well. Add the yogurt and egg yolks only and mix well with a fork until well combined. It will look like small crumbles.

Lightly dust flour on a work surface and remove the dough from the bowl. Knead the dough a few times until it is smooth and tacky, but not sticky, 15 to 20 turns (it should not leave dough on your hand when you pull away).

Divide into 4 equal portions and roll each portion into a rope ¾ inch thick. Join the ends of the rope to form bagels. Brush the top with the egg whites and sprinkle both sides with seasoning of your choice.

Place a piece of air fryer parchment inside an air fryer basket to avoid sticking. Place the bagels in the basket and fry at 280°F until golden, 16 to 17 minutes. (No need to flip.)

Set the bagels aside to cool.

MEANWHILE, FOR THE SANDWICHES: Heat a large nonstick skillet over medium heat and spray with oil. Add the eggs and season with the salt and black pepper to taste. Cook the eggs, scrambling with a wooden spoon, until just set, about 2 minutes. Set aside.

Cut the bagels in half horizontally and then assemble the sandwiches by layering a slice of ham on each side, then the eggs and cheese.

Per Serving (1 sandwich) | Calories 445 | **Protein 32 g** | Carbohydrate 34 g | Fiber 2 g | Sugars 3 g | Fat 20 g | Saturated Fat 8 g | Cholesterol 496 mg | Sodium 918 mg

SERVES 4

YOGURT EGG BAGELS

1¼ cups (6.25 ounces) unbleached all-purpose flour, whole wheat, or gluten-free flour, plus more for dusting

2 teaspoons baking powder

¾ teaspoon kosher salt

¾ cup 0% Greek yogurt (not regular yogurt, it will be too sticky), preferably Stonyfield or Fage

2 large eggs, separated, whites and yolks lightly beaten separately

Optional toppings: Everything bagel seasoning, sesame seeds, poppy seeds, onion flakes, or garlic flakes

SANDWICHES

Olive oil spray

8 large eggs, beaten

⅛ teaspoon kosher salt

Freshly ground black pepper

4 ounces thinly sliced reduced-sodium deli ham

4 slices cheddar cheese

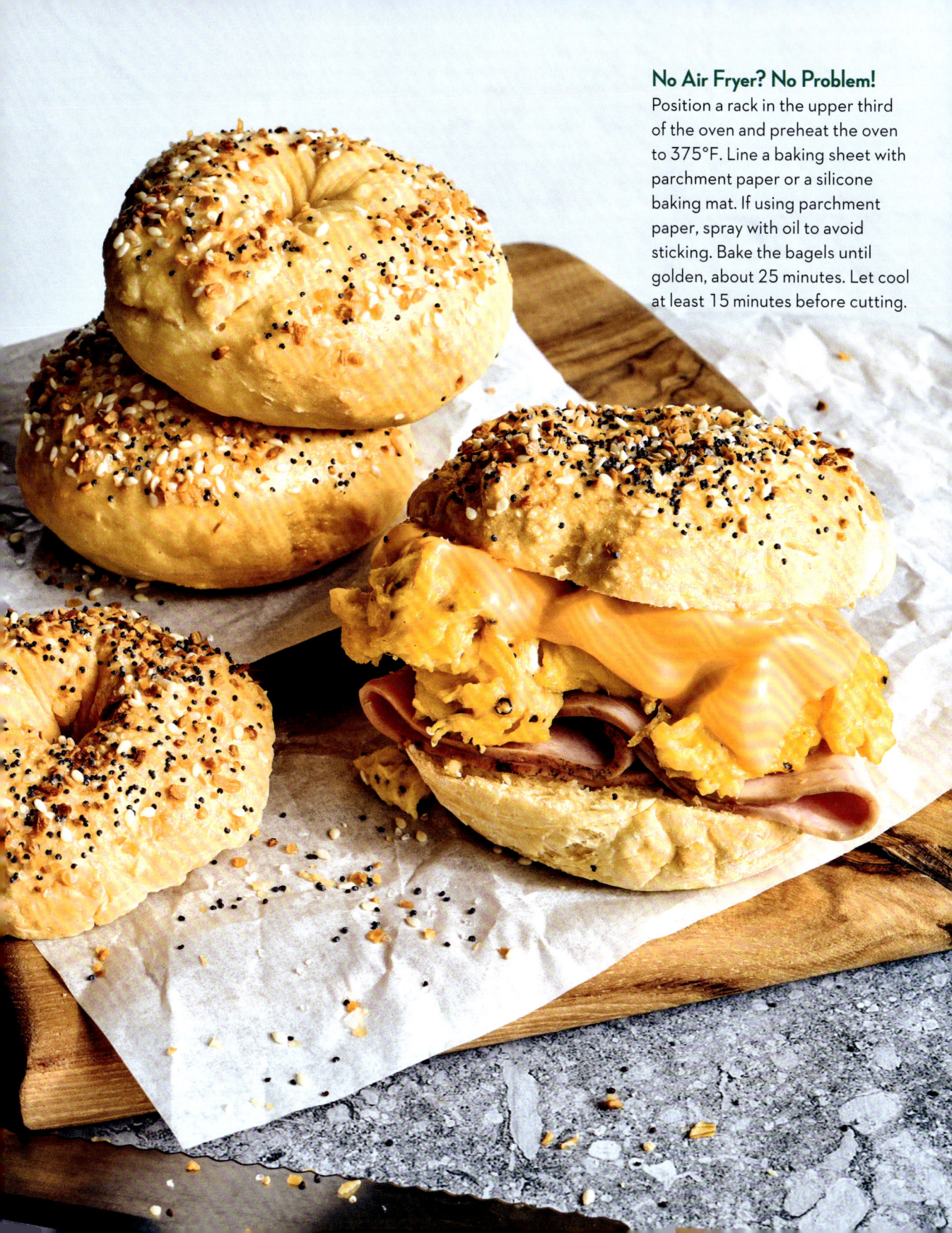

No Air Fryer? No Problem!

Position a rack in the upper third of the oven and preheat the oven to 375°F. Line a baking sheet with parchment paper or a silicone baking mat. If using parchment paper, spray with oil to avoid sticking. Bake the bagels until golden, about 25 minutes. Let cool at least 15 minutes before cutting.

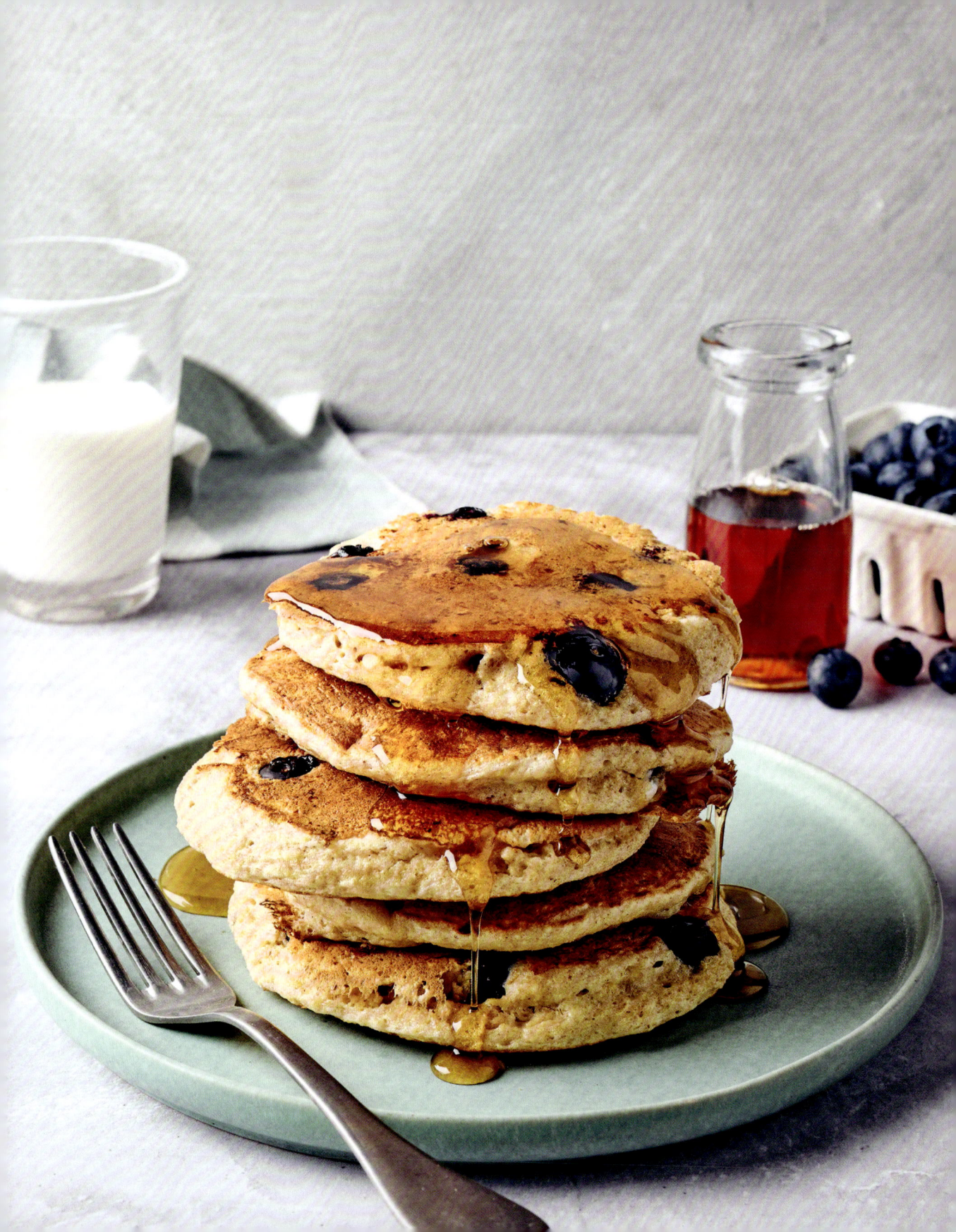

BLUEBERRY-LEMON COTTAGE CHEESE OAT PANCAKES

This dish satisfies my weekend craving for pancakes, while still being both high in protein and fiber! I tested this out on my cousins and aunt and they loved it! I love the texture from the oat bran, but if you want smoother pancakes, you can blend the cottage cheese and oat bran together before mixing with the remaining ingredients. The whole batch is one serving, but I honestly can't finish this whole stack of pancakes at one time, so I usually eat half with eggs, and heat up the other half the next day. The recipe is super easy to scale up to feed more if needed, and it can be meal prepped for the week.

In a medium bowl, whisk together the oats, oat flour, baking powder, and salt.

In a large bowl, beat the egg whites with a hand mixer until fluffy, 30 to 60 seconds, then mix in the cottage cheese, vanilla, sweetener (if using), and lemon zest. Add the oat mixture and gently fold in to combine.

Spray a large nonstick or griddle with oil and heat over medium-low heat.

In batches as needed, pour ¼ cup of the pancake mixture into the skillet. Arrange a few blueberries on top. Cook on medium-low until the bottom browns, 2 to 3 minutes. Flip and cook until golden and cooked through in the center, an additional 2 to 3 minutes. Repeat with the remaining batter.

Serve topped with your favorite fruit compote or syrup, if desired.

SERVES 1

⅓ cup high-protein oat bran cereal or high-protein oatmeal* (such as Bob's Red Mill High Fiber Oat Bran Hot Cereal)

⅓ cup oat flour*

¼ teaspoon baking powder

Pinch of kosher salt

½ cup egg whites

⅓ cup 2% cottage cheese

½ teaspoon vanilla extract

1 tablespoon monk fruit or sweetener of choice (optional)

Grated zest of ½ lemon

Coconut oil or olive oil spray

½ cup blueberries, fresh or thawed frozen

Fruit compote or syrup (optional), for serving

*Read the label to be sure this product is gluten-free.

Perfect Pairings
I love topping this with Wholesome Yum Zero Sugar Maple Syrup, or I make a super-easy blueberry sauce by warming up frozen wild blueberries in the microwave for 1 minute and then pouring them over the pancakes.

Per Serving (4 pancakes) | Calories 473 | **Protein 35 g** | Carbohydrate 69 g | Fiber 13 g | Sugars 12 g | Fat 7 g | Saturated Fat 1.5 g | Cholesterol 10 mg | Sodium 622 mg

ENCHILADA BREAKFAST CASSEROLE

This Mexican breakfast casserole is so good, and it's perfect for make-ahead breakfast meal prep, but you can also enjoy this for lunch or dinner. It's so versatile! Swap the ground chicken for turkey breakfast sausage or leave the meat out and double the egg and egg whites to keep it vegetarian. I love using my homemade enchilada sauce (recipe on my blog), but you can always use store-bought in a pinch.

Preheat the oven to 350°F. Spray a 9 × 13-inch baking dish with oil.

Heat a large skillet over high heat and spray with oil. Add the ground chicken, 1 teaspoon salt, and the cumin and cook, breaking it up until cooked through, about 5 minutes. Transfer to a large bowl and set aside.

Add the olive oil to the skillet and reduce the heat to medium. Add the bell peppers, scallions, and a pinch of salt and cook until tender, 3 to 5 minutes. Reduce the heat to medium-low.

Add the whole eggs, egg whites, and ¼ teaspoon salt and cook, stirring, until just set, about 2 minutes. Transfer to the bowl with the cooked chicken and stir in ½ cup of the enchilada sauce.

Spread ½ cup of the enchilada sauce on the bottom of the prepared baking dish, then top with 6 tortillas, overlapping as needed. Add half of the egg-chicken mixture, ½ cup of the enchilada sauce, and 1 cup of the cheese. Repeat with the remaining 6 tortillas, chicken-egg mixture, 1 cup enchilada sauce, and 1 cup cheese.

Cover with foil and bake for 30 minutes. Remove the foil and bake until the cheese is melted and bubbling, 10 more minutes. Garnish with the jalapeño slices and more scallions. Cut into 6 pieces and serve.

TO MEAL PREP: Divide into 6 meal-prep containers. Keep covered and refrigerate up to 4 days.

TO FREEZE: Divide into 6 freezer-safe meal-prep containers. Freeze for up to 3 months. To reheat, transfer to the refrigerator or reheat from frozen in 30-second intervals until heated through.

SERVES 6

Cooking oil spray

1 pound ground chicken breast, preferably organic

Kosher salt

1 teaspoon ground cumin

2 teaspoons extra-virgin olive oil

1 red bell pepper, finely diced

1 green bell pepper, finely diced

4 scallions, chopped, plus more for garnish

6 large eggs

4 large egg whites

2½ cups red enchilada sauce (homemade or store-bought from two 10-ounce cans)

12 extra-thin corn tortillas, such as Mission

2 cups shredded reduced-fat Mexican cheese blend (I like Sargento)

1 jalapeño, thinly sliced, for garnish

Perfect Pairings
Serve it with slices of avocado and sour cream.

Per Serving (1 piece) | Calories 407 | **Protein 43 g** | Carbohydrate 26 g | Fiber 5.5 g | Sugars 7 g | Fat 16 g | Saturated Fat 6.5 g | Cholesterol 246 mg | Sodium 1,205 mg

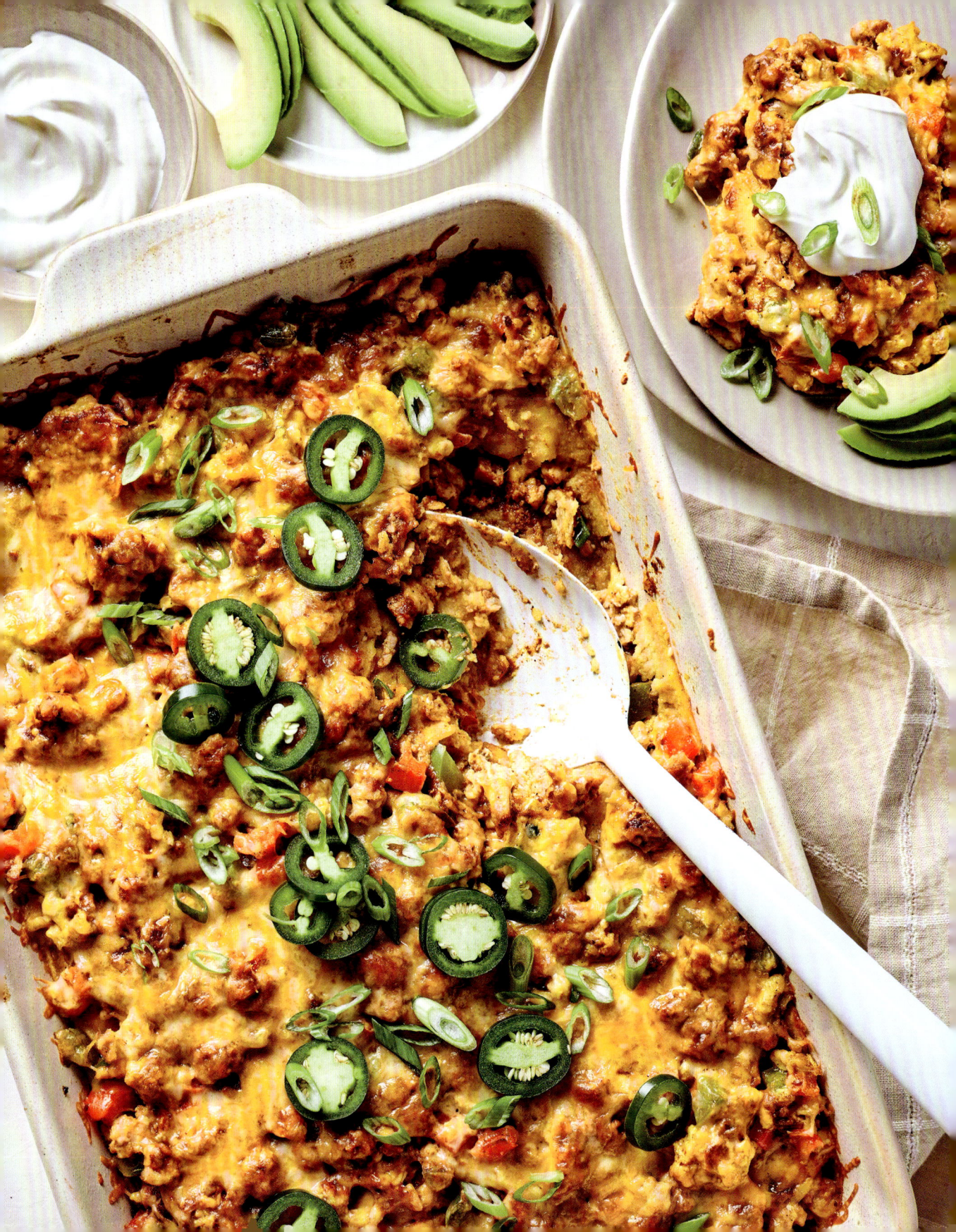

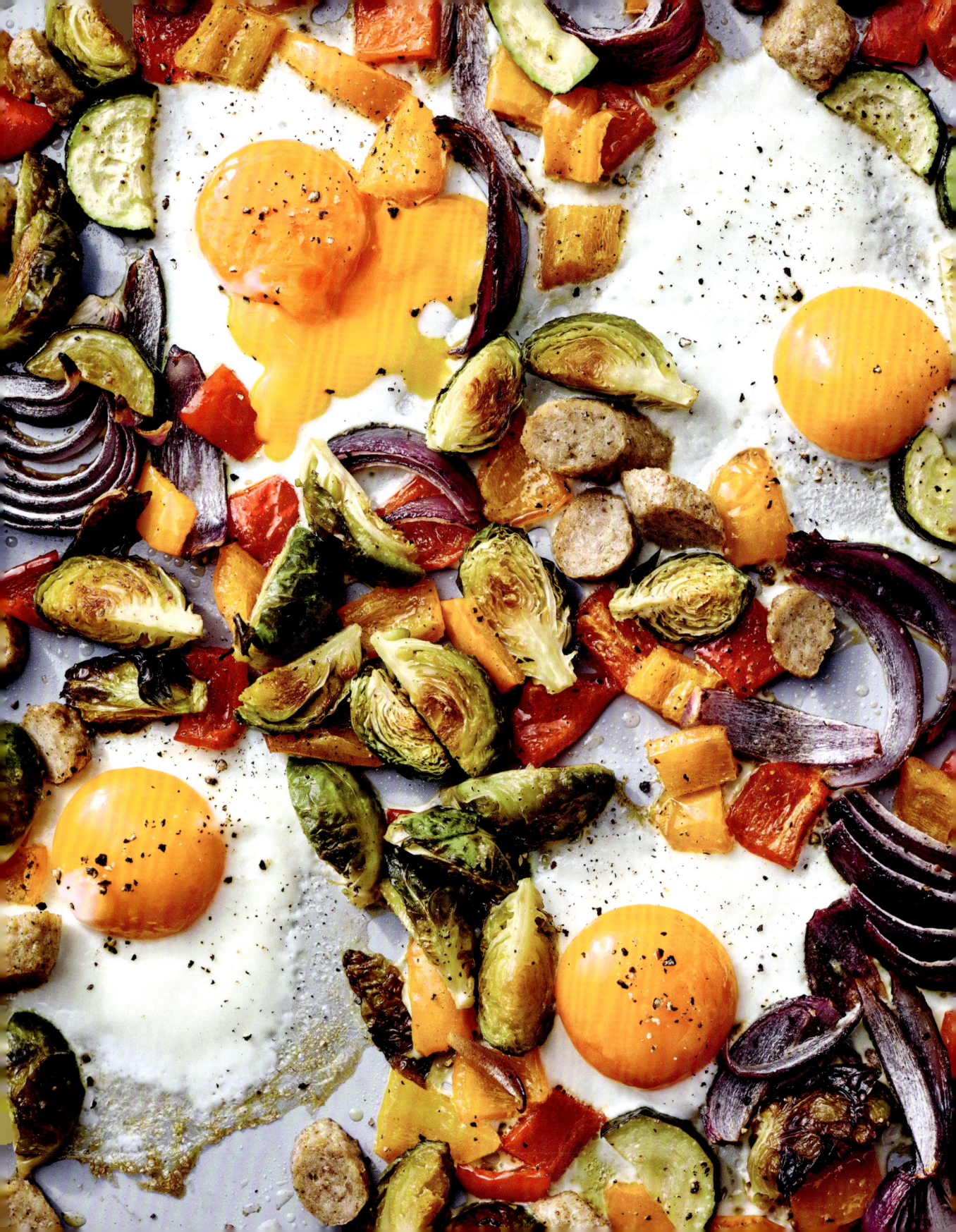

SHEET PAN BREAKFAST

with Veggie Hash

I love having roasted veggies with my eggs, so this easy sheet pan breakfast is a winner because it's a one and done! Use whatever chopped seasonal veggies you like plus breakfast sausage, then nestle in the eggs and bake until the yolks are jammy. It's a delicious breakfast that can really be eaten any time of the day. In fact, if you love breakfast for dinner, this would be the perfect meal.

Preheat the oven to 425°F. Adjust two racks in the center of the oven. Spray two sheet pans with oil to coat the entire surface.

Divide the cut vegetables between the two pans and arrange in a single layer without overcrowding. Drizzle with olive oil and season with ¾ teaspoon kosher salt and black pepper to taste.

Roast for 15 minutes. Remove from the oven, toss the veggies, and add the breakfast sausage. Return to the oven and roast until the vegetables are tender, another 10 to 15 minutes. Remove from the oven but leave the oven on.

Create 8 wells in the veggies for the eggs. Carefully crack one egg at a time into a small bowl and pour into a well (this helps keep the eggs from breaking). Return the pans to the oven and bake until the egg whites have set and the yolks are cooked to your desired amount, 6 to 8 minutes.

Serve immediately.

TIP: For variations, you can use finely diced butternut squash or sweet potatoes in place of the peppers and zucchini. To make it vegetarian, use vegan sausage instead.

SERVES 4

Olive oil spray

12 ounces Brussels sprouts, trimmed and quartered

1 red bell pepper, cut into ½-inch pieces

1 orange bell pepper, cut into ½-inch pieces

1 large zucchini, sliced into half-moons ½ inch thick

1 small red onion, cut into 8 wedges

1 tablespoon extra-virgin olive oil

¾ teaspoon kosher salt

Freshly ground black pepper

12 frozen turkey or chicken breakfast sausage links (I like Applegate), cut into ½-inch-thick rounds (8.5 ounces total)

8 extra-large eggs

Per Serving (2 eggs + 3 sausage links + generous ¾ cup vegetables) | Calories 358 | **Protein 30 g** | Carbohydrate 18 g | Fiber 5.5 g | Sugars 8 g | Fat 20 g | Saturated Fat 6 g | Cholesterol 462 mg | Sodium 840 mg

EGG WHITE COTTAGE CHEESE MUFFINS
with Turkey Bacon

These easy egg white muffins are a real hit on my Skinnytaste website! Inspired by my friend Raquel, they're loaded with cottage cheese, turkey bacon, bell pepper, broccoli, scallions, and shallots, all baked in a muffin tin and topped with a little cheddar. They're perfect to meal prep on the weekends so you can have a quick breakfast on the go all week.

Preheat the oven to 350°F. Spray 12 cups of a nonstick muffin tin very generously with oil (not nonstick spray) so the eggs don't stick.

In a medium skillet, heat the oil over medium-low heat. Add the shallots, scallions, and bell pepper and sauté until tender, 5 to 6 minutes. Add the broccoli and set aside.

Meanwhile, in a large bowl, combine the egg whites, cottage cheese, garlic powder, and seasoning salt.

Stir the veggies into the egg white/cottage cheese mixture. Line each muffin cup with a half slice of turkey bacon around the edges and pour in the egg mixture, about 1/3 cup each. Top with the shredded cheddar.

Bake until set, about 25 minutes. Remove from the muffin cups and serve.

TIP: Swap the turkey bacon for Tofurky smoky maple bacon to make it vegetarian.

SERVES 4

Olive oil spray

1½ teaspoons extra-virgin olive oil

¼ cup chopped shallots or red onion

¼ cup chopped scallions

1 medium orange or red bell pepper, chopped

½ cup chopped steamed fresh broccoli or thawed frozen

1 (16-ounce) carton egg whites

1 (5.3-ounce) container 2% cottage cheese (a little over ½ cup), drained

½ teaspoon garlic powder

¼ teaspoon seasoning salt (such as adobo)

6 slices Applegate uncured turkey bacon, cut in half

¼ cup shredded sharp cheddar cheese

Per Serving (3 egg muffins) | Calories 201 | **Protein 30 g** | Carbohydrate 8 g | Fiber 2 g | Sugars 4 g | Fat 8 g | Saturated Fat 2.5 g | Cholesterol 43 mg | Sodium 672 mg

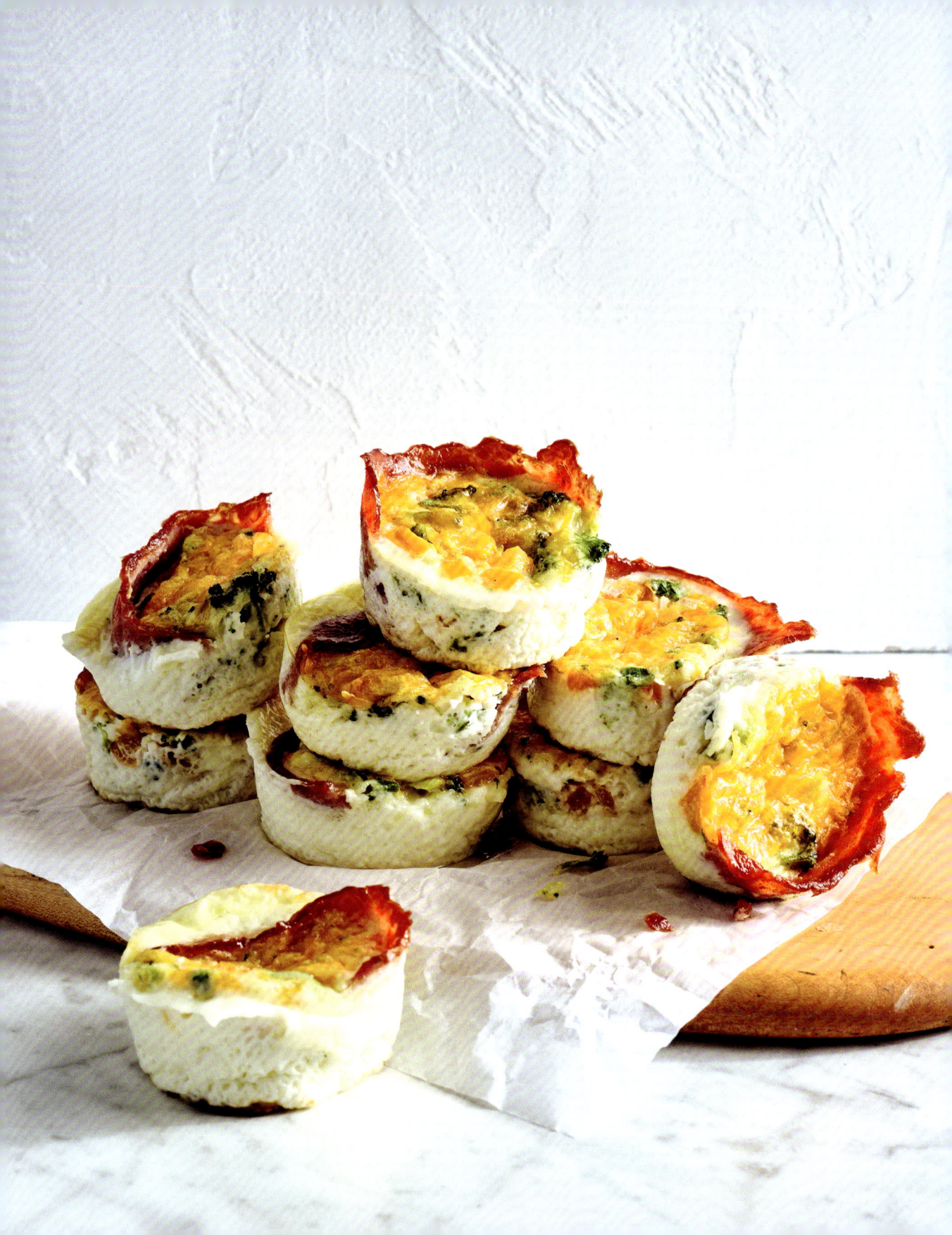

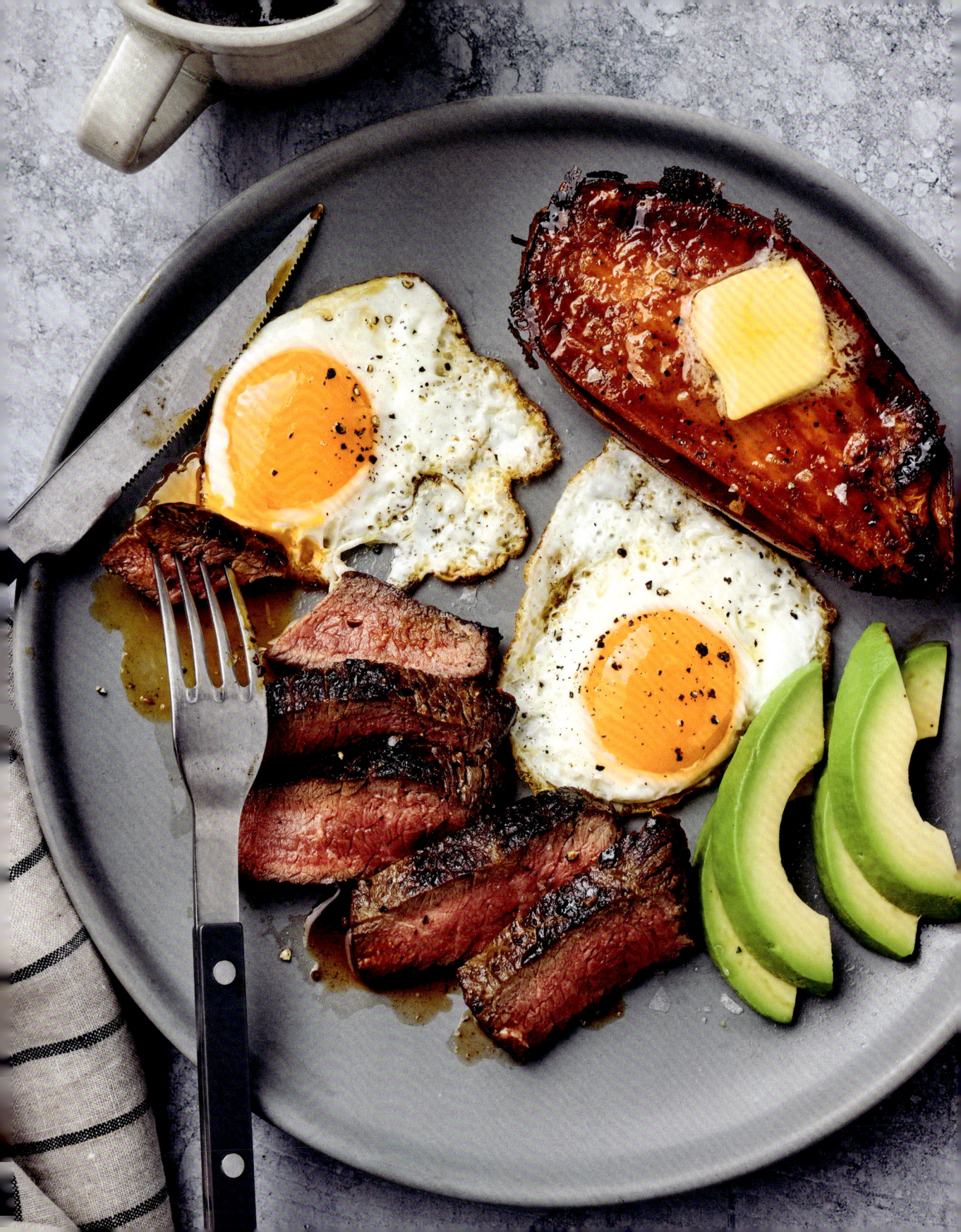

STEAK & EGGS

Sink your fork into this protein-packed plate filled with juicy steak, golden fried eggs, and roasted sweet potato goodness. This breakfast will absolutely keep you satisfied until lunch! My aunt, who works with me at Skinnytaste, avoids gluten and dairy, so I'm always mindful of creating anti-inflammatory meals she can enjoy. I also wanted to craft a high-protein breakfast that didn't rely on cottage cheese or egg whites to hit the protein mark. This dish strikes the perfect balance of protein, carbs, and healthy fats to kick-start your day—and it's downright delicious!

Preheat your oven to 400°F. Line a baking sheet with parchment paper or aluminum foil for easy cleanup.

Season the steak with ¼ teaspoon salt and black pepper to taste.

Spray the cut sides of the potato with olive oil and sprinkle with a pinch each of salt and pepper. Place the sweet potato halves cut-side down on the baking sheet and roast until the thickest part is tender when pierced with a fork, 30 to 35 minutes.

Heat a medium cast-iron skillet over high heat. When hot, spray with oil and add the steak to the pan. Once you've put it down, don't move it for at least 3 minutes, then flip it over. Reduce the heat to medium-high and cook an additional 3 minutes, or until the internal temperature reads 130°F for medium-rare, or longer as needed. (The steak will continue to cook 5 degrees while it rests.) If you like your steak more well done, cook for another minute on each side for medium.

Heat a medium nonstick skillet over medium heat and spray with oil. Gently add your eggs and reduce the heat to medium-low. Cover and cook until the yolk is still runny but the whites are cooked through, 2 to 3 minutes. Slice the steak and plate alongside the eggs, sweet potato half, and avocado. Add the butter to the sweet potato and season everything with salt and pepper to taste. Serve immediately.

TIP: You can add more veggies like sautéed mushrooms, grilled asparagus, or wilted spinach.

Per Serving | Calories 441 | **Protein 39 g** | Carbohydrate 20 g | Fiber 4.5 g | Sugars 6 g | Fat 23 g | Saturated Fat 7 g | Cholesterol 451 mg | Sodium 445 mg

SERVES 2

8 ounces sirloin steak or strip steak, trimmed of fat

Kosher salt

Freshly ground black pepper

Olive oil spray

1 medium sweet potato, about 6 ounces sliced in half lengthwise

4 large eggs

2 ounces sliced avocado (about ½ small Hass)

½ teaspoon unsalted butter or nondairy butter

QUICK-FIX LUNCHES

Let's face it—lunch is often the most overlooked meal of the day. Whether you're juggling work, errands, kids, or just life in general, it can be tempting to grab something quick (and often unsatisfying), or to just skip lunch altogether. But a high-protein lunch doesn't have to be complicated or time-consuming.

This chapter is all about embracing the "lazy girl" approach to lunch: simple, satisfying meals that come together quickly and still pack in plenty of protein to keep you energized for the rest of the day. These recipes are designed with busy schedules in mind, featuring minimal prep, easy cleanup, and ingredients you probably already have on hand.

From protein-packed salads and wraps to one-bowl meals and reheatable options you can meal prep ahead of time, these lunches prove that fueling your body doesn't have to mean sacrificing time or flavor. Many of these dishes can be made in under 15 minutes, like the Spicy Tuna Queso Melt (page 79), and others are perfect for prepping the night before, like one of my favorite go-tos, Choose-Your-Adventure Protein Sheet Pan Bake (page 80), so all you have to do is grab and go.

Whether you're working from home, heading to the office, or just trying to keep up with a packed schedule, these recipes will help you stay on track, feel full, and keep lunch stress-free. Because we're all busy, but we still deserve a delicious, protein-packed lunch.

CHICKEN AVOCADO SALAD CHIP DIP

This quick-to-prepare lunch is perfectly balanced with healthy fats from the avocado, protein from the chicken, cucumber for texture, and crackers for crunch. My sister-in-law got me hooked on eating chicken salad with Mary's Gone Crackers Super Seed crackers—so delish. The trick to making the dip creamy without adding too much mayo is using a little chicken broth, and it works great! You can also make this using leftover roasted chicken breast or a rotisserie chicken breast.

Chop the chicken really fine so it has the texture of canned tuna and transfer it to a medium bowl. Add the cucumber, avocado, onion, chicken broth, mayo, and salt. Stir until creamy and mixed well. Scoop it up with the crackers and enjoy.

TIP: If you want to meal prep this, you can easily double the recipe and add the avocado just before serving.

SERVES 1

3 ounces cooked boneless, skinless chicken breast, preferably organic

¼ cup finely chopped Persian (mini) cucumber

1 ounce diced avocado (about ¼ small Hass)

2 tablespoons chopped red onion or scallions

3 tablespoons chicken broth*

1 tablespoon plus 1 teaspoon mayonnaise (I like Hellmann's)

⅛ teaspoon kosher salt, plus (optional) more to taste

10 gluten-free crackers (I like Mary's Gone Crackers Super Seed)

*Read the label to be sure this product is gluten-free.

Per Serving (1 bowl + 10 crackers) | Calories 446 | **Protein 33 g** | Carbohydrate 19 g | Fiber 5 g | Sugars 1 g | Fat 27 g | Saturated Fat 4.5 g | Cholesterol 106 mg | Sodium 622 mg

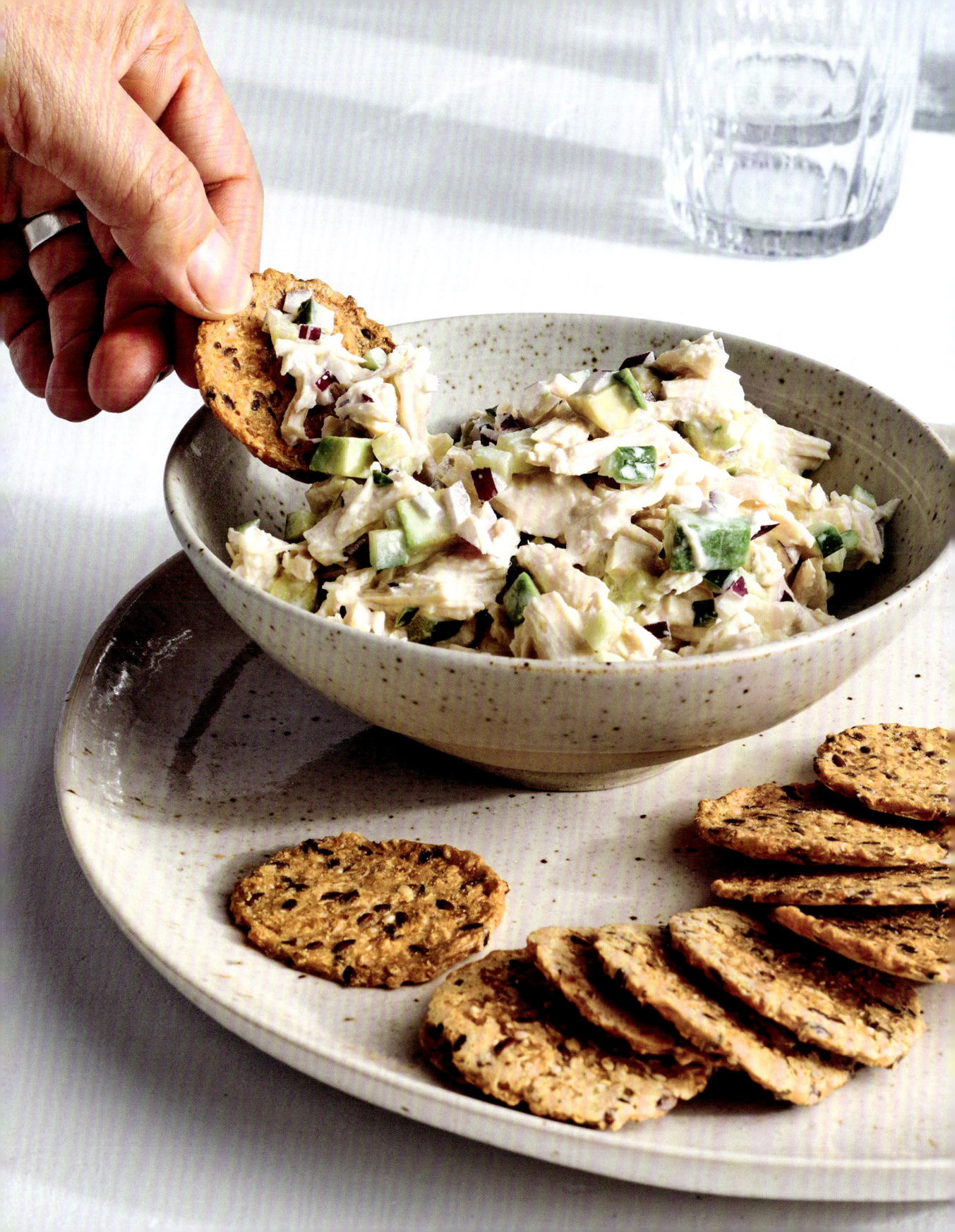

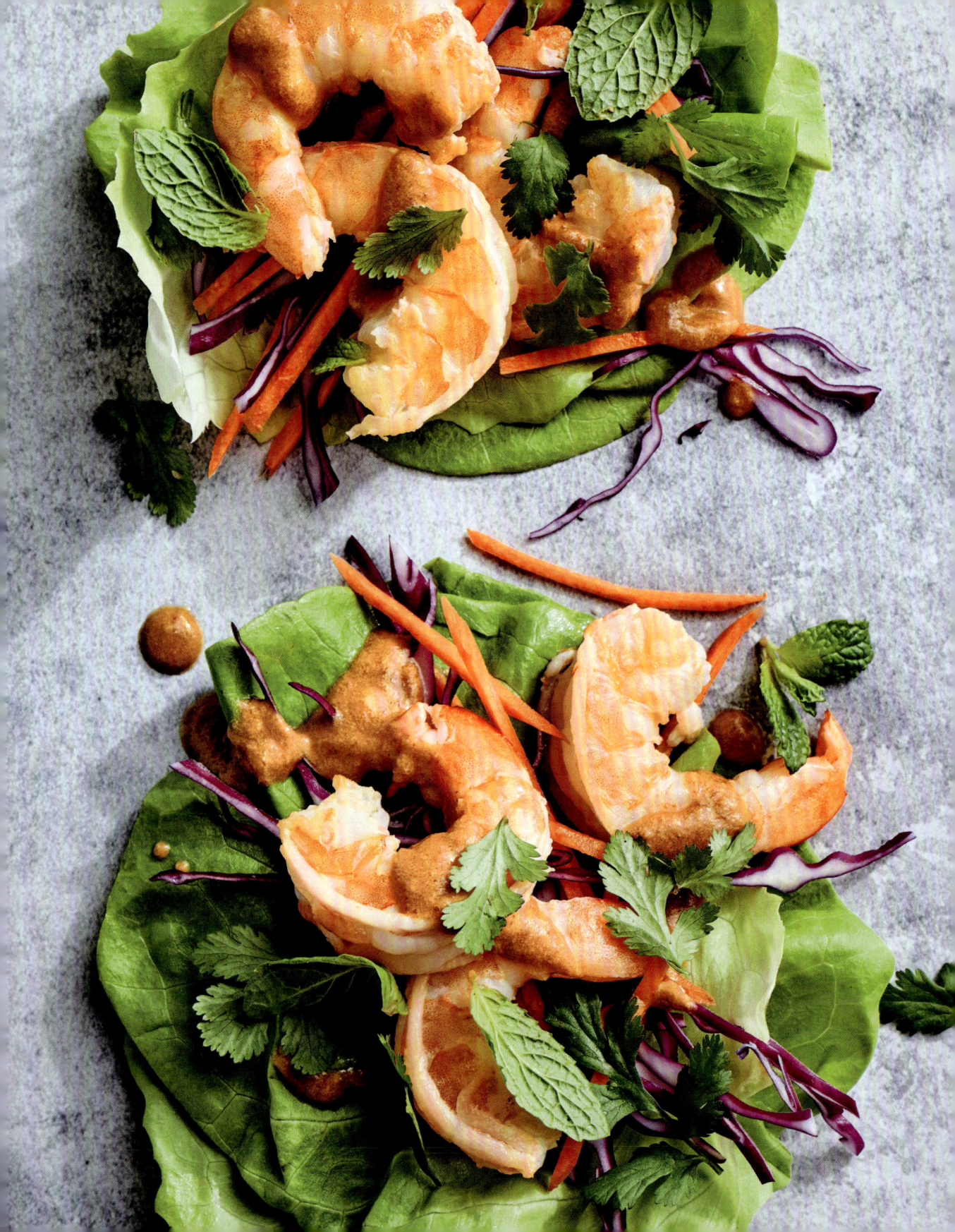

SHRIMP SUMMER ROLL LETTUCE WRAPS

I created this tasty quick lunch one day after a summer party when I had leftover shrimp cocktail in the fridge. I love making traditional shrimp summer rolls, but they take a lot of time because the rice paper can be difficult to work with. These lettuce wraps are the perfect solution! They're made with everything I put in my shrimp summer rolls sans the rice paper! It's a great way to use up the mint that grows wild in my summer garden.

MAKE THE HOISIN PEANUT SAUCE: In a small bowl, stir together the hoisin, peanut butter, and ginger along with enough hot tap water to make the sauce smooth and easy to drizzle.

ASSEMBLE THE LETTUCE WRAPS: Stack 2 lettuce leaves on a plate or cutting board, top with 3 pieces of shrimp, ¼ cup each of the carrots and cabbage, and drizzle with the sauce. Top with 3 mint leaves and some cilantro or basil. Repeat with the remaining lettuce, shrimp, and toppings.

Enjoy.

SERVES 1

HOISIN PEANUT SAUCE

1 tablespoon hoisin sauce*

1 tablespoon smooth unsweetened peanut butter

¼ teaspoon grated fresh ginger or paste

2½ to 3 tablespoons very hot tap water

LETTUCE WRAPS

6 large butter lettuce leaves

9 peeled cooked jumbo shrimp (about 4 ounces)

¾ cup shredded carrots

¾ cup shredded red cabbage

9 fresh mint leaves

¼ cup loosely packed fresh cilantro leaves or basil

*Read the label to be sure this product is gluten-free.

Per Serving | Calories 312 | **Protein 31 g** | Carbohydrate 26 g | Fiber 6.5 g | Sugars 13 g | Fat 11 g | Saturated Fat 1.5 g | Cholesterol 193 mg | Sodium 696 mg

SPICY SALMON HAND ROLLS

Have some leftover salmon from dinner or a can of salmon in the cupboard? Turn it into a spicy salmon salad and serve it in a seaweed sheet with rice and cucumbers for a quick and easy lunch! It's a little messy to eat since it's loosely folded like a taco rather than rolled like sushi, but it's seriously delicious nonetheless.

In a small bowl, combine the salmon, mayo, Sriracha, scallion whites and light-green parts, and a pinch of salt and mix well.

To build the hand rolls, place a sheet of seaweed in one hand, top with a spoonful of rice, then the salmon salad, cucumbers, and scallion greens. Drizzle with soy sauce and more Sriracha (for a spicier hit), if desired. Form a loose roll and eat and repeat. Enjoy with edamame on the side.

SERVES 1

1 (5-ounce) can water-packed skinless wild pink salmon, drained, or 5 ounces cooked salmon

1 tablespoon Kewpie mayonnaise

1 teaspoon Sriracha sauce, plus more (optional) for serving

1 scallion, thinly sliced, dark green portion kept separate

Kosher salt

1 (0.14-ounce) individual packet toasted nori seaweed snack sheets

½ cup cooked brown rice, heated

1 Persian (mini) cucumber, halved lengthwise and cut into thin strips

Reduced-sodium soy sauce or gluten-free tamari (optional), for serving

⅓ cup shelled edamame

Per Serving | Calories 452 | **Protein 41 g** | Carbohydrate 34 g | Fiber 8 g | Sugars 4 g | Fat 17 g | Saturated Fat 2.5 g | Cholesterol 110 mg | Sodium 731 mg

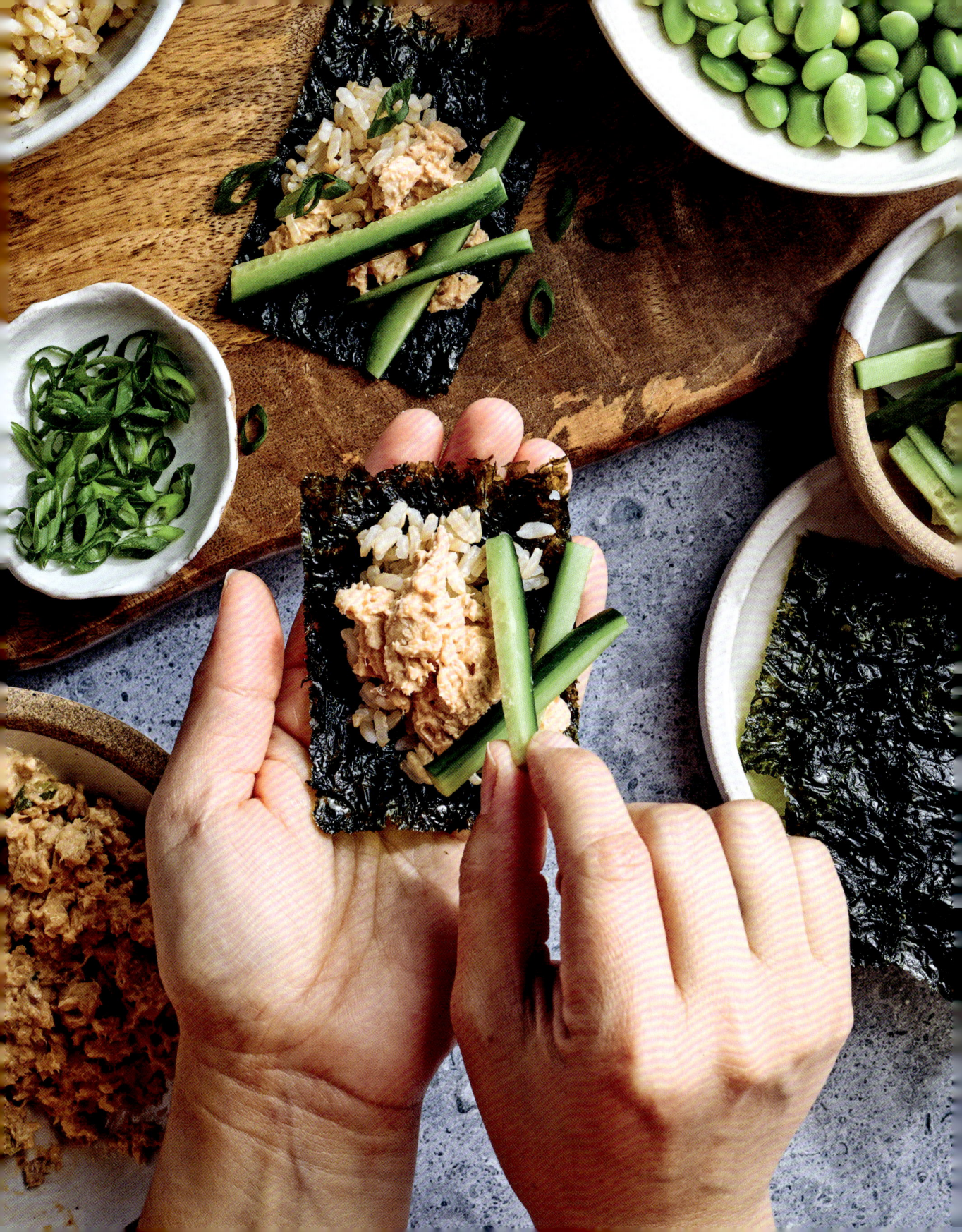

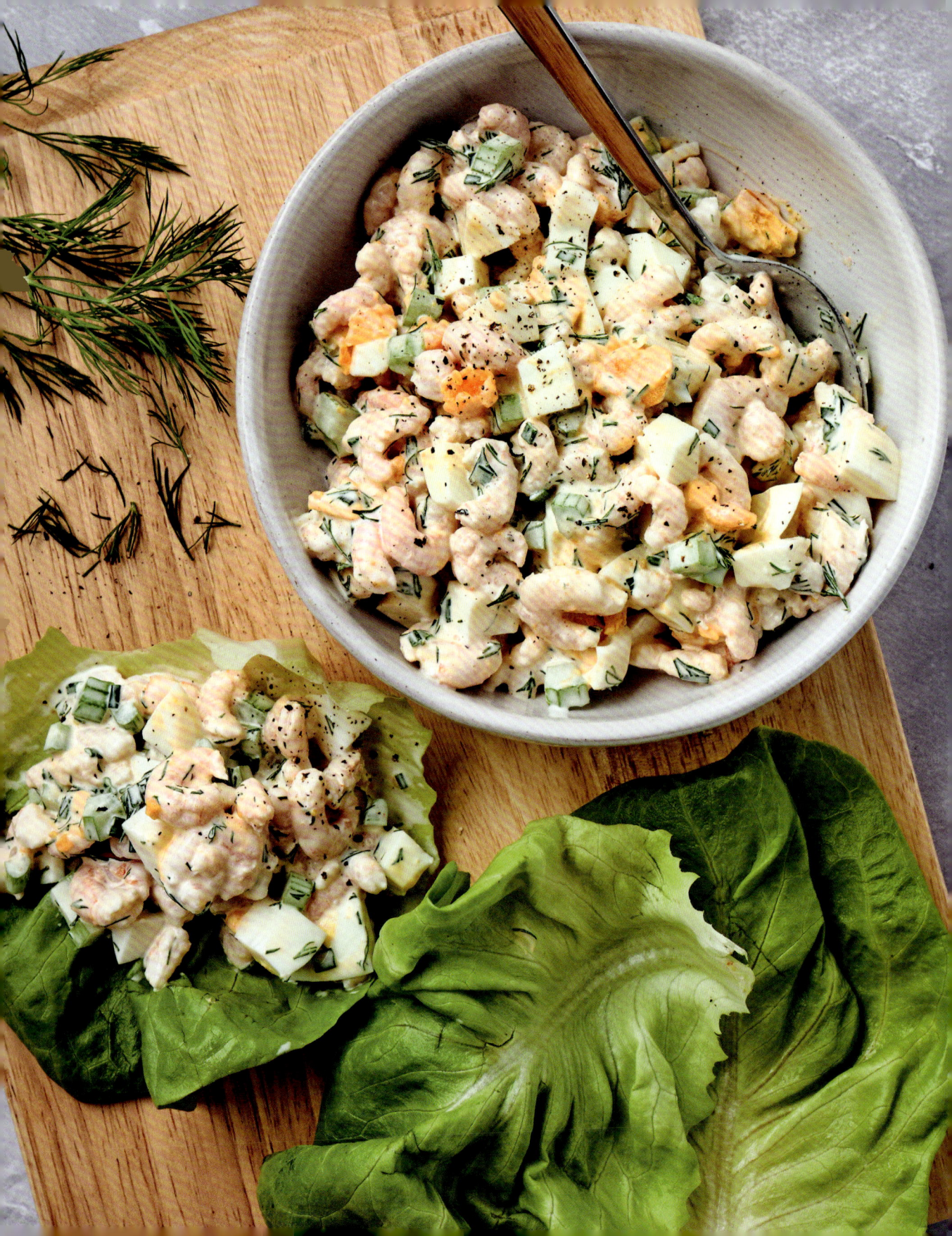

CHILLED SHRIMP SALAD
with Eggs

When I worked in New York City many years ago, I would order shrimp salad with hard-boiled eggs from a nearby deli for lunch nearly every week! It was a surprising but delicious combo, and now I make this tasty salad at home with precooked shrimp and eggs, and it comes together in just minutes. It's hard to stop yourself from eating this right out of the bowl, but it really tastes best after letting it chill in the fridge for at least an hour. It's a perfect summer salad. I love serving it in butter leaf lettuce, but it's also delicious on toasted sourdough bread.

In a medium bowl, combine the shrimp, eggs, mayo, celery, chives, and dill. Refrigerate for 1 hour or until chilled. Enjoy served in lettuce leaves. This will last in the fridge for up to 3 days.

TIP: If the shrimp are small, leave them whole, and if large, you can cut them into smaller pieces.

SERVES 2

½ pound peeled and deveined cooked shrimp

2 hard-boiled eggs, chopped

¼ cup mayonnaise

¼ cup chopped celery

3 tablespoons chopped fresh chives

3 tablespoons chopped fresh dill

Butter lettuce leaves

Per Serving (1 generous cup) | Calories 392 | **Protein 31 g** | Carbohydrate 3 g | Fiber 1 g | Sugars 1 g | Fat 29 g | Saturated Fat 5 g | Cholesterol 389 mg | Sodium 514 mg

SPINACH EGG WRAPS

If you've tried the popular egg wraps from Trader Joe's, you're going to love my copycat version! I live too far from TJs to go on a regular basis, so I decided to re-create their egg wraps on my own, and, well, they came out perfect. The combination of egg whites and whole eggs provides a good amount of protein, and the oat flour adds a bit of structure to the wraps, making them stronger than an omelet. I added a little spinach for some extra nutrients.

In a blender, combine the egg whites, whole eggs, oat flour, spinach, and salt and blend until the mixture is smooth, about 1 minute.

Heat a 10-inch nonstick skillet over medium-low heat and lightly spray with olive oil. When hot, pour in about ⅓ cup of the egg mixture. Quickly swirl the skillet to spread the egg mixture into a thin, even layer, forming a round. Cook until the edges start to lift and the bottom is set, 1 to 2 minutes.

Carefully flip the wrap using a spatula and cook just until set, another 30 seconds. Transfer the cooked wrap to a plate and cover it with a clean kitchen towel to keep it warm and pliable. Repeat the process with the remaining egg mixture, making sure to lightly coat the skillet with oil spray before cooking each wrap.

Once all the wraps are cooked, you can use them immediately or let them cool completely and store them in an airtight container in the refrigerator for up to 1 week. To serve, transfer a wrap to a plate, add your desired fillings, and carefully roll it up.

MAKES 6 WRAPS

1¼ cups egg whites

2 large eggs

1½ tablespoons oat flour*

½ cup baby spinach, loosely packed

¼ teaspoon kosher salt

Olive oil spray

Fillings of your choice (see Variations)

*Read the label to be sure this product is gluten-free.

Variations
These egg wraps are so versatile! You can eat them hot or cold, and fill them with anything you like to hit 30 grams of protein. Here are some of my favorite fillings:

Turkey breast + arugula + mustard

Roasted red pepper hummus + veggies

Roast beef + cheese + mayo + arugula

Turkey + bacon + lettuce + tomato

Tuna salad + avocado

Lox + cream cheese + cucumber

Chicken + avocado + sautéed peppers and onions

Per Serving (2 unfilled wraps) | Calories 117 | **Protein 16 g** | Carbohydrate 4 g | Fiber 0.5 g | Sugars 1 g | Fat 4 g | Saturated Fat 1 g | Cholesterol 124 mg | Sodium 314 mg

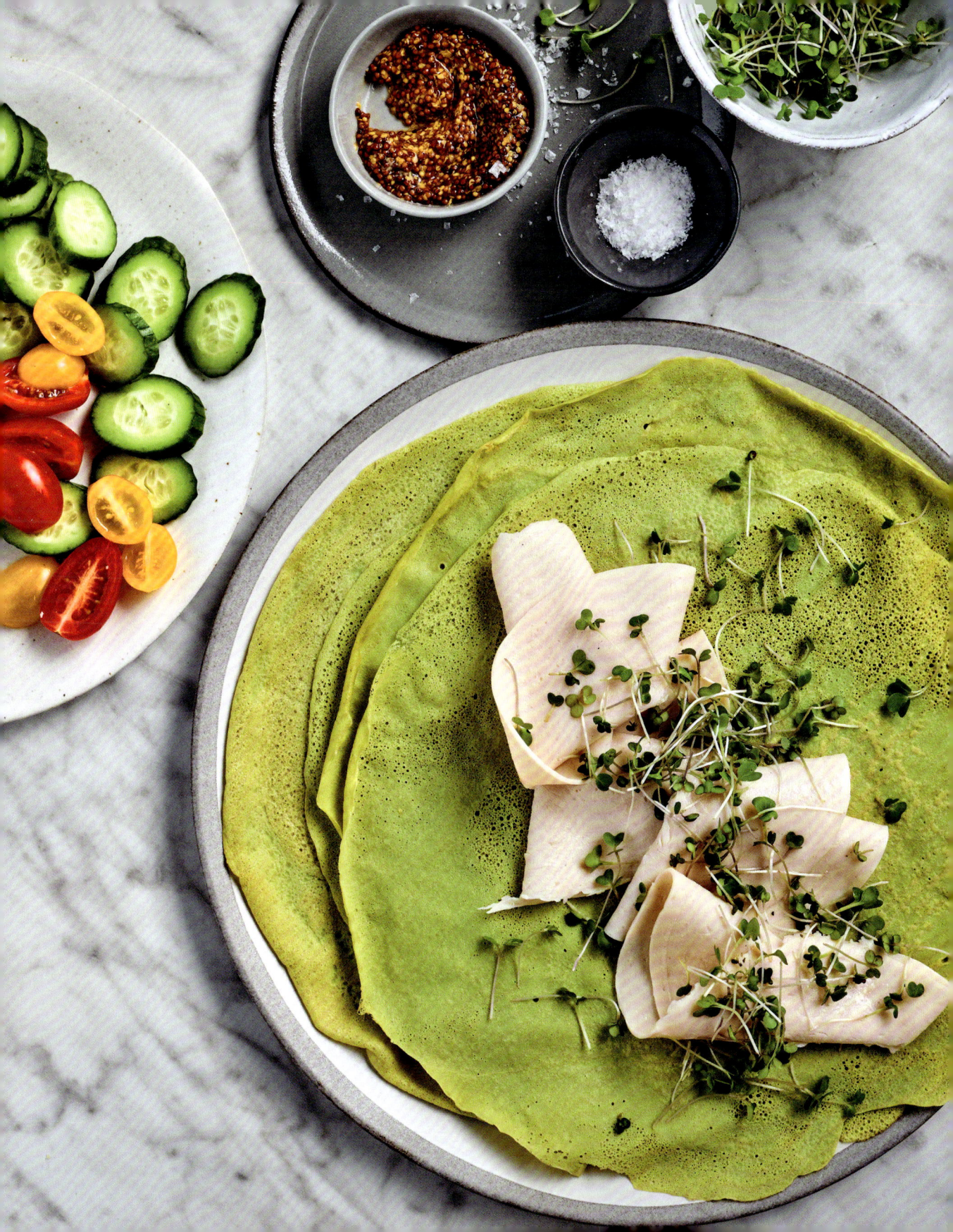

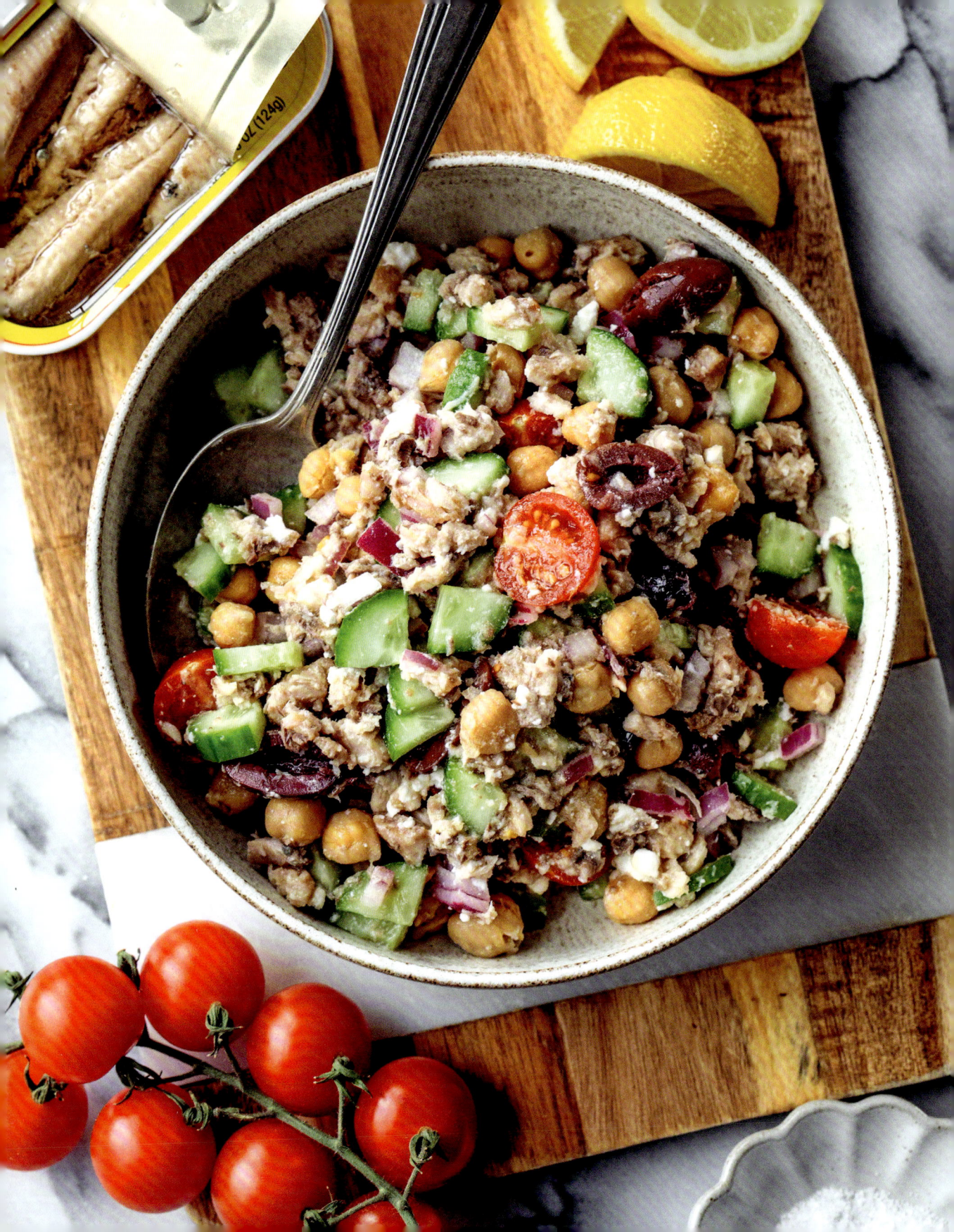

MEDITERRANEAN SARDINE SALAD

Did you know that a small can of sardines contains the highest concentration of heart-healthy omega-3s of any fish? My doctor inspired me to eat more sardines because of their cardiovascular and cognitive health benefits. They're high in protein and healthy fats, and since they're so tiny, they are known for having low mercury levels. To make sardines extra tasty, I love combining them with Mediterranean ingredients like cucumbers, tomatoes, olives, and feta cheese. It's the perfect lunch that's on the table in under 15 minutes, and it can easily be doubled for meal prep.

In a medium bowl, combine the sardines, chickpeas, cucumber, tomatoes, onion, olives, oil, lemon juice, vinegar, feta, and salt and gently toss. Taste for salt and adjust as needed.

TIP: If making this ahead or doubling for meal prep, this can be refrigerated for up to 3 days.

SERVES 1

1 (4.4-ounce) tin skinless, boneless sardines in olive oil (I like Mina), drained and chopped

½ cup drained canned chickpeas or cannellini beans

1 Persian (mini) cucumber, chopped

¼ cup halved cherry tomatoes

¼ cup chopped red onion

2 tablespoons halved kalamata olives

1 teaspoon extra-virgin olive oil

Juice of ½ lemon

½ teaspoon red wine vinegar

½ ounce feta cheese, crumbled (omit for dairy-free)

Pinch of kosher salt

Per Serving | Calories 410 | **Protein 31 g** | Carbohydrate 29 g | Fiber 6 g | Sugars 8 g | Fat 22 g | Saturated Fat 5.5 g | Cholesterol 48 mg | Sodium 934 mg

TUNA MACARONI SALAD

I often eat this delicious tuna salad for lunch because it comes together in minutes, and it's made with ingredients I almost always have in my pantry. It's also easy to modify this recipe using whatever you have on hand. You can swap out capers for kalamata olives and cucumber for chopped cherry tomatoes or just use a handful of baby arugula instead.

Bring a medium pot of generously salted water to a boil. Once boiling, add the pasta and cook according to the package directions. Drain in a colander.

Meanwhile, in a medium bowl, combine the tuna, red onion, olive oil, vinegar, capers, and caper brine and mix well.

Rinse the macaroni in the colander under cold water and drain, then add to the bowl and toss to combine. Stir in the cucumber and dill and season with a pinch of salt and black pepper to taste. Enjoy at room temperature or chilled.

TIP: You can double or triple this for meal prep for the week. It can be refrigerated for up to 4 days.

SERVES 1

Kosher salt

2 ounces high-protein farfalle or elbow macaroni (I like Barilla) or a gluten-free high-protein pasta

1 (3-ounce) packet water-packed light tuna (I like Safe Catch), drained

2 tablespoons chopped red onion

1 tablespoon extra-virgin olive oil

½ teaspoon red wine vinegar

1 tablespoon capers

1 teaspoon caper brine

1 Persian (mini) cucumber, diced

½ teaspoon chopped fresh dill

Freshly ground black pepper

Per Serving | Calories 427 | **Protein 35 g** | Carbohydrate 43 g | Fiber 5 g | Sugars 4 g | Fat 15 g | Saturated Fat 2 g | Cholesterol 40 mg | Sodium 554 mg

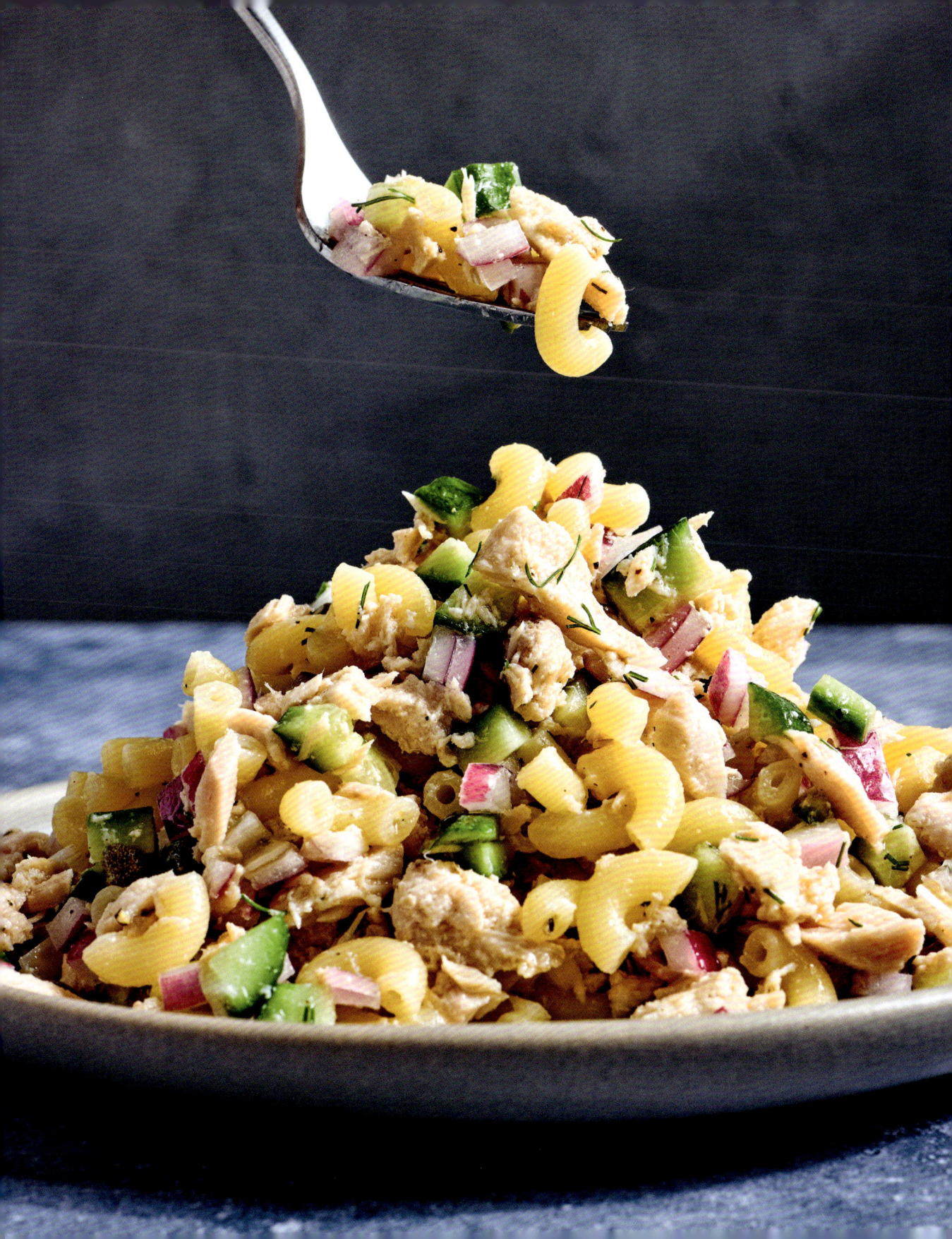

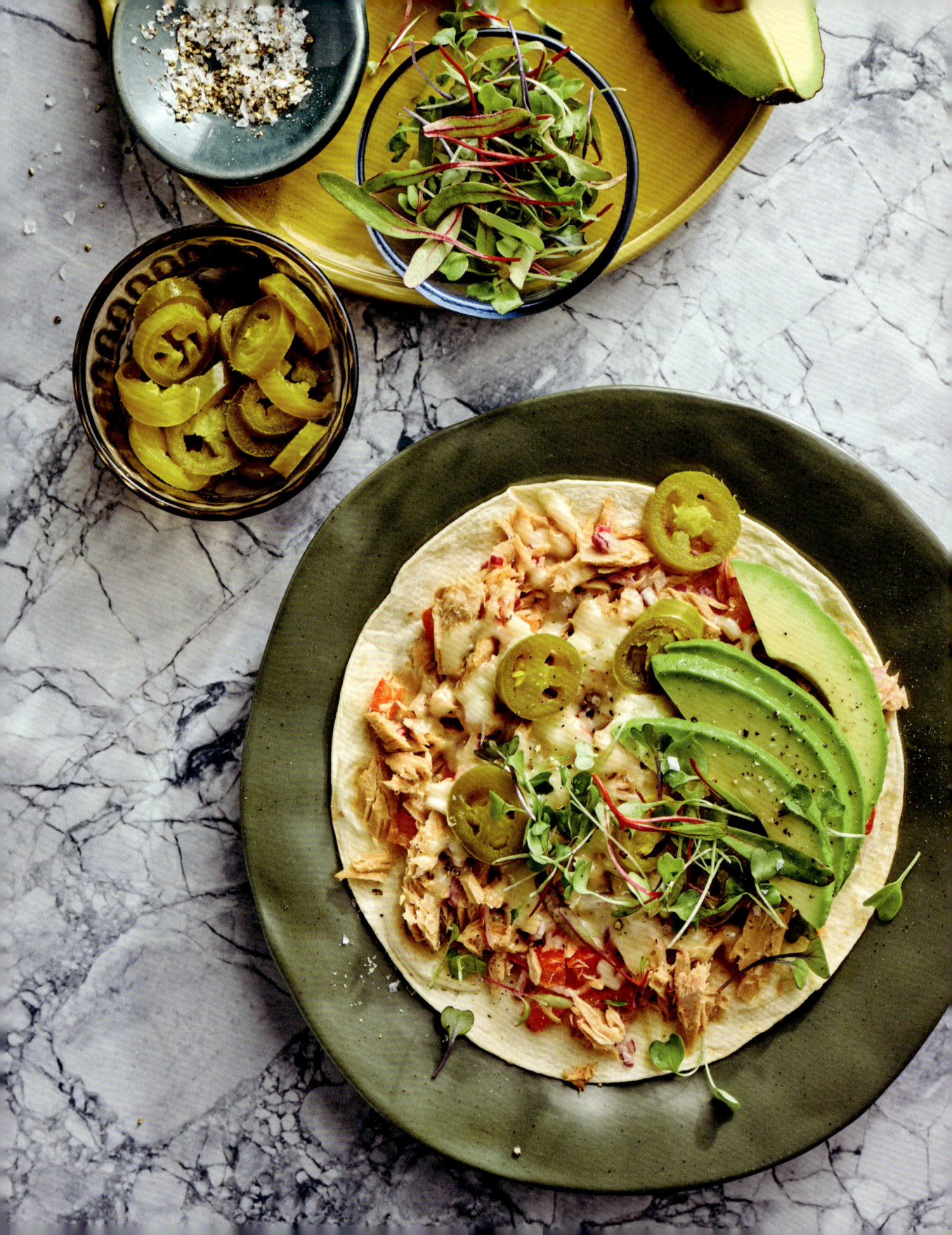

SPICY TUNA QUESO MELT

Here's a lunch that's ready in less than 10 minutes and is perfect if you enjoy a spicy kick! Serving this spicy tuna melt open-faced on a tortilla adds a bold, fun, Mexican-inspired twist. The tortilla crisps up beautifully as it cooks, making this an easy handheld sandwich-meets-quesadilla. It's simple to prepare for a quick lunch or snack and easy to customize with any protein. If you have leftover chicken breast, feel free to use that instead of the tuna!

———————

In a small bowl, combine the tuna, hot sauce, red onion, and tomato.

Heat a large skillet over medium heat until hot, then spray with oil. Add the tortilla and cook until toasted on the bottom, about 1 minute. Flip and reduce the heat to medium-low. Add the tuna on top, then sprinkle with the cheese and top with the jalapeño slices. Cover and cook until the cheese is melted, about 2 minutes.

Serve topped with the avocado and garnish with microgreens (if using).

SERVES 1

1 (3-ounce) packet water-packed wild tuna (I like Safe Catch), drained

½ teaspoon Frank's RedHot sauce

1 tablespoon diced red onion

2 tablespoons diced seeded tomato

Olive oil spray

1 large (7½- to 8½-inch) soft flour tortilla, such as Mission Carb Balance, or Siete almond flour tortilla

1 ounce shredded pepper jack cheese or nondairy cheddar (I like Violife)

5 pickled jalapeño slices

1 ounce sliced avocado (about ¼ small Hass)

Microgreens (optional), for garnish

Perfect Pairings
I try to get 1 cup of vegetables with every meal. For this dish, I love serving it with an easy side like a basic cabbage slaw using shredded cabbage, dressed with a little olive oil, lime juice, salt, and pepper. A simple green salad with tomatoes and cucumbers would also be great.

Per Serving | Calories 341 | **Protein 37 g** | Carbohydrate 26 g | Fiber 17 g | Sugars 2 g | Fat 16 g | Saturated Fat 7.5 g | Cholesterol 70 mg | Sodium 958 mg

CHOOSE-YOUR-ADVENTURE PROTEIN SHEET PAN BAKE

Sheet pan bakes are my go-to for meal-prepping lunches and for easy weeknight dinners. The possibilities are endless with the combinations of protein, veggies, and spices you can use. **THE FORMULA HERE IS EASY: Choose your protein, choose 2 cups of veggies, add some aromatics, and then toss with oil, salt, and your seasoning of choice. Into the oven it goes, and you're done!** You can mix and match and create so many different meals.

SERVES 1

CHOOSE 1 LEAN PROTEIN

6 ounces boneless, skinless chicken breast, cut into ½-inch cubes

6 ounces boneless, skinless chicken thighs, cut into 1-inch cubes

7 ounces tofu, drained and cut into ½-inch cubes

6 ounces boneless white fish fillet

6 ounces salmon, cut into 1-inch cubes

6 ounces peeled and deveined shrimp

CHOOSE 2 CUPS NON-STARCHY VEGGIES
(Feel free to mix and match as long as you have 2 cups total)

Broccoli florets

Cauliflower florets

Brussels sprouts, halved or quartered

Asparagus, cut into 1-inch pieces

Green beans, ends trimmed

Mushrooms, halved

Bell peppers, cut into 1-inch pieces

Zucchini, cut into ½-inch cubes

Grape or cherry tomatoes

½ cabbage wedge, quartered

ADD THE AROMATICS

½ cup chopped red onion, yellow onion, or shallot

1 garlic clove, chopped

TOSS WITH

1 teaspoon extra-virgin olive oil or avocado oil

¼ teaspoon kosher salt

Freshly ground black pepper

ADD SPICES AND SEASONINGS (OPTIONAL)

Garlic powder

Onion powder

Sweet paprika

Dried or fresh herbs

Chili powder

Curry powder

SERVE WITH

½ cup of your favorite grains or legumes

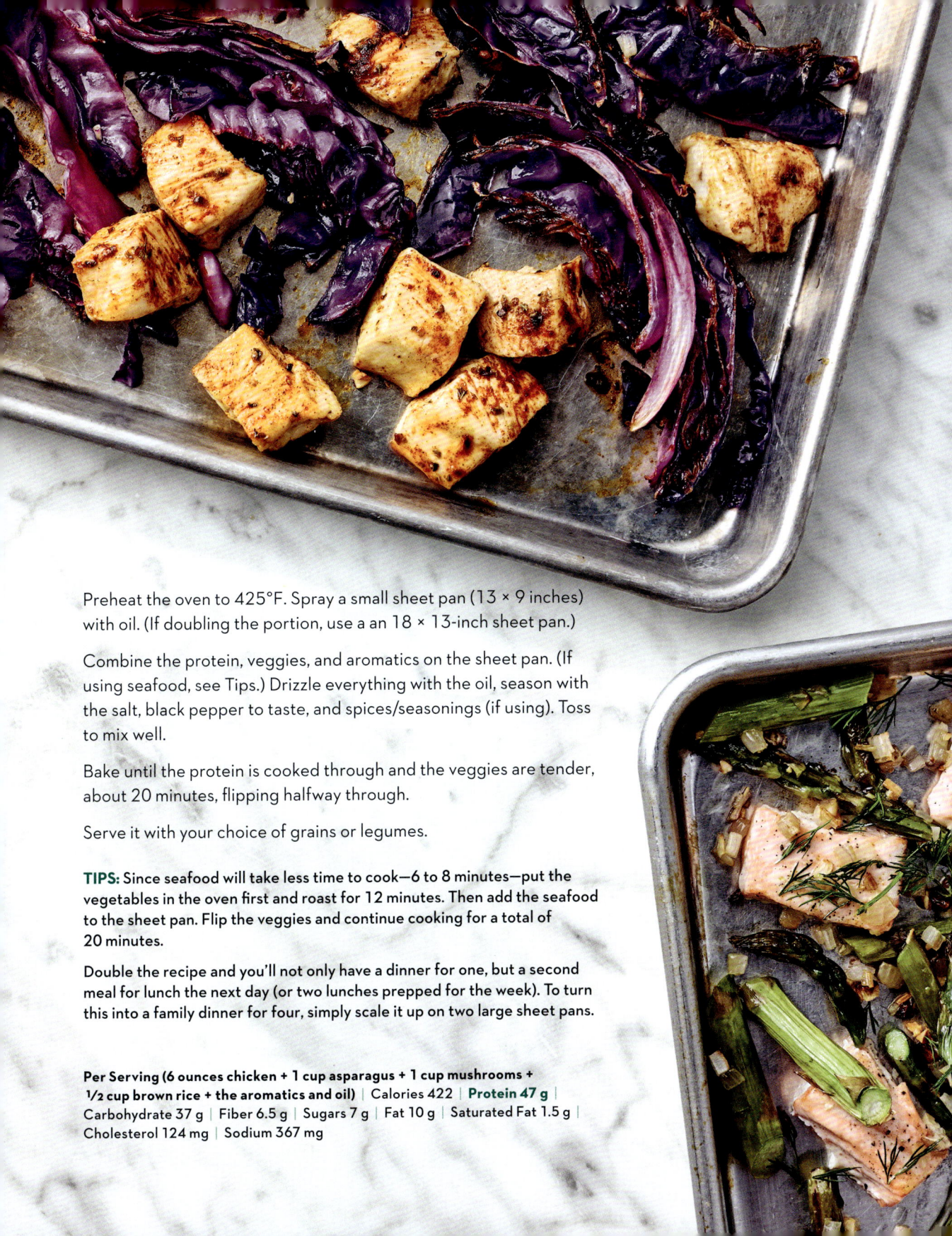

Preheat the oven to 425°F. Spray a small sheet pan (13 × 9 inches) with oil. (If doubling the portion, use a an 18 × 13-inch sheet pan.)

Combine the protein, veggies, and aromatics on the sheet pan. (If using seafood, see Tips.) Drizzle everything with the oil, season with the salt, black pepper to taste, and spices/seasonings (if using). Toss to mix well.

Bake until the protein is cooked through and the veggies are tender, about 20 minutes, flipping halfway through.

Serve it with your choice of grains or legumes.

TIPS: Since seafood will take less time to cook—6 to 8 minutes—put the vegetables in the oven first and roast for 12 minutes. Then add the seafood to the sheet pan. Flip the veggies and continue cooking for a total of 20 minutes.

Double the recipe and you'll not only have a dinner for one, but a second meal for lunch the next day (or two lunches prepped for the week). To turn this into a family dinner for four, simply scale it up on two large sheet pans.

Per Serving (6 ounces chicken + 1 cup asparagus + 1 cup mushrooms + ½ cup brown rice + the aromatics and oil) | Calories 422 | **Protein 47 g** | Carbohydrate 37 g | Fiber 6.5 g | Sugars 7 g | Fat 10 g | Saturated Fat 1.5 g | Cholesterol 124 mg | Sodium 367 mg

AIR FRYER CRISPY CHICKEN PATTY SANDWICHES

This is a cross between a "fried" chicken sandwich and a chicken burger. It's so flavorful and juicy, and there's even some hidden cauliflower rice inside, but I promise you can't taste it! My husband, Tommy, loved these sandwiches and doesn't like cauliflower. I went classic with the toppings—cheese, mayo, lettuce, and tomato—but you can also add pickles, spicy mayo, barbecue sauce, or any other sandwich topping you like.

——————

MAKE THE CHICKEN PATTIES: In a large bowl, combine the chicken, cauliflower rice, salt, onion powder, garlic powder, and black pepper and mix well. With wet hands, form the mixture into 4 round flattened patties about ½ inch thick and 4 inches across. Place on a large plate and freeze for 30 to 40 minutes to firm up so they don't fall apart when you bread them.

Meanwhile, set up a dredging station in two shallow bowls: Beat the egg in one bowl and place the panko in a second bowl.

Dip the partially frozen patties in the egg, then transfer to the panko and turn to coat, gently pressing to adhere.

Spray the tops of the patties with oil and add the breaded patties to the air fryer basket in a single layer. Cook at 400°F until golden and cooked through, 12 to 13 minutes, flipping halfway and spraying the other side with oil.

ASSEMBLE THE SANDWICHES: Place a slice of cheese on each patty and close the air fryer basket to melt the cheese with the residual heat, about 1 minute.

Meanwhile, lightly toast the buns. Spread 1 tablespoon mayonnaise on the bottoms of the buns. Top with the chicken, butter lettuce, and tomato.

TIP: Don't use 100% ground breast meat here, as it will be too dry. Use a mix of dark meat or 92% lean ground chicken.

Per Serving (1 sandwich) | Calories 480 | **Protein 36 g** | Carbohydrate 28 g | Fiber 3 g | Sugars 6 g | Fat 26 g | Saturated Fat 9.5 g | Cholesterol 176 mg | Sodium 908 mg

SERVES 4

CHICKEN PATTIES

1 pound ground chicken (92% lean; see Tip), preferably organic (I like Bell & Evans)

½ cup frozen cauliflower rice

¾ teaspoon kosher salt

¾ teaspoon onion powder

¾ teaspoon garlic powder

⅛ teaspoon freshly ground black pepper

1 large egg

1 cup seasoned panko bread crumbs, regular or gluten-free

Olive oil spray

SANDWICHES

4 slices American, cheddar, or nondairy cheese

4 (100-calorie) burger buns or gluten-free buns

4 tablespoons light mayonnaise

8 butter lettuce leaves

4 thin tomato slices

No Air Fryer? No Problem!

Place the patties on a sheet pan sprayed with oil and then spray the tops with oil. Bake in a preheated 450°F oven until golden and cooked through, about 20 minutes, flipping halfway. Add the cheese and cook until melted, about 1 minute.

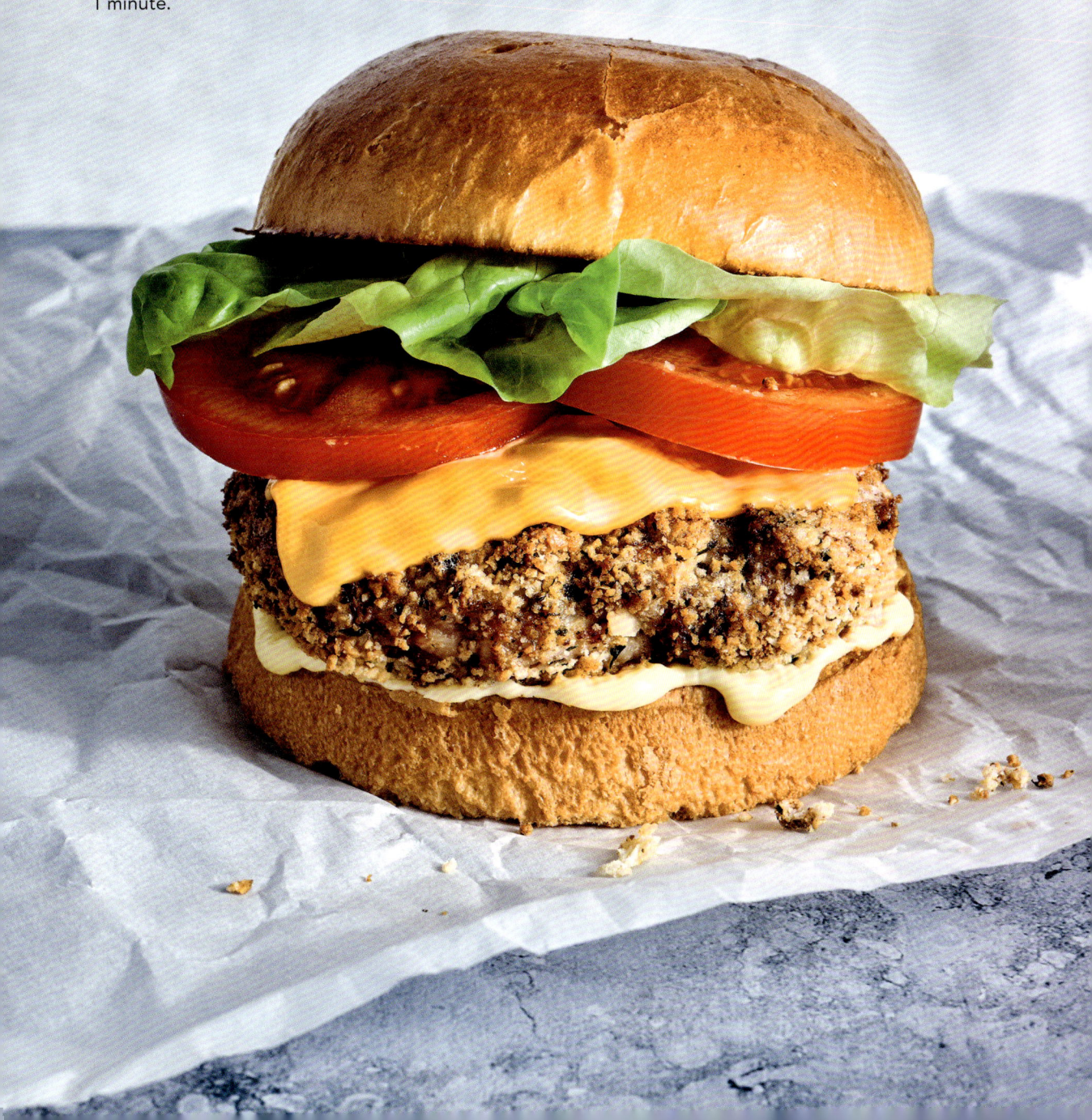

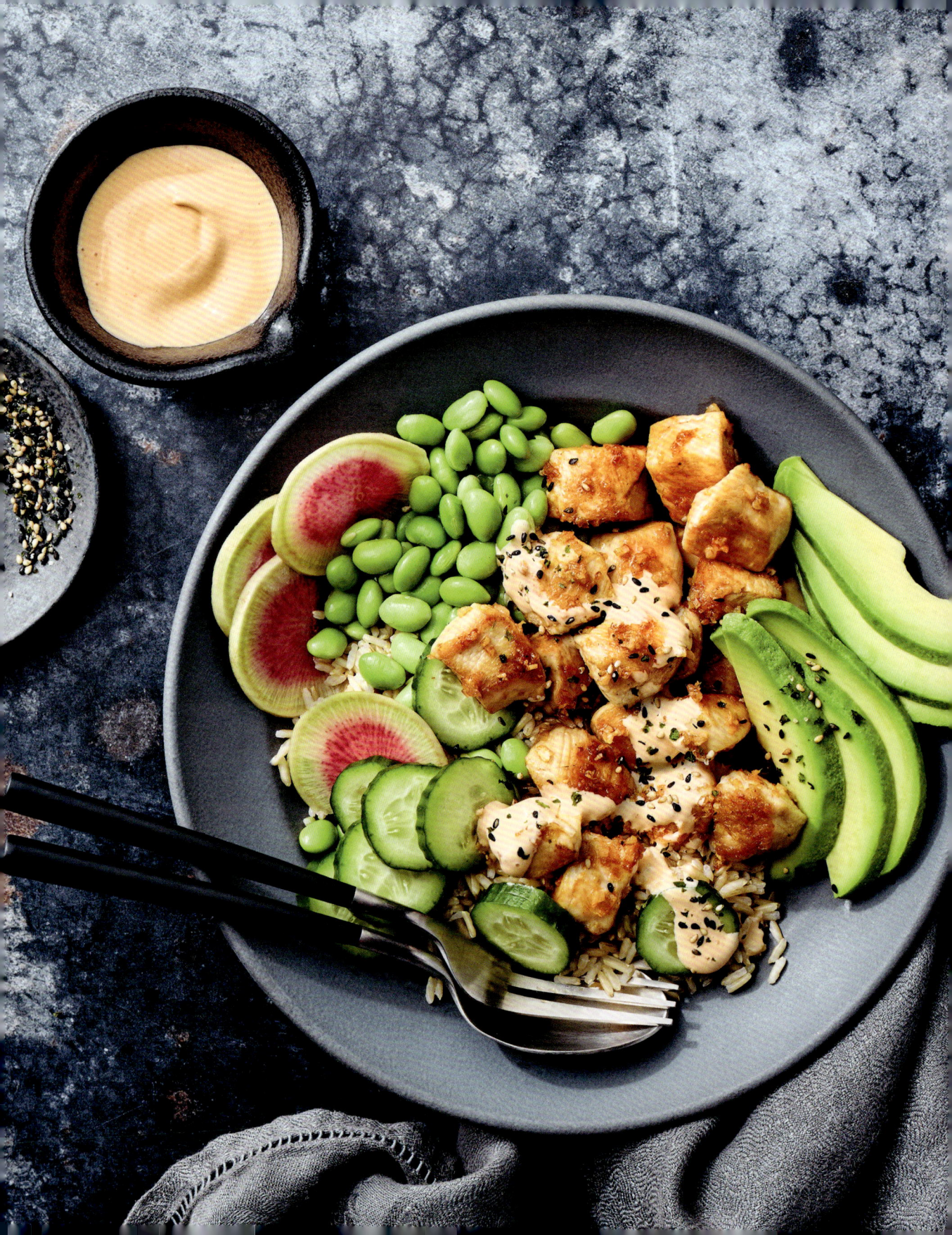

SPICY CHICKEN POKE BOWL

Chicken breast is a great lean protein option, but it's kinda boring, so I'm always looking for creative ways to make it taste delicious. Since I love all the flavors of a tuna poke bowl, I decided to try it with chicken, and the result is this beautiful dish loaded with flavor, color, and nutrition! It's also incredibly customizable—add more veggies like carrots or radishes, swap the chicken for tofu or tempeh, play around with different grains, or leave them out altogether and serve it over salad or cauliflower rice.

In a small bowl, combine the mayo and ½ teaspoon of the Sriracha and set aside. If you want to make this easier to drizzle, add a drop of water.

Season the chicken with the salt. In a medium skillet, heat the sesame oil over medium heat. Add the garlic and sauté until fragrant, 30 to 60 seconds. Add the chicken and cook, turning halfway, until almost cooked through in the center, about 4 minutes. Stir in the ginger and cook until the chicken is completely cooked through, about 1 more minute. Remove from the heat and stir in the remaining ¼ teaspoon Sriracha.

Spoon the rice and edamame into a shallow bowl. Top with the chicken, cucumber, and avocado and drizzle with the soy sauce and spicy mayo. If desired, garnish with sesame seeds or furikake.

SERVES 1

1 teaspoon Kewpie mayonnaise

¾ teaspoon Sriracha sauce

6 ounces boneless, skinless chicken breast, preferably organic, cut into ½-inch cubes

¼ teaspoon kosher salt

1 teaspoon toasted sesame oil

2 garlic cloves, minced

½ teaspoon grated fresh ginger, or to taste

¾ cup cooked brown rice or quinoa, warm

¼ cup shelled edamame, thawed if frozen

1 Persian (mini) cucumber, sliced

1 ounce sliced avocado (about ¼ small Hass)

1 teaspoon reduced-sodium soy sauce or gluten-free tamari

Sesame seeds or furikake (optional), for garnish

Per Serving | Calories 546 | **Protein 48 g** | Carbohydrate 45 g | Fiber 9 g | Sugars 3 g | Fat 19 g | Saturated Fat 2.5 g | Cholesterol 132 mg | Sodium 680 mg

10-MINUTE MEAL PREP DECONSTRUCTED FRIED RICE BOWLS

This dish is like fried rice, but even simpler and more customizable—hence the name! I find myself making this whenever I have a package of ground turkey or chicken in the house. I toss in whatever fresh or frozen veggies I have on hand, scramble an egg in the same skillet, and serve it over rice. It works with ground chicken, turkey, or pork and any fresh or frozen veggies, from peas and carrots to zucchini.

Heat a large nonstick skillet over medium-high heat and spray with oil. Add the ground meat and scallion whites and cook, breaking up the meat, until no longer pink, about 5 minutes. Push the turkey to the side of the pan and add 1 teaspoon of the sesame oil and the eggs to the empty part. Scramble until just cooked, about 1 minute, then mix in with the turkey.

Add the frozen mixed veggies, remaining 1 teaspoon sesame oil, the soy sauce, and 2 to 3 tablespoons water, to make it saucy or more as needed if it's too dry. Reduce the heat to medium, cover, and cook until heated through, 3 to 4 minutes.

To serve, divide the rice among four containers and top with the meat and veggie mixture and scallion greens. Refrigerate for up to 4 days.

SERVES 4

Olive oil spray

1 pound ground turkey or chicken (93% lean)

2 scallions, chopped, white and green parts kept separate

2 teaspoons toasted sesame oil

2 large eggs

2 cups frozen vegetables of your choice (or use a combo of two: peas and carrots, chopped broccoli, corn, frozen mixed vegetables)

3 tablespoons reduced-sodium soy sauce or gluten-free tamari, plus more (optional) for serving

3 cups cooked sticky rice or frozen brown rice, warmed

Per Serving (1 cup turkey and veggies + ¾ cup rice) | Calories 398 | **Protein 30 g** | Carbohydrate 37 g | Fiber 4 g | Sugars 0 g | Fat 15 g | Saturated Fat 3.5 g | Cholesterol 177 mg | Sodium 577 mg

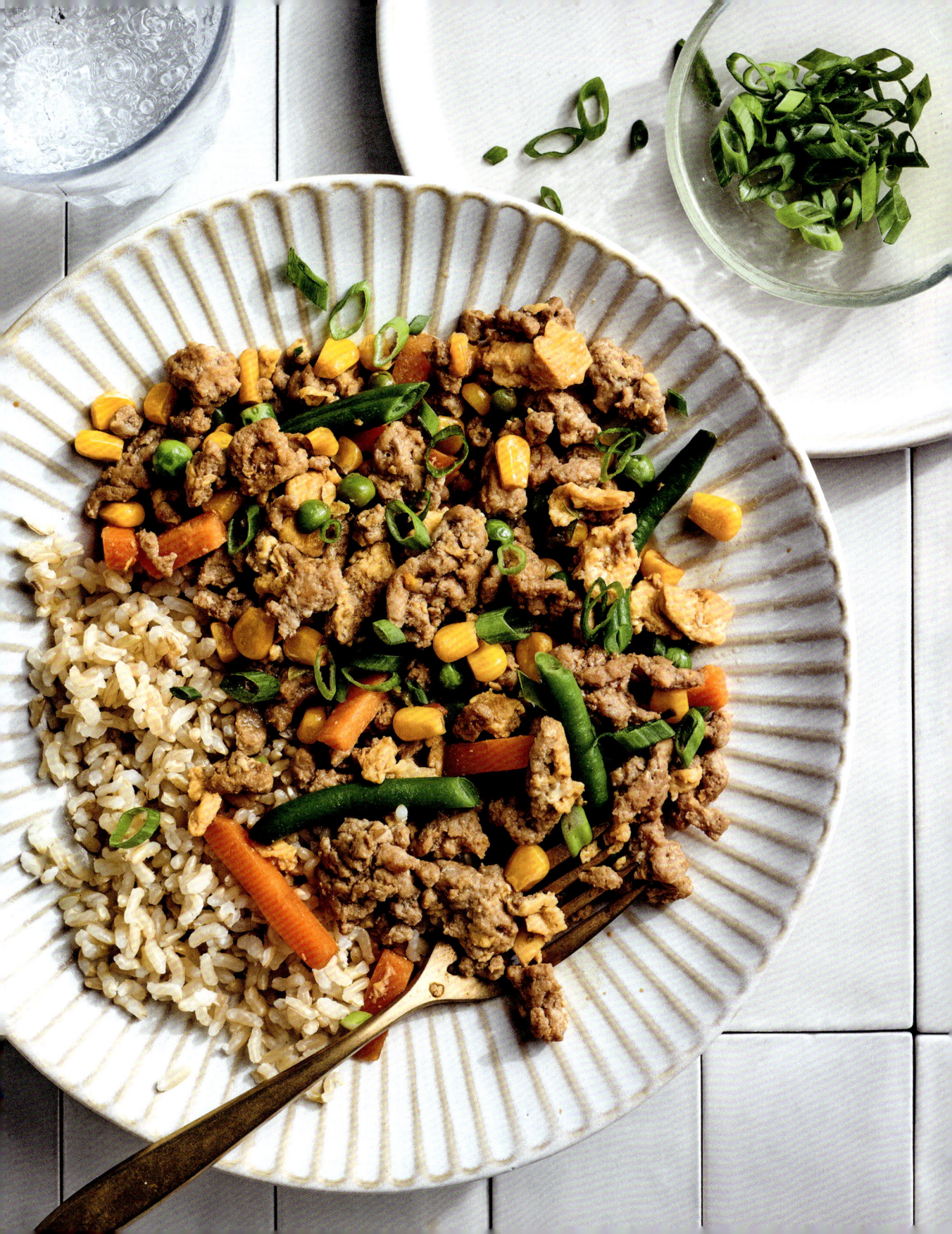

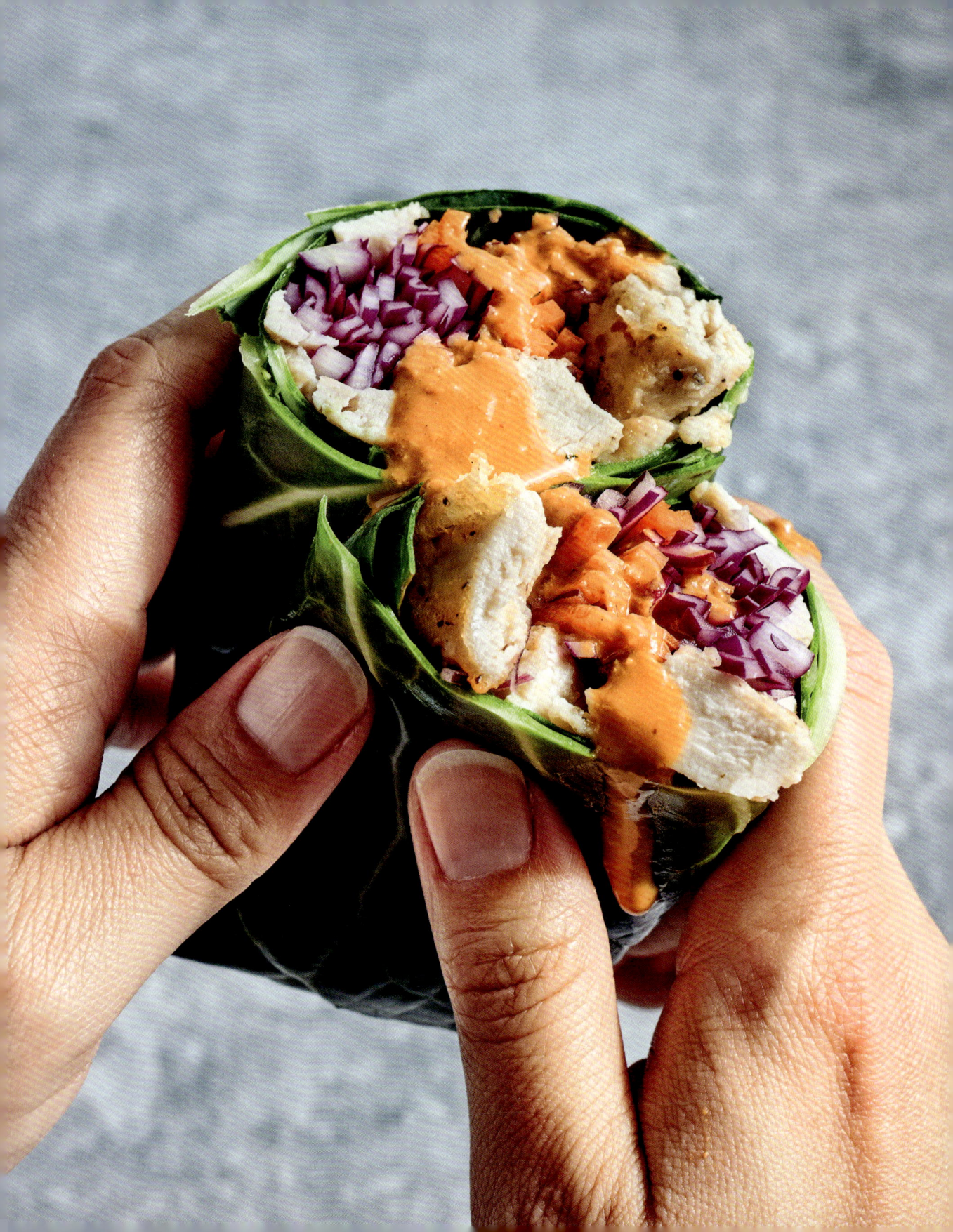

CHICKEN COLLARD WRAP

with Peanut Sesame Dipping Sauce

I love using collard greens as sandwich wraps—they're fresh, healthy, and require no cooking! They're a fantastic alternative to processed supermarket wraps, and can create a tasty handheld salad. I fill them with everything from egg salad and tuna to hummus and more. These chicken collard wraps have a summer roll vibe. They're packed with fresh and flavorful ingredients with lots of texture, like cabbage and carrots, and in my opinion, the light peanut dressing is the star of the show, it's that good!

Remove the stems of the collards and then stack the leaves. Place the chicken in the center and top with the cabbage, carrots, and red onion. Tightly roll up the wrap like a burrito.

MAKE THE PEANUT SESAME DIPPING SAUCE: In a small bowl, combine the peanut butter powder, rice vinegar, 1 tablespoon water, the Sriracha, maple syrup, sesame oil, ginger paste, and salt and mix until smooth.

Serve the sauce alongside the wrap for dipping.

TIP: If you want to meal prep, double the recipe. They can be refrigerated for up to 3 days.

SERVES 1

2 large or 3 medium collard leaves

4 ounces chopped cooked chicken breast, from a rotisserie chicken or leftovers

⅓ cup shredded red cabbage

2 tablespoons shredded carrots

2 tablespoons thinly sliced red onion

PEANUT SESAME DIPPING SAUCE

2 tablespoons PBfit peanut butter powder

1 tablespoon seasoned rice vinegar

1 to 2 teaspoons Sriracha sauce (omit of you don't like spice)

1 teaspoon maple syrup or sugar-free maple-flavored syrup

1 teaspoon toasted sesame oil

½ teaspoon ginger paste

Pinch of kosher salt

Per Serving (1 wrap + 3½ tablespoons sauce) | Calories 314 | **Protein 35 g** | Carbohydrate 24 g | Fiber 4.5 g | Sugars 15 g | Fat 10 g | Saturated Fat 1.5 g | Cholesterol 83 mg | Sodium 858 mg

ITALIAN ROAST BEEF SUB SALAD

During my college years, Subway was my go-to lunch on a budget, and I always ordered the roast beef sandwich piled high with all the fixings—lettuce, tomatoes, banana peppers, black olives, red onions, and their MVP vinaigrette. This Subway-inspired dish brings back those memories, but trust me, you won't miss the bread! This salad is perfect for meal prep, too—just double the recipe and keep the dressing separate so you can toss it in right before eating.

———————

In a small bowl, whisk together the olive oil, vinegar, Italian seasoning, garlic, salt, and pepperoncini brine.

In a medium bowl, combine the lettuce. roast beef, cheese, tomatoes, red onion, olives, and pepperoncini.

When ready to eat, drizzle in the dressing and toss to coat. Enjoy immediately.

TIP: I love this with roast beef because it has fewer processed ingredients than most deli meats (you can also use leftover roast beef), but feel free to swap it for turkey or your favorite sandwich meat.

SERVES 1

2 teaspoons extra-virgin olive oil

2 teaspoons red wine vinegar

⅛ teaspoon Italian seasoning

½ small garlic clove, minced

Pinch of kosher salt

1 teaspoon pepperoncini brine

2 cups chopped iceberg or romaine lettuce

4 ounces cooked roast beef (I like it medium-rare), chopped

2 tablespoons shredded part-skim mozzarella cheese, provolone, or nondairy cheese

4 cherry tomatoes, chopped

2 tablespoons sliced red onion

2 tablespoons sliced black olives

1 tablespoon sliced pickled pepperoncini or banana peppers

Per Serving | Calories 448 | **Protein 42 g** | Carbohydrate 11 g | Fiber 3 g | Sugars 6 g | Fat 26 g | Saturated Fat 8 g | Cholesterol 120 mg | Sodium 597 mg

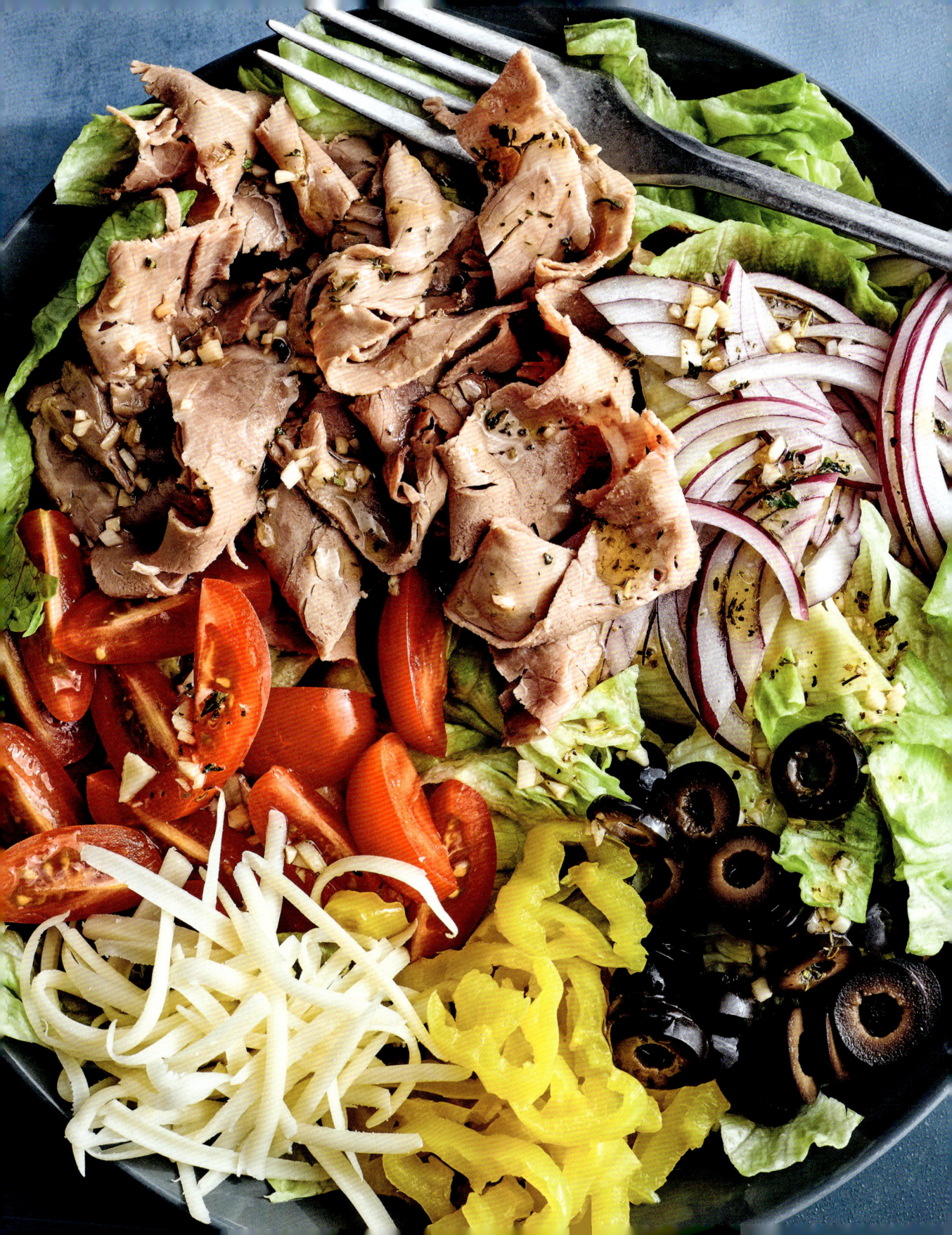

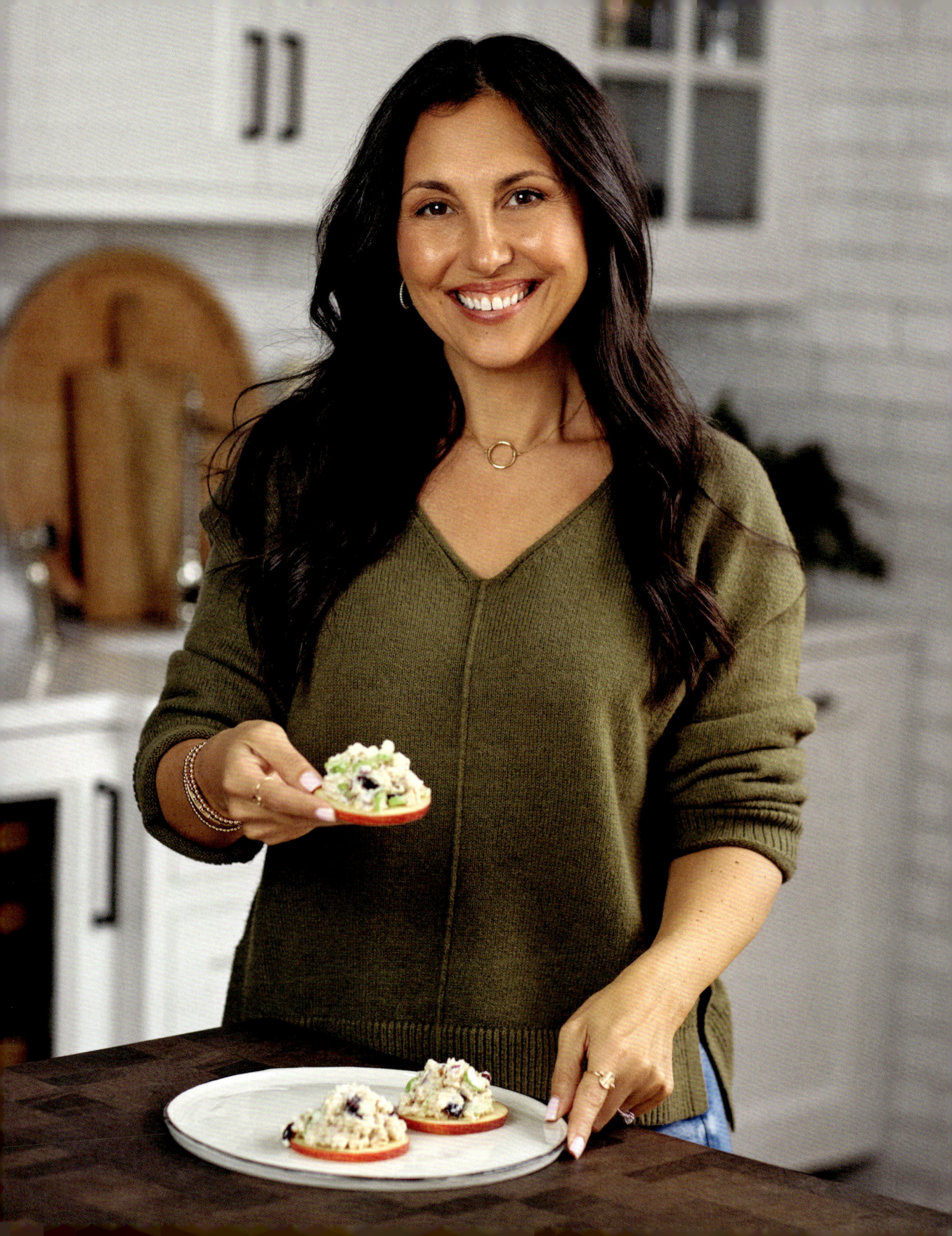

CRANBERRY CHICKEN SALAD ON APPLE SLICES

If you're a chicken salad fan, you're going to love this refreshing recipe that is as nutritious as it is delicious. Each bite has the perfect mix of sweet, tart, and crunch—it's become my go-to lunch whenever I have leftover chicken or turkey. Adding a little broth to the chicken salad helps to make it moist, without adding a lot of mayo. To meal prep, just store the chicken salad in a separate container and, for best results, slice the apple right before eating or toss with a little lemon juice.

In a medium bowl, combine the chicken. celery, mayo, chicken broth, cranberries, and onion and stir until combined. Season with a pinch of salt and black pepper to taste.

When ready to eat, slice the apples into ¼-inch-thick slices and remove the seeds. (I use a piping tip to cut them out.) Spoon a generous amount of chicken salad onto each apple slice and enjoy!

TIP: One of the great things about this recipe is how versatile it is. You can easily customize it to suit your taste preferences. Not a fan of chicken? Try using leftover turkey or tuna. Like green apples? Use them instead, or try this on sliced pears.

SERVES 2

8 ounces cooked chicken breast, from a rotisserie chicken or leftovers, shredded or diced

¼ cup sliced celery

3 tablespoons mayonnaise

¼ cup chicken broth*

1 tablespoon dried cranberries

1 tablespoon chopped red onion

Kosher salt

Freshly ground black pepper

2 sweet red apples

*Read the label to be sure this product is gluten-free.

Per Serving (1 apple + 1 generous cup salad) | Calories 452 | **Protein 36 g** | Carbohydrate 31 g | Fiber 5 g | Sugars 23 g | Fat 21 g | Saturated Fat 3.5 g | Cholesterol 104 mg | Sodium 317 mg

BUFFALO CHICKEN RICE BOWLS

I often find myself craving these Buffalo bowls! This recipe is one of the top twenty most popular recipes on my entire Skinnytaste website for good reason. These bowls are not only high in protein and packed with fiber, they're also absolutely delicious and are perfect for meal prep. Chicken breast, black beans, and brown rice are smothered in hot sauce and topped with cheese and scallions—it's fast, filling, and packed with flavor!

In a medium saucepan, heat the oil over medium-low heat. Add the onion and cook until lightly caramelized, about 5 minutes.

Stir in the black beans, paprika, cumin, and salt and cook for 3 to 4 minutes to heat through.

Meanwhile, heat a large skillet over high heat. Spray with oil and add the chicken. Cook until browned and cooked through in the center, about 5 minutes. Transfer to a medium bowl and toss with the Buffalo sauce.

Dividing evenly, spoon the rice into each of four bowls and top with beans, cheese, and chicken. (If eating right away, I like to melt the cheese by heating the bowls in the microwave for 30 seconds.) Top with the scallions and serve. (If meal-prepping, they can be refrigerated for up to 4 days and frozen for up to 3 months.)

SERVES 4

1 teaspoon extra-virgin olive or canola oil

½ cup diced red onion

1 cup canned no-salt-added black beans,* rinsed and drained

½ teaspoon sweet paprika

½ teaspoon ground cumin

¼ teaspoon kosher salt

Olive oil spray

3 boneless, skinless chicken breasts (8 ounces each), preferably organic, cut into ½-inch cubes

½ cup Buffalo sauce, such as Frank's RedHot

3 cups cooked brown rice

½ cup shredded reduced-fat cheddar, jack, or nondairy cheese

¼ cup chopped scallions

*Read the label to be sure this product is gluten-free.

Perfect Pairings
If you want more veggies, swap the rice for cauliflower rice, add corn to the rice, top with avocado, or serve it with cucumber sticks or a salad on the side.

Per Serving (1 bowl) | Calories 461 | **Protein 49 g** | Carbohydrate 45 g | Fiber 6 g | Sugars 1 g | Fat 10 g | Saturated Fat 2.5 g | Cholesterol 134 mg | Sodium 1,387 mg

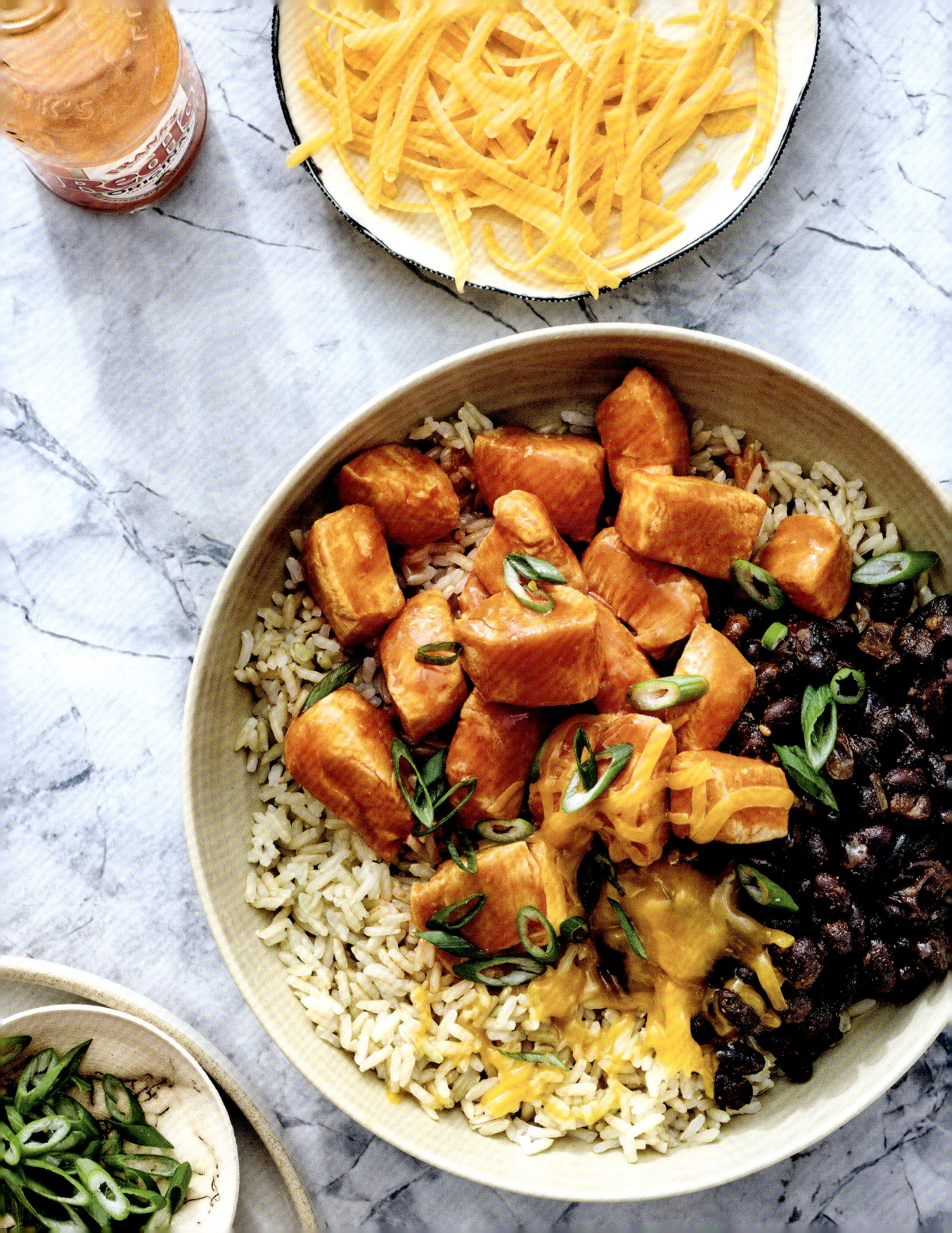

SNACKING WITH PURPOSE

Snacking often gets a bad rap, but when it's done right, it can be a powerful tool to keep your energy up and your hunger in check. For me, snacks are an essential part of hitting my daily protein goals without feeling like I have to cram everything into my main meals. The key is snacking *with intention*.

This chapter is all about purposeful snacking—options that aren't just tasty but also packed with 10 to 20 grams of protein to help you power through your day. Whether you're battling midafternoon cravings, need a quick pick-me-up, or want something satisfying after dinner, these recipes and ideas will keep you on track without compromising flavor or convenience.

You'll find everything from protein-packed dips like Yogurt Taco Dip (page 102), to easy grab-and-go bites like the quick Protein Picnic Boxes (page 109) and even sweet treats like Peanut Butter Chocolate Protein Bars (page 113) that deliver on both satisfaction and nutrition. These snacks are simple to make, perfect for meal prep, and will make you rethink the role of snacking in your daily routine.

Snacking doesn't have to be mindless—it can be purposeful, nourishing, and, most important, enjoyable. With each snack delivering 10 to 20 grams of protein, you can fuel your day without missing a beat.

NO-BAKE COTTAGE CHEESE CHEESECAKE BOWL

with Strawberries

I was actually attempting to make something else entirely when I accidentally created this strawberry cottage cheese bowl that tastes just like cheesecake! If you don't mind the texture of cottage cheese (I don't), then you can skip the blending step and just mix the ingredients together instead. You can play around with different fruits; crushed pineapple would also work well.

In a mini food processor or blender, combine the cottage cheese, sweetener, vanilla, and lemon zest and whip until smooth. Transfer to a serving bowl and top with strawberries and sprinkle with graham crackers and/or honey, if desired.

SERVES 1

1 (5.3-ounce) container low-fat (2%) cottage cheese (I like Good Culture)

1½ teaspoons monk fruit sweetener or sugar

¼ teaspoon vanilla extract

⅛ teaspoon grated lemon zest

½ cup sliced strawberries

Crushed graham crackers and/or honey (optional), for topping

Per Serving | Calories 139 | **Protein 20 g** | Carbohydrate 11 g | Fiber 1.5 g | Sugars 8 g | Fat 4 g | Saturated Fat 2 g | Cholesterol 21 mg | Sodium 465 mg

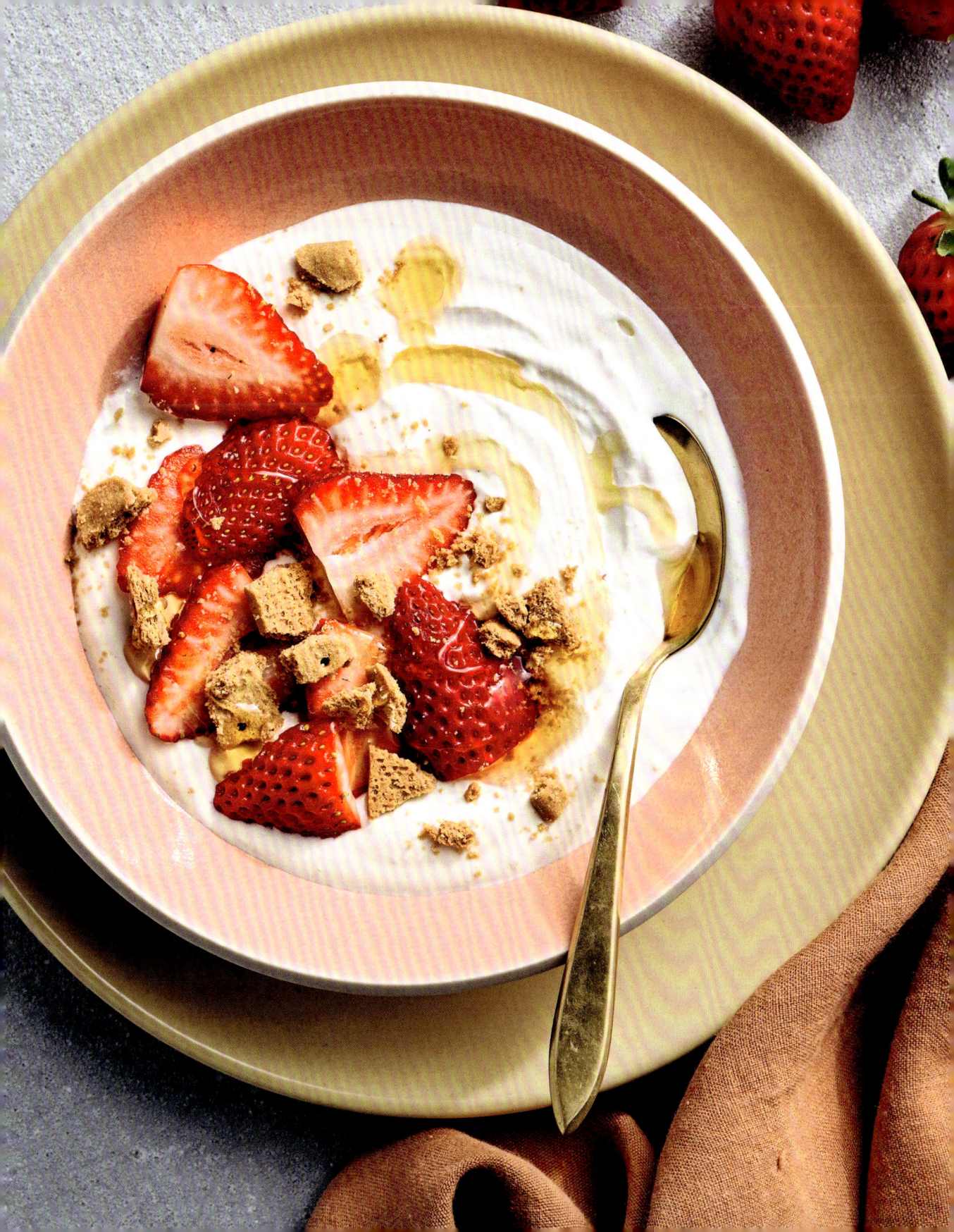

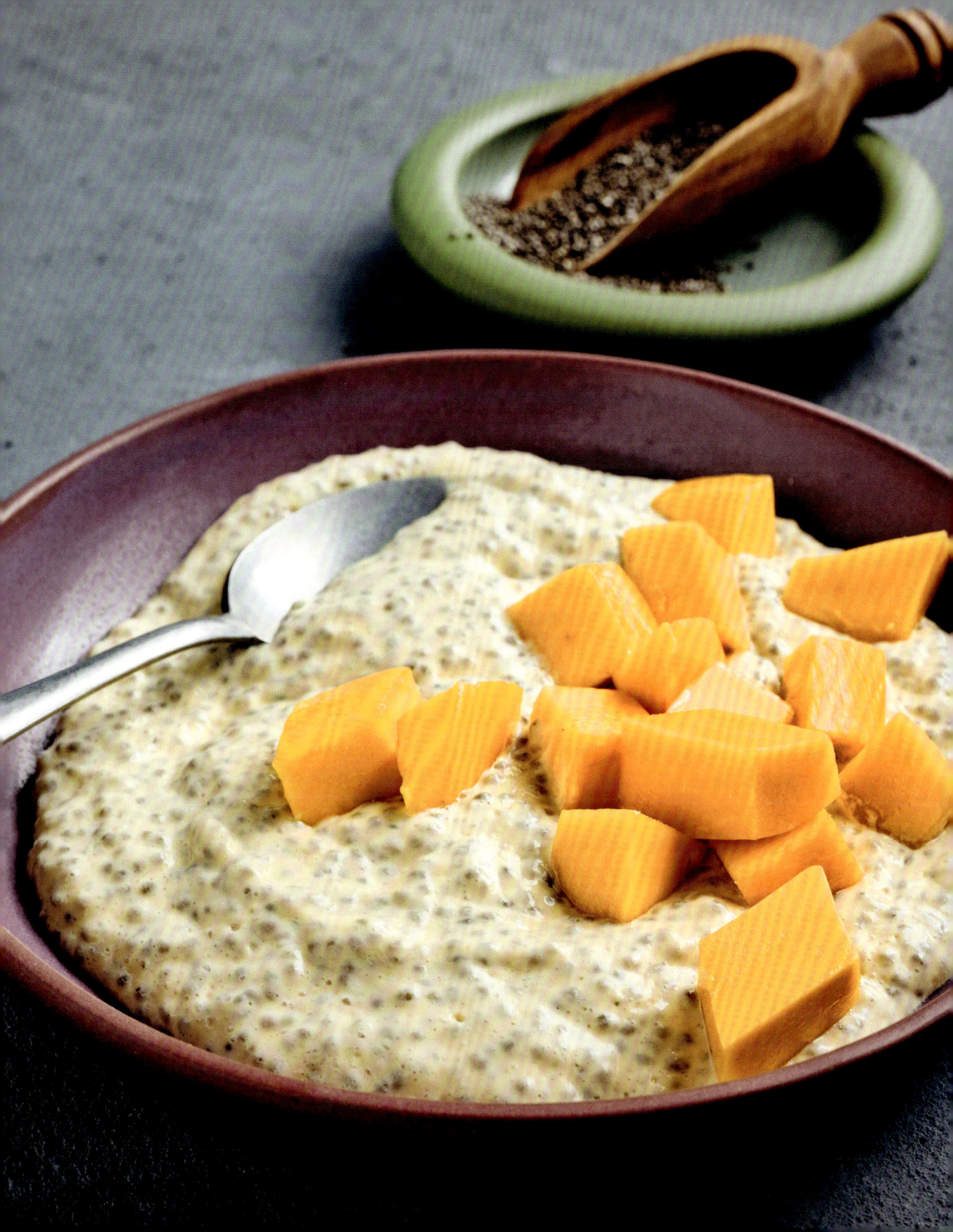

MANGO YOGURT CHIA PUDDING

I try to eat chia seeds every day because they're super nutritious and packed with fiber! Adding yogurt to chia pudding makes it creamy and adds extra protein, while fresh fruits bring nutrients and sweetness. I really love ripe mango and I think it's the perfect fruit for this pudding, but if you don't like mangoes, in-season fruit like sweet summer peaches would work great, too.

In a blender, combine the yogurt, milk, ¼ cup of the mango, and sweetener and puree until smooth. Pour the mixture into a small bowl and whisk in the chia seeds. Let sit for 10 minutes, then whisk again. Cover and refrigerate for 6 to 8 hours or overnight.

Serve topped with the remaining ½ cup mango.

TIP: Any yogurt can be used, but I've been loving Oikos Pro, which has 20 grams of protein per serving. Ratio is another brand that tastes great. Double or triple this recipe if you want to meal prep—they will last up to 4 days in the refrigerator.

SERVES 1

½ cup high-protein vanilla yogurt, such as Oikos Pro

½ cup 2% milk or milk of choice

¾ cup diced mango

1 teaspoon monk fruit sweetener, stevia, sugar, honey, or maple syrup

2 tablespoons chia seeds

Per Serving | Calories 364 | **Protein 24 g** | Carbohydrate 43 g | Fiber 10 g | Sugars 27 g | Fat 12 g | Saturated Fat 3 g | Cholesterol 23 mg | Sodium 100 mg

YOGURT TACO DIP

Here's a scaled-down high-protein version of a dip I've been making for years for parties. My daughter Karina gave it the nickname "The Stuff" because she loves it, and the name has stuck all these years. It's so simple to whip up, and it's great with chips (I like it with Quest Loaded Taco Tortilla-Style protein chips) or crudités, such as carrot sticks, cucumber sticks, and mini bell peppers. It tastes amazing!

In a bowl or glass meal-prep container, mix the yogurt, salsa, and taco seasoning until smooth. Top with the shredded lettuce, cheese, and tomatoes.

SERVES 1

½ cup plain high-protein yogurt, such as Oikos Pro

⅓ cup jarred chunky mild salsa (I like Tostitos)

½ teaspoon taco seasoning

¼ cup shredded iceberg or romaine lettuce

1 tablespoon shredded cheddar cheese

2 tablespoons diced tomato

Per Serving | Calories 165 | **Protein 20 g** | Carbohydrate 8 g | Fiber 1.5 g | Sugars 6 g | Fat 5 g | Saturated Fat 1.5 g | Cholesterol 24 mg | Sodium 607 mg

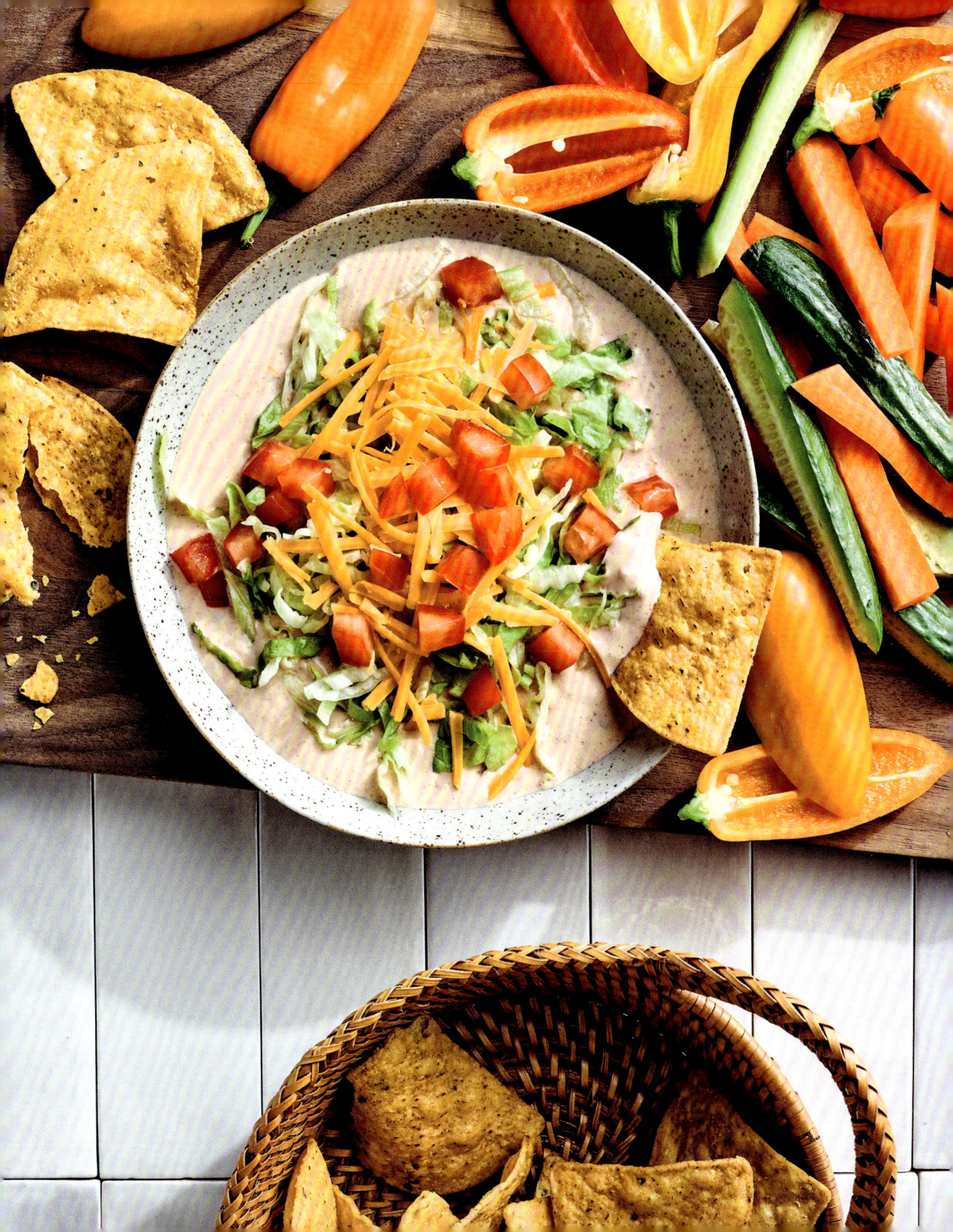

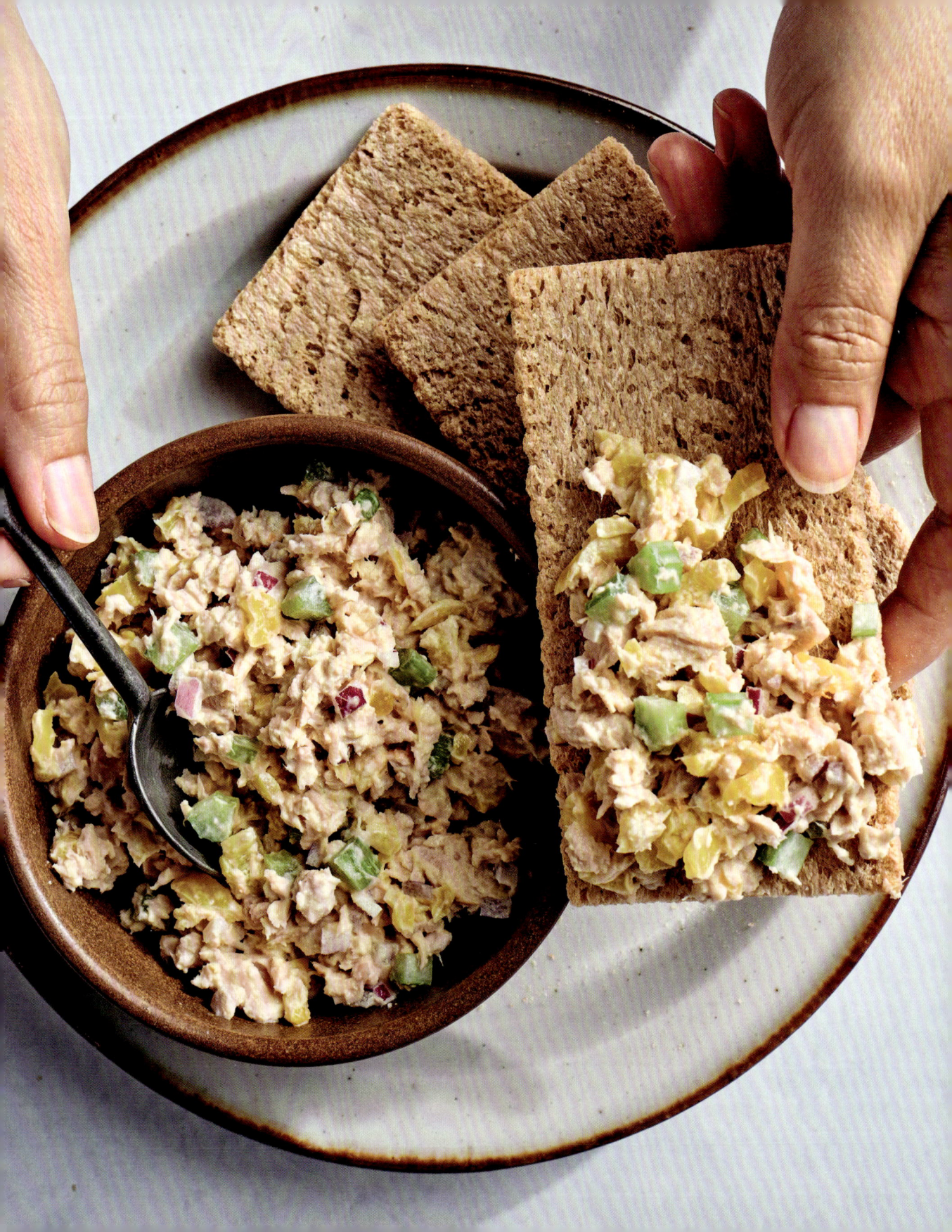

ZESTY BANANA PEPPER TUNA SALAD

with Crackers

Tuna salad with crackers is one of my go-to high-protein snacks because I always have everything in my kitchen I need to whip this up in just minutes. Adding jarred banana peppers (I love their tangy pickled crunch) to the tuna salad really takes this snack to another level! Look for high-quality wild-caught tuna and multigrain crackers with lots of texture, such as Wasa Crisp'n Light 7 Grains Crispbreads.

In a medium bowl, combine the tuna, banana peppers, brine, red onion, celery, and mayo and mix to combine. Serve on Wasa Crispbread or your favorite crackers.

TIP: Pepperoncini can be used in place of banana peppers; however, pepperoncini tend to be spicier, so be sure to adjust the amount as needed. You can double or triple the tuna salad and refrigerate it for up to 4 days.

SERVES 1

1 (3-ounce) packet water-packed wild tuna

¼ cup jarred mild banana pepper rings, chopped

1 teaspoon banana pepper brine

1 tablespoon chopped red onion or scallion

1 tablespoon chopped celery

1 tablespoon mayonnaise

2 Wasa Crisp'n Light 7 Grains Crispbreads or gluten-free crackers

Per Serving | Calories 257 | **Protein 26 g** | Carbohydrate 14 g | Fiber 2 g | Sugars 4 g | Fat 11 g | Saturated Fat 1.5 g | Cholesterol 45 mg | Sodium 400 mg

PEANUT BUTTER YOGURT DIP
with Apples

I love discovering quick and easy snack options that not only keep me full but also taste amazing! Yogurt makes a great high-protein base, while powdered peanut butter adds an extra boost of protein. Apples provide fiber, sweetness, and crunch. You can also swap in bananas, or simply enjoy it by the spoonful. An extra drizzle of peanut butter on top or some chocolate shavings are great ideas, too.

In a small bowl, stir together the yogurt and peanut butter powder and mix well. Serve with the apple wedges.

TIP: To make this nut-free, use a seed butter such as Wowbutter.

SERVES 1

½ cup nonfat vanilla Greek yogurt, such as Oikos Triple Zero, or nondairy yogurt of your choice

2 tablespoons peanut butter powder, such as PBFit

1 medium apple, sliced into wedges

Per Serving | Calories 248 | **Protein 18 g** | Carbohydrate 40 g | Fiber 5 g | Sugars 24 g | Fat 2 g | Saturated Fat 0 g | Cholesterol 7 mg | Sodium 136 mg

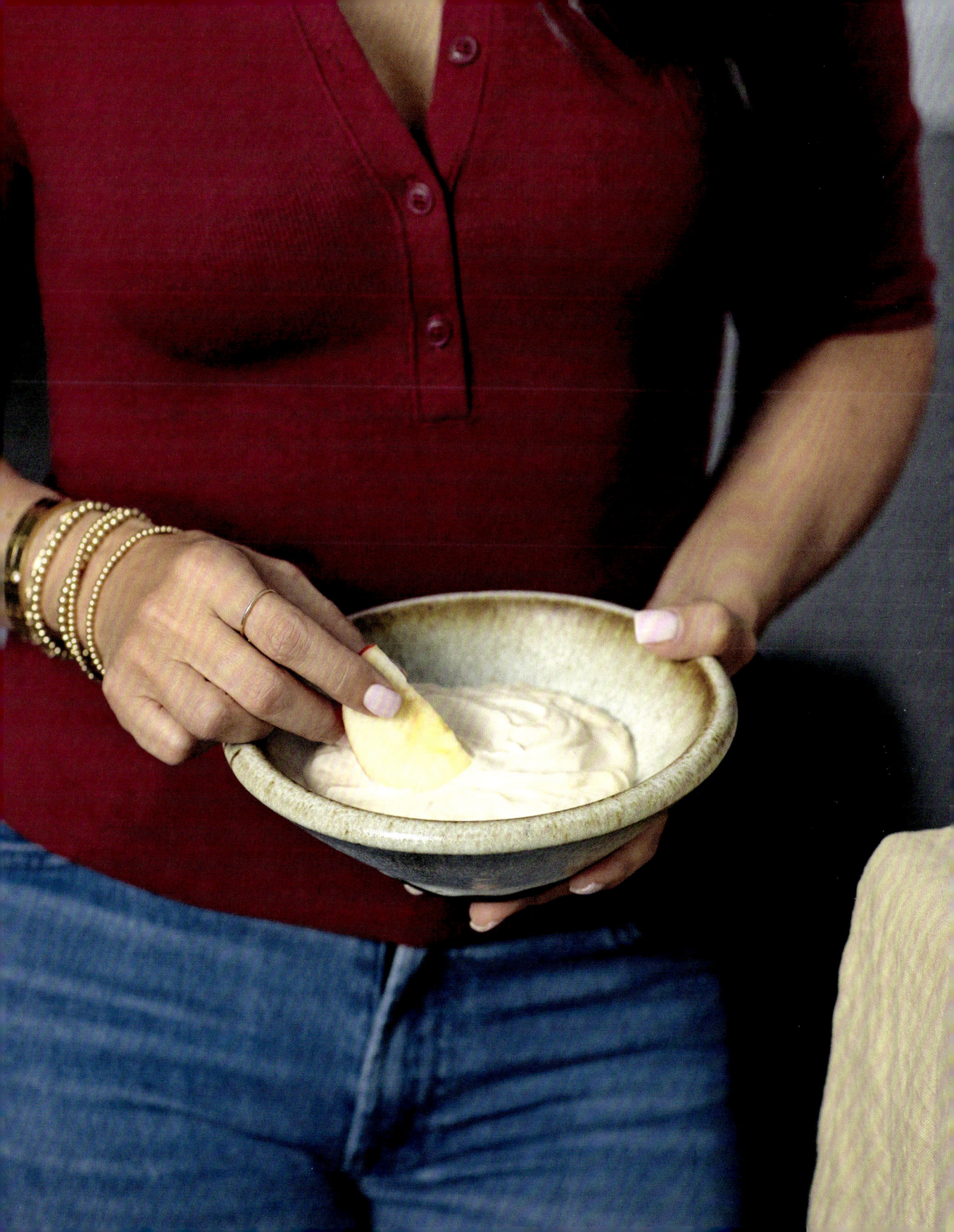

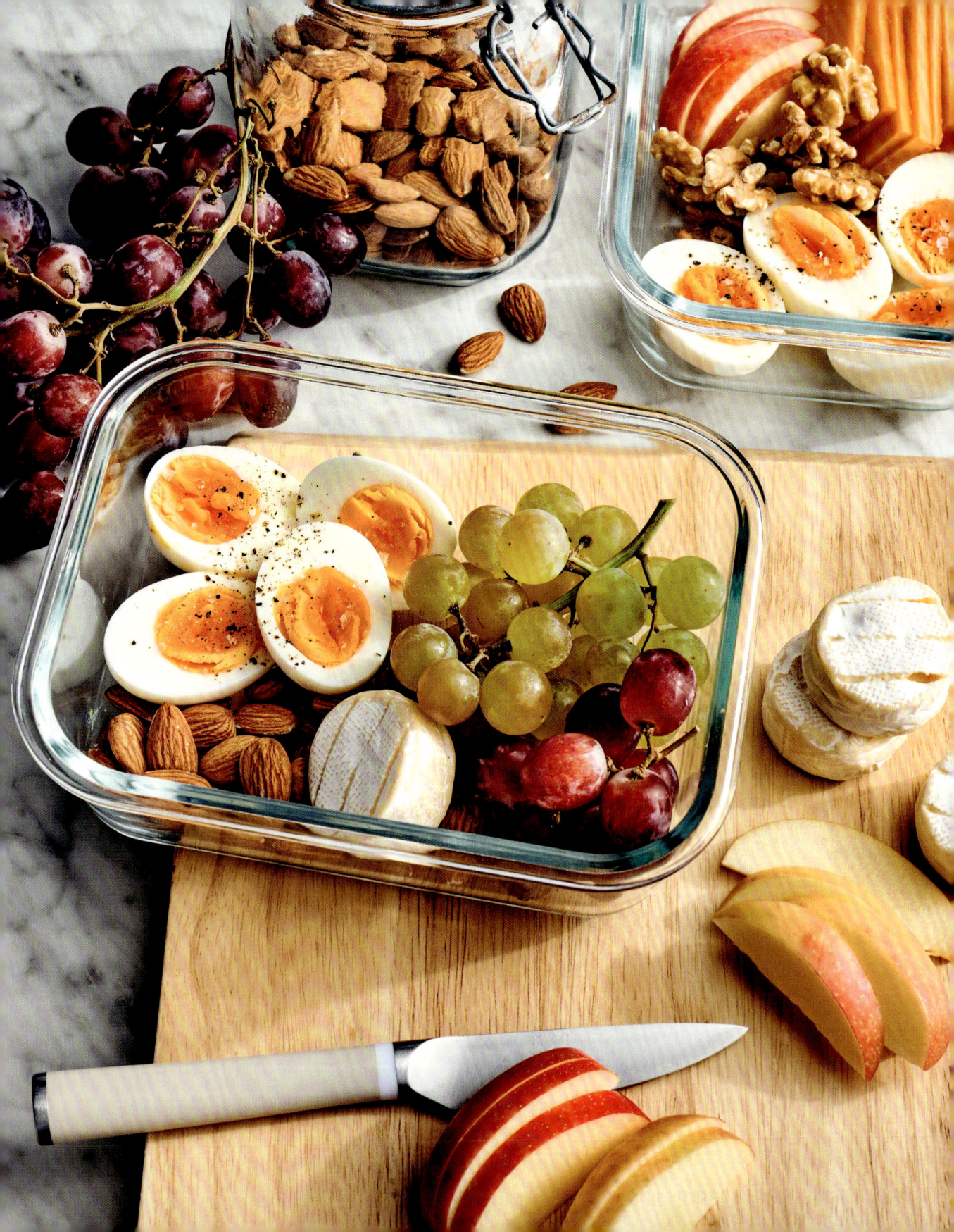

PROTEIN PICNIC BOXES

The simplest snacks are often the best! Having healthy premade (and homemade!) snack boxes in your fridge is perfect for quick bites between meals, for road trips, or for post-workout snacks. Hard-boiled eggs are the perfect convenient, protein-packed option. For a simple, nutritious snack, I pair the eggs with Brie bites for extra protein, fresh grapes for a sweet touch, and almonds for crunch. These boxes are easily customizable—swap in seasonal fresh fruit or dried options like figs, and change up the cheese or leave it out if you're dairy-free. You can also add veggies like sugar snap peas or cucumbers, or some prosciutto or roast beef for an extra protein boost. See below for even more great ideas!

———————

Place the eggs in a medium pot and add cold water to cover by about 1 inch. Bring to a boil over medium-high heat. When the water boils, remove from the heat and cover for 20 minutes (they will continue to cook). Drain and rinse the eggs under cold water until cooled, then peel right away.

Divide the eggs, mini Brie bites, grapes, and almonds among four meal-prep containers. Refrigerate for up to 4 days.

TIP: When I make hard-boiled eggs, I use the raw eggs that have been sitting in my fridge the longest because they are easier to peel once hard-boiled.

MAKES 4 PICNIC BOXES

8 large eggs

4 (0.9-ounce) Brie bites (I like Supreme or Ile de France)

40 red or green grapes (or a mix of both)

32 almonds

Variations
There are so many other yummy combos of cheese, fruit, and nuts that you can swap in when making your own protein picnic boxes! Here are a few other options to try:

Eggs + goat cheese + figs + pistachios

Eggs + cheddar + apples + walnuts

Eggs + blue cheese + pears + pecans

Eggs + Gruyère + cherries + cashews

Eggs + mozzarella + plums + pine nuts

Per Serving (1 snack box) | Calories 306 | **Protein 19 g** | Carbohydrate 13 g | Fiber 1.5 g | Sugars 9 g | Fat 21 g | Saturated Fat 7.5 g | Cholesterol 392 mg | Sodium 303 mg

FALL HARVEST JARS

After a fun day of apple picking with my family, I found myself with more apples than I knew what to do with. Naturally, I created some new recipes including these yummy jars filled with shredded apples, crunchy granola, yogurt, and cinnamon. They're the perfect healthy make-ahead snack or light breakfast. My daughter Karina loves them, and they stay fresh in the fridge for up to 3 days.

In a small bowl, combine the brown sugar and cinnamon.

Divide the yogurt among four mason jars or meal-prep bowls and add the raisins. Top with the apples, then the brown sugar mixture and granola. Refrigerate for up to 4 days.

TIP: You can use any type of apple—if you prefer a tart flavor, go for green apples, and if you're after something sweeter, Honeycrisp is a great choice.

SERVES 4

2 teaspoons monk fruit brown sugar or very loosely packed brown sugar

1½ teaspoons ground cinnamon

4 cups high-protein vanilla yogurt, such as Oikos Pro, or nondairy yogurt

¼ cup golden raisins

1½ cups coarsely grated apples (about 2 medium)

½ cup gluten-free granola (I like Purely Elizabeth)

Per Serving (1 jar or bowl) | Calories 333 | **Protein 33 g** | Carbohydrate 39 g | Fiber 2.5 g | Sugars 21 g | Fat 6 g | Saturated Fat 2 g | Cholesterol 27 mg | Sodium 126 mg

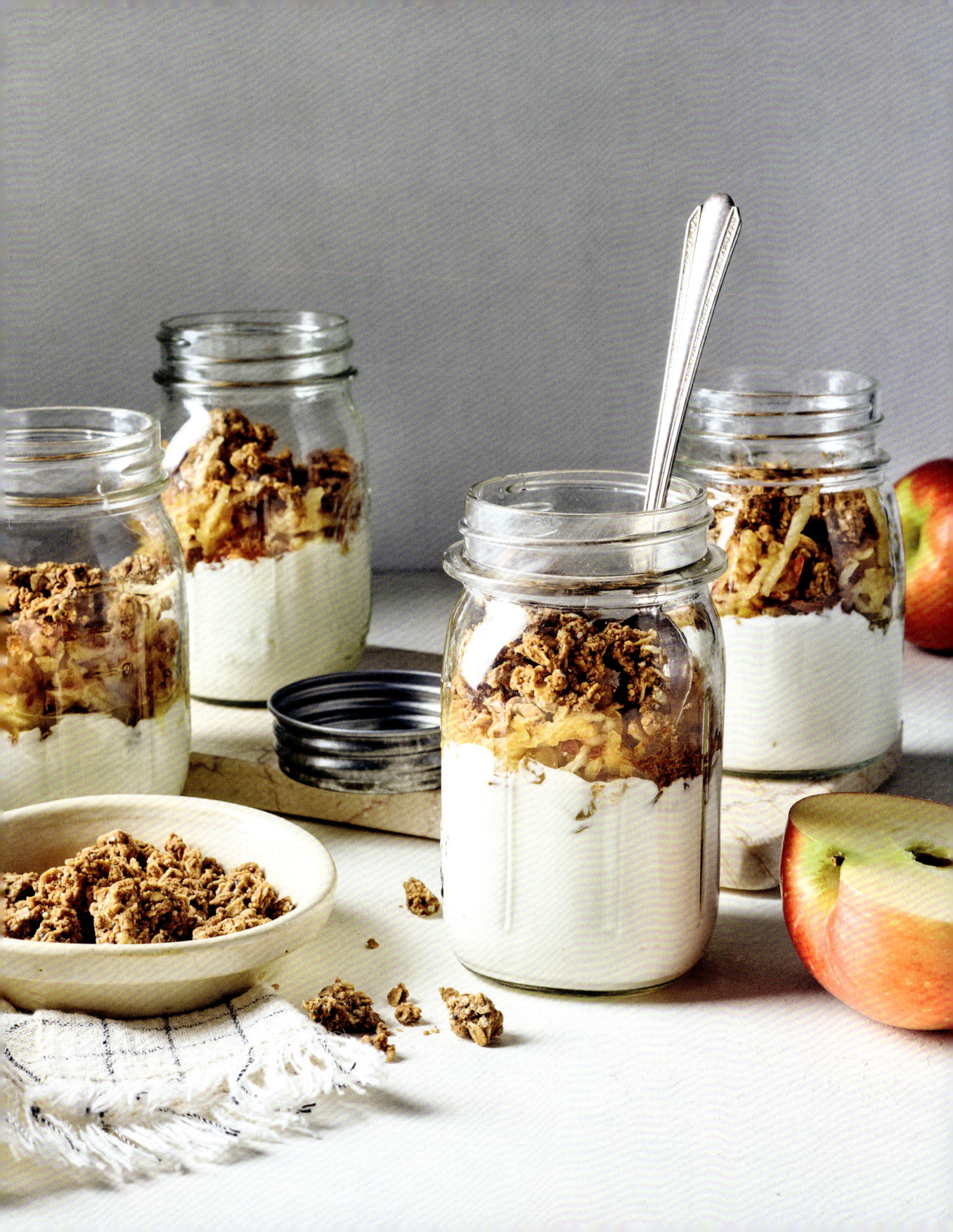

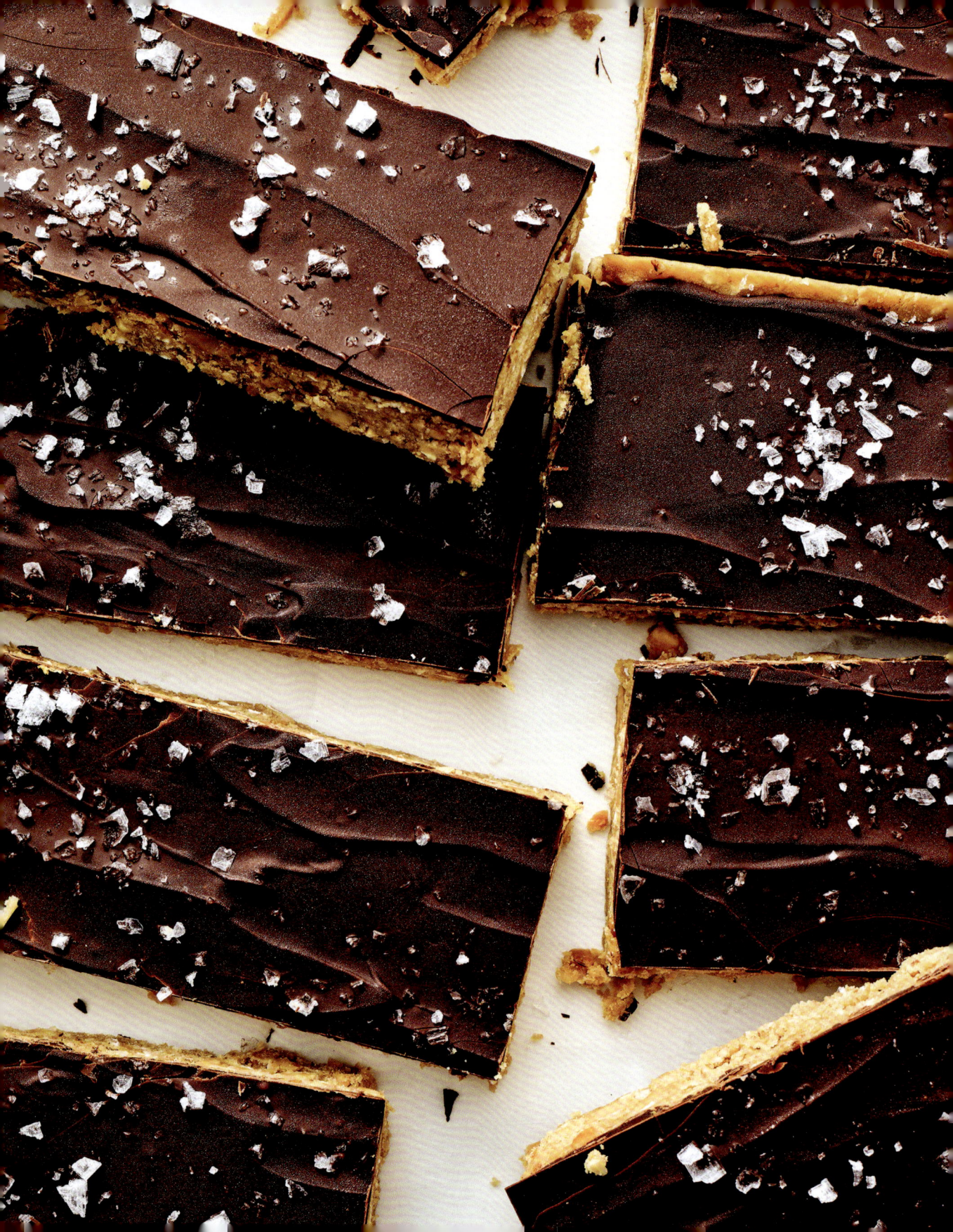

PEANUT BUTTER CHOCOLATE PROTEIN BARS

These no-bake, refrigerator protein bars are one of my go-to snacks because they're incredibly easy to make. I usually keep a batch in my fridge, ready to grab whenever I want a healthy treat. With 14 grams of protein, they make an ideal post-workout snack, a midday pick-me-up, or an end-of-the-day treat. For an extra protein boost, I use a blend of unflavored pea protein powder and collagen, and trust me, you'll never know it's there.

Line an 8 × 8 glass or metal pan with parchment paper with overhang and set aside.

In a mini food processor or blender, pulse the oats until they resemble coarse sand. Transfer to a large bowl.

Add the protein powder, collagen, and crispy rice cereal and whisk together to evenly combine. Add the syrup, vanilla, peanut butter, 4 to 5 tablespoons water (enough to make it smooth), and salt and mix with a spatula until thoroughly combined. Transfer the mixture to the prepared pan and press and spread evenly with your hands or the back of a dry measuring cup.

In a small microwave-safe bowl, melt the chocolate in 30-second increments on 50% power, mixing after each minute, until melted, about 2 minutes total. Once fully melted, spread the chocolate evenly over the peanut butter mixture. Sprinkle with the flaky sea salt, if using. Refrigerate for at least 2 hours (the longer the better).

Once set, cut the bars in a 5-by-2 grid into 10 rectangles each measuring about 4 × 1½ inches. Store in the refrigerator wrapped in plastic for up to 1 week or freeze for up to 3 months.

TIP: I tested this with pure pea protein powder and Truvani unflavored plant protein and had success with both. Bob's Red Mill sells a one-ingredient protein oats with 50 percent more protein than regular oats grown from a special hull-less variety. You can use regular oats here too, if that's all you have.

MAKES 10 BARS

½ cup organic protein oats* (I like Bob's Red Mill)

½ cup unflavored pea protein powder

¼ cup unflavored collagen peptides or vegetarian collagen peptide powder

½ cup crispy brown rice cereal, such as Nature's Path Organic

¼ cup sugar-free maple-flavored syrup, such as Wholesome Yum

1 teaspoon vanilla extract

1 cup unsweetened crunchy peanut butter

½ teaspoon kosher salt

¼ cup dark chocolate chips (1½ ounces) or dairy-free chocolate chips

Sea salt flakes (optional), for topping

*Read the label to be sure this product is gluten-free.

Per Serving (1 bar) | Calories 247 | **Protein 14 g** | Carbohydrate 20 g | Fiber 3 g | Sugars 6 g | Fat 15 g | Saturated Fat 3.5 g | Cholesterol 0 mg | Sodium 167 mg

CHOCOLATE EDAMAME BARK

This edamame bark is the ultimate late-night snack for those moments when a chocolate craving strikes. I'll admit, I wasn't sure if edamame would pair well with chocolate, but let's be real—chocolate-covered anything is almost always a win, and this combo does not disappoint! Here's why it works: Edamame packs more protein than peanuts or even chickpeas. So I melted some chocolate and mixed it with roasted edamame, a staple in my pantry. The result? A ridiculously simple, two-ingredient snack that satisfies your sweet tooth and delivers nearly 10 grams of protein per serving. Perfect for people like me who crave a little chocolate before bed.

SERVES 8

1 cup (6 ounces) sugar-free semisweet chocolate chips, such as Lakanto

1½ cups salted dry-roasted edamame

Line a large sheet pan with parchment paper or a silicone baking mat.

Place the chocolate in a microwave-safe medium bowl and melt in the microwave in 30-second increments, stirring after each, until completely melted, 1½ to 2 minutes total. (Be careful not to overdo it or the chocolate will scorch.)

Add the edamame to the chocolate and stir. Using a spatula, scoop every last bit of the chocolate edamame onto the parchment on the baking sheet and spread into an even layer.

Put in the freezer and allow it to harden for at least 15 minutes. Once it becomes solid, cut it into 8 pieces. Store in the fridge or freezer.

TIP: I used sugar-free chocolate here, but you can use whatever chocolate you like. If you're dairy-free, use dairy-free chips instead.

Per Serving (1 piece) | Calories 166 | **Protein 10 g** | Carbohydrate 17 g | Fiber 8 g | Sugars 0.5 g | Fat 10 g | Saturated Fat 5 g | Cholesterol 0 mg | Sodium 103 mg

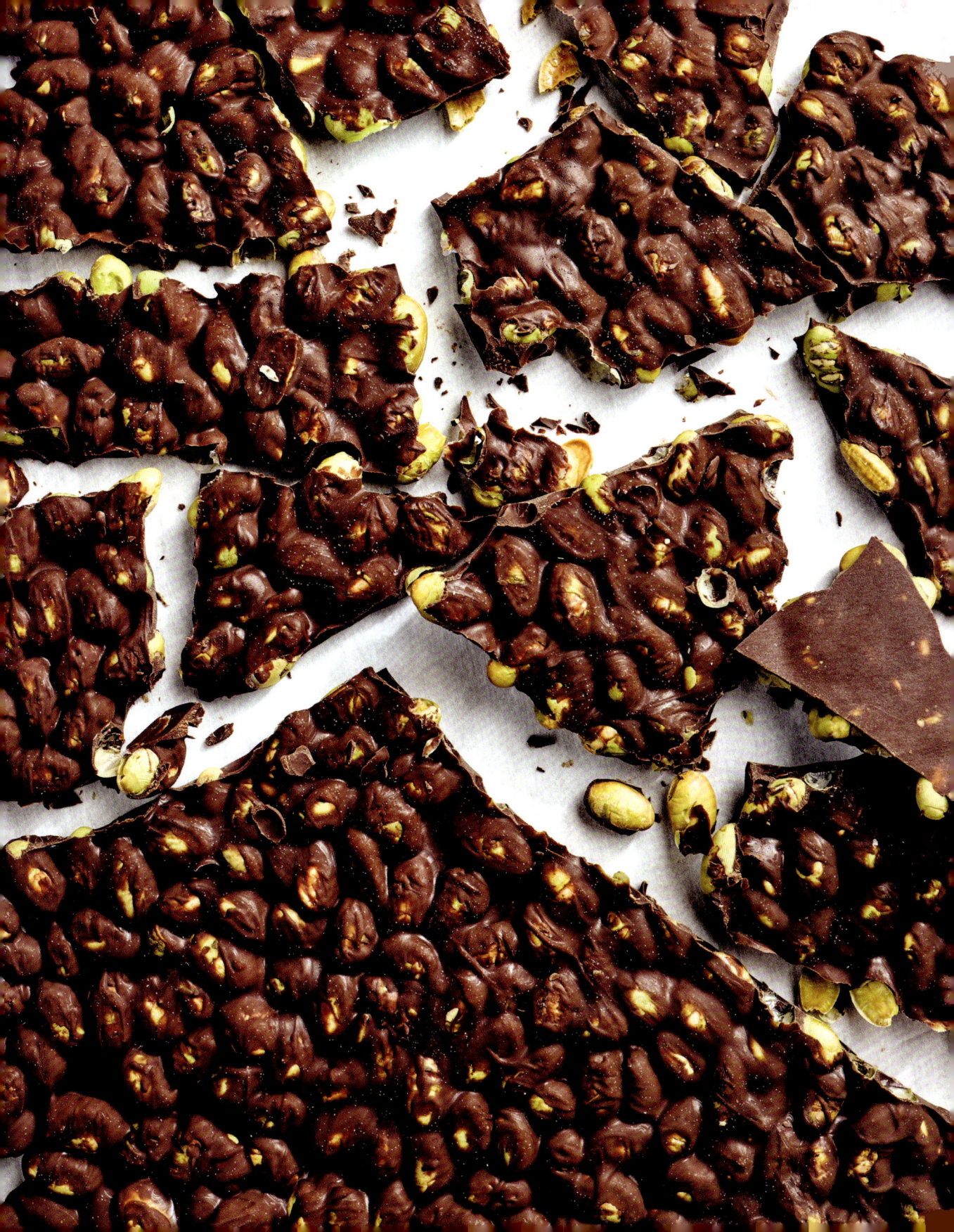

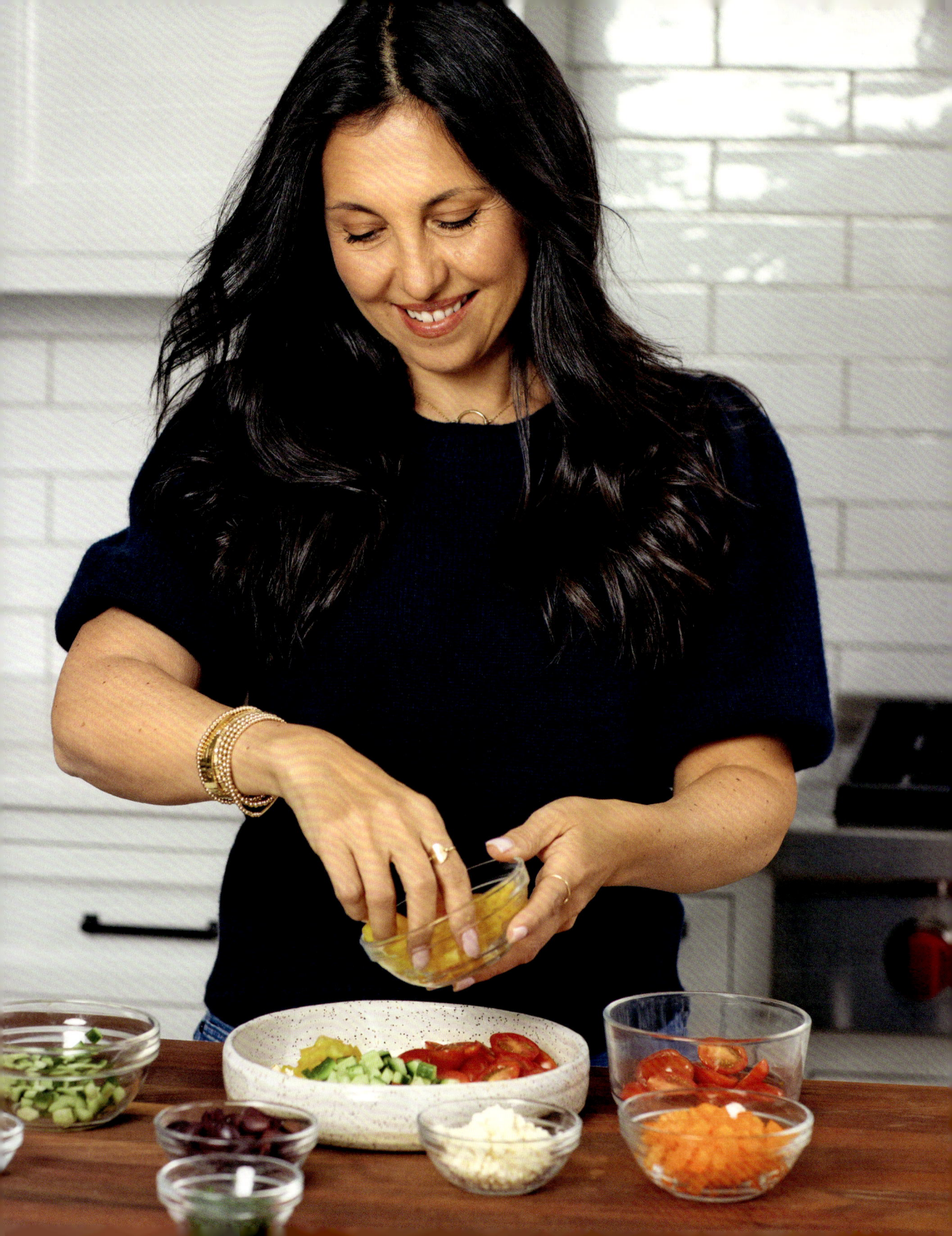

GREEK COTTAGE CHEESE BOWL

This savory cottage cheese bowl is inspired by a Greek salad with tomatoes, cucumbers, bell pepper, kalamata olives, feta, and fresh dill. It couldn't be simpler to whip up—just chop the veggies and mix everything together in a bowl. It's fast, delicious, and packed with protein. Plus, it's great for meal prep—just keep the components separate until you're ready to eat. This recipe has become a fan favorite on my Skinnytaste website, where I recommend increasing the cottage cheese to 1 cup for a satisfying breakfast. As a snack, ¾ cup is just the right amount. One reader raved, "I'd give this recipe a ten if I could! I eat it nearly daily for breakfast!" I hope you love it, too!

In a serving bowl, mix the cottage cheese with 1½ teaspoons of the fresh dill. Top with the cherry tomatoes, cucumbers, and bell pepper. Season with the salt and pepper. Top with the olives, feta, and remaining 1½ teaspoons dill. Drizzle with the olive oil and serve.

SERVES 1

¾ cup 2% cottage cheese

1 tablespoon chopped fresh dill

¼ cup cherry tomatoes, quartered

¼ cup chopped Persian (mini) cucumbers

¼ cup diced yellow or orange bell pepper

Pinch each of kosher salt and freshly ground black pepper

2 tablespoons chopped pitted kalamata olives

1 tablespoon crumbled feta cheese

½ teaspoon extra-virgin olive oil

Per Serving | Calories 205 | **Protein 23 g** | Carbohydrate 10 g | Fiber 2 g | Sugars 8 g | Fat 10 g | Saturated Fat 4 g | Cholesterol 31 mg | Sodium 816 mg

MIGHTY MEATLESS MEALS

This chapter was by far the most challenging for me to create. Getting 30 grams of protein in a meal is simple when meat or seafood is involved, but achieving that with vegetarian ingredients? Not so much. It took a lot of testing and experimenting and a bit of creativity to find combinations that worked, *and* tasted amazing.

The key was to lean on high-protein plant-based ingredients like tofu, edamame, peas, lentils, and cottage cheese (yes, it's a vegetarian powerhouse!) to build meals that are satisfying, nourishing, and protein-packed. I often like to eat vegetarian in my house and try to have a few plant-based meals per week. Through this cookbook creation process, I realized that vegetarian cooking offers endless possibilities for creativity and flavor, proving it can be just as satisfying and enjoyable as meals with meat.

In this chapter, you'll find recipes that prove plant-based meals don't have to sacrifice flavor or protein. From comforting pastas like Lasagna Roll-Ups with Cottage Cheese (page 136) to one-bowl meals like Lentil Chili (page 128, these dishes are designed to deliver at least 30 grams of protein per serving without relying on meat.

Whether you're vegetarian, looking to incorporate more meatless meals into your week, or simply up for the challenge of powering up with plants, I hope you find this chapter helpful.

FUGAZZA (WHITE ONION) PERSONAL PIZZA

Fugazza is a popular Argentinian-style pizza topped with *tons* of onions, mozzarella, and dried oregano. My friend Mariella, who was born in Argentina, introduced me to this veggie pie, and it quickly became my family's favorite pizza! The amount of onions may seem like overkill, but trust me, as they soften and char, they mix beautifully with the melted cheese. My secret ingredient to making this decadent pizza lighter and higher in protein is cottage cheese! I use it to make the high-protein thin crust, and I mix even more cottage cheese with the Pecorino, mozzarella, and onion topping. My daughter Madison devoured this pizza, and she had no idea it was made with cottage cheese!

Preheat the oven to 500°F. Place a sheet pan or pizza steel in the oven to get hot.

Meanwhile, in a small bowl, mix the flour with ¼ cup of the cottage cheese. Knead the dough until very smooth, then transfer to a floured surface. Flour the rolling pin to prevent sticking and roll out the dough to form a thin 8-inch pizza crust. Poke holes all around the crust with a fork to prevent air pockets.

Use oven mitts to remove the hot sheet pan from the oven and carefully place the pizza crust on top. Return to the oven and parbake the dough until slightly golden, 3 to 4 minutes. Remove from the oven but leave the oven on.

Spread the remaining ⅓ cup cottage cheese over the crust. Top with 1 tablespoon of the Pecorino cheese, half of the onions, the mozzarella, and the oregano. Add the rest of the onions, drizzle with the olive oil, season with the salt. Finish with the remaining 1 teaspoon Pecorino.

Return to the oven and bake until the mozzarella is melted and the onions and Pecorino are golden and browned on top, about 8 minutes. Serve immediately.

SERVES 1

¼ cup self-rising flour, plus more for dusting

1 (5.3-ounce) container low-fat (2%) cottage cheese (I like Good Culture), drained well

1 tablespoon plus 1 teaspoon grated Pecorino Romano cheese

½ cup thinly sliced yellow onion (about ½ small)

¼ cup shredded mozzarella cheese

⅛ teaspoon dried oregano

1 teaspoon extra-virgin olive oil

⅛ teaspoon kosher salt

Per Serving | Calories 385 | **Protein 32 g** | Carbohydrate 32 g | Fiber 1 g | Sugars 7 g | Fat 16 g | Saturated Fat 7.5 g | Cholesterol 49 mg | Sodium 1,244 mg

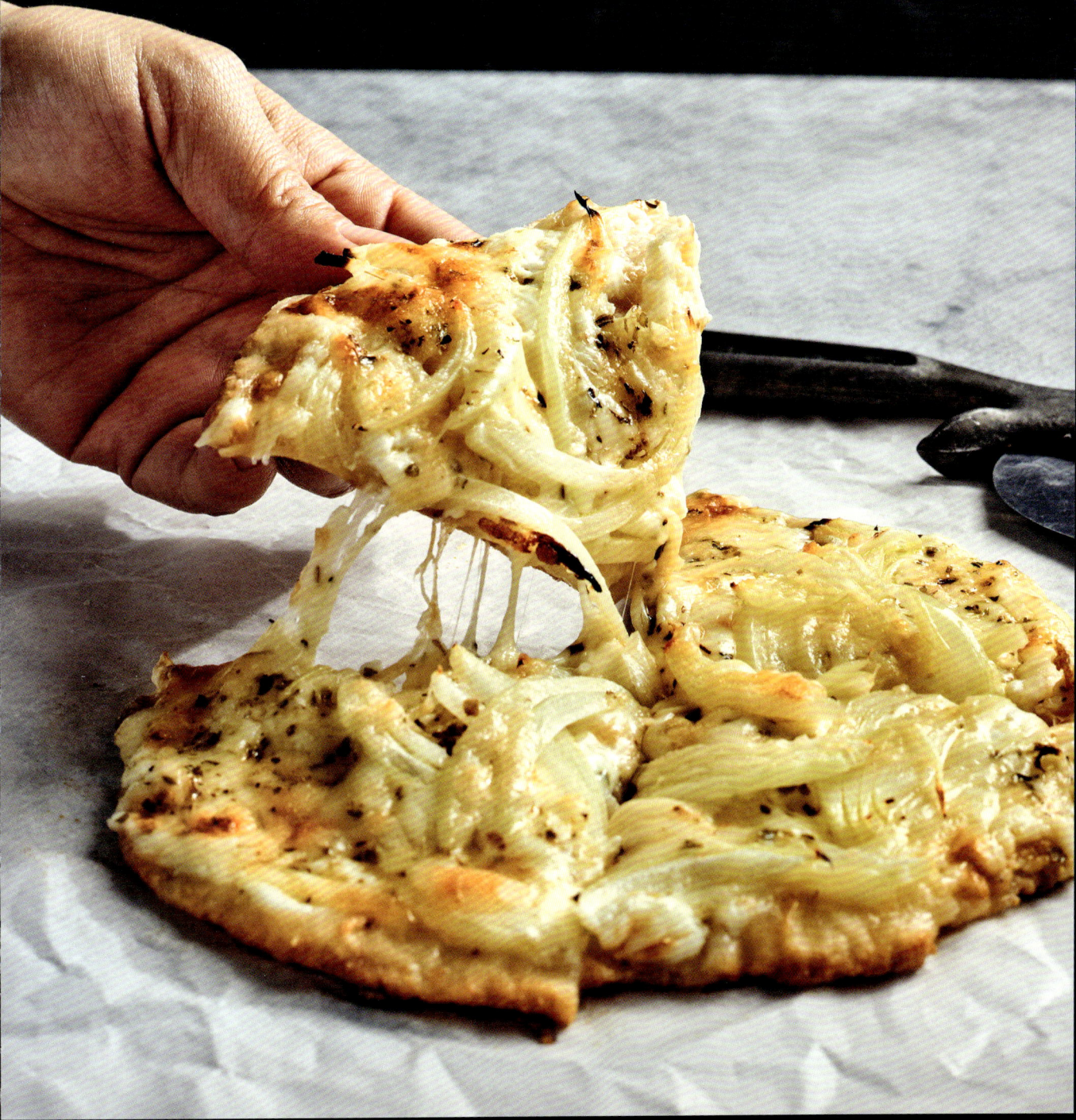

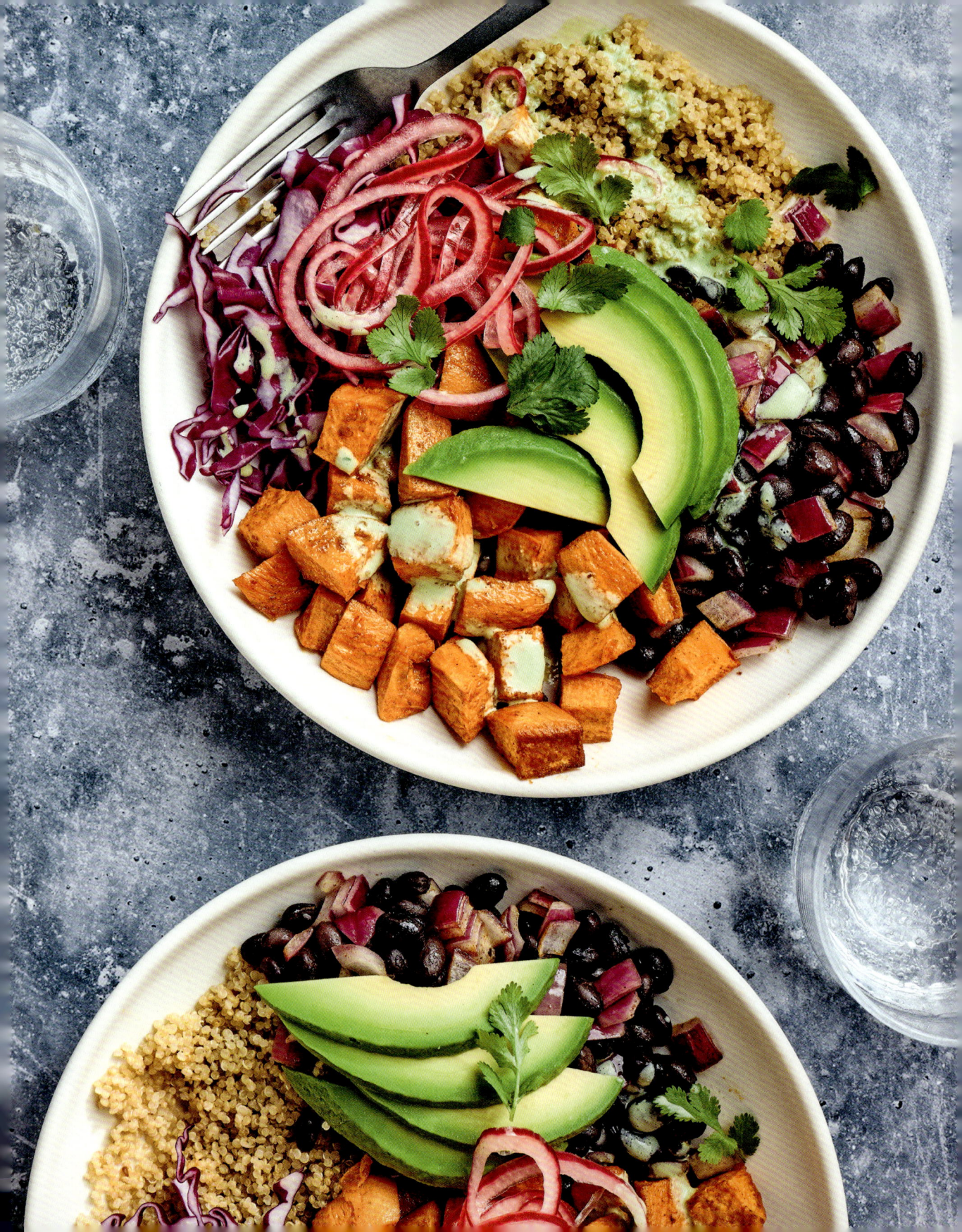

BLACK BEAN QUINOA BOWLS

Eating a high-protein vegetarian diet can be challenging, but here's one easy way to make it work. Combine black beans, which are rich in protein, nutrients, and fiber, with quinoa, one of the few grain-based proteins that is a complete protein (a complete protein contains all nine essential amino acids that the body can't make). The yogurt-based dressing adds even more protein, creating a delicious and nutritious bowl.

MAKE THE QUICK-PICKLED ONIONS: Place the onions in a heatproof bowl. In a small saucepan, combine the vinegar, ⅓ cup water, the sugar, and salt and bring to a boil over medium heat until the sugar dissolves, about 2 minutes. Pour the liquid over the onions and set aside to cool. Refrigerate for 30 minutes while preparing the rest of the recipe. The longer they sit, the more flavor they will have.

ROAST THE SWEET POTATOES AND BLACK BEANS: Adjust the oven racks in the center and bottom third of the oven and preheat to 425°F. Spray two large sheet pans with oil.

In a large bowl, toss the sweet potato with the olive oil and season with the garlic powder, ½ teaspoon of the paprika, and ¼ teaspoon of the salt. Spread them in an even layer on the prepared sheet pan and roast on the center rack, flipping halfway, until tender and golden and browned on the edges, 25 to 30 minutes.

At the same time, on the second sheet pan, toss together the onion, black beans, and remaining 1 teaspoon paprika and ¼ teaspoon salt. Spray with oil and roast until the onions are cooked and the beans are heated through, 10 to 15 minutes.

MEANWHILE, MAKE THE CREAMY JALAPEÑO SAUCE: In a blender, combine the yogurt, jalapeño, lime juice, garlic cloves, cilantro, and the salt and blend until smooth. Taste for salt and adjust if needed.

ASSEMBLE THE BOWLS: Divide the quinoa into each of four bowls. Top with ¾ cup roasted black bean/onion mixture, ½ cup sweet potatoes, ¼ cup cabbage, and 1 ounce avocado. Serve each with ⅓ cup jalapeño sauce and garnish with the pickled onions and cilantro.

Per Serving (1 bowl) | Calories 634 | **Protein 30 g** | Carbohydrate 106 g | Fiber 22 g | Sugars 12 g | Fat 11 g | Saturated Fat 1.5 g | Cholesterol 3 mg | Sodium 791 mg

SERVES 4

QUICK-PICKLED ONIONS

1 medium red onion, thinly sliced into rounds

½ cup apple cider vinegar

1 tablespoon sugar

1 teaspoon kosher salt

POTATOES AND BEANS

Olive oil spray

2 medium sweet potatoes, peeled and cut into cubes

2 teaspoons olive oil

½ teaspoon garlic powder

1½ teaspoons sweet paprika

½ teaspoon kosher salt

1 small red onion, chopped

2 (15-ounce) cans black beans,* drained and rinsed

CREAMY JALAPEÑO SAUCE

1 cup 0% Greek yogurt or nondairy yogurt

1 jalapeño

2 tablespoons fresh lime juice

2 garlic cloves

¼ cup chopped cilantro

¼ teaspoon kosher salt

ASSEMBLY

3½ cups cooked quinoa

1 cup shredded red cabbage

4 ounces diced avocado

Chopped fresh cilantro leaves

*Read the label to be sure this product is gluten-free.

EGG CURRY with Yogurt Naan

The combination of tomatoes and eggs is a naturally tasty union as evidenced by dishes all over the world, such as Middle Eastern shakshuka. This rich and flavorful Indian egg curry, made with hard-boiled eggs simmered in a spiced tomato-based sauce, takes this combo to a whole other level!

In a large heavy skillet, heat the oil over medium heat. Add the cinnamon sticks and let them sizzle for 1 minute. Reduce the heat to medium-low, add the onions, and cook, stirring often so they don't burn, until they are caramelized and light brown, about 18 minutes.

Stir in the garlic and ginger and cook, stirring, until fragrant, another 2 minutes. Stir in the cardamom, coriander, cumin, and turmeric. Add the diced tomatoes, salt, and 1 cup water. Bring to a boil, then cover and simmer on low, stirring occasionally, until thickened, about 15 minutes.

Discard the cinnamon and add the garam masala and cooked eggs to the pan, stirring gently to coat the eggs. Cook until the eggs are warmed, 3 to 4 minutes. Garnish with cilantro and serve with naan.

Per Serving (3 eggs + ¾ cup sauce) | Calories 364 | **Protein 22 g** | Carbohydrate 20 g | Fiber 5 g | Sugars 8 g | Fat 22 g | Saturated Fat 5.5 g | Cholesterol 558 mg | Sodium 849 mg

SERVES 4

2 tablespoons avocado oil

2 small cinnamon sticks

2 medium yellow onions, finely chopped

6 garlic cloves, finely chopped

2 tablespoons grated fresh ginger, or paste

1 teaspoon ground cardamom

1 teaspoon ground coriander

½ teaspoon ground cumin

½ teaspoon ground turmeric

2 (14.5-ounce) cans petite diced tomatoes

1 teaspoon kosher salt

½ teaspoon garam masala

12 hard-boiled eggs, peeled

Chopped fresh cilantro, for garnish

4 Yogurt Naan (recipe follows)

YOGURT NAAN

In a large bowl, combine the flour, salt, and yogurt. Mix well with a fork until combined. Use your hands to knead the mixture until smooth and form it into a large ball. Divide the dough into 4 equal portions and roll each into a ball. Lightly flour a clean work surface. Dust a rolling pin with flour and roll each portion into a thin oval shape.

Heat a nonstick skillet over medium heat. When hot, place the rolled-out dough on the skillet and cook until browned on the bottom, about 3 minutes. Flip and cook until browned on the other side, about 2 minutes more. Repeat until all the naan bread is cooked.

Once cooked, lightly brush the tops with the melted butter.

Per Serving (1 naan) | Calories 175 | **Protein 10 g** | Carbohydrate 31 g | Fiber 0 g | Sugars 2 g | Fat 1 g | Saturated Fat 1 g | Cholesterol 7 mg | Sodium 580 mg

MAKES 4 NAAN

1⅓ cups self-rising flour, plus more for dusting

¼ teaspoon kosher salt

1 cup fat-free Greek yogurt or nondairy Greek yogurt, such as Kite Hill

1½ teaspoons melted butter or nondairy butter

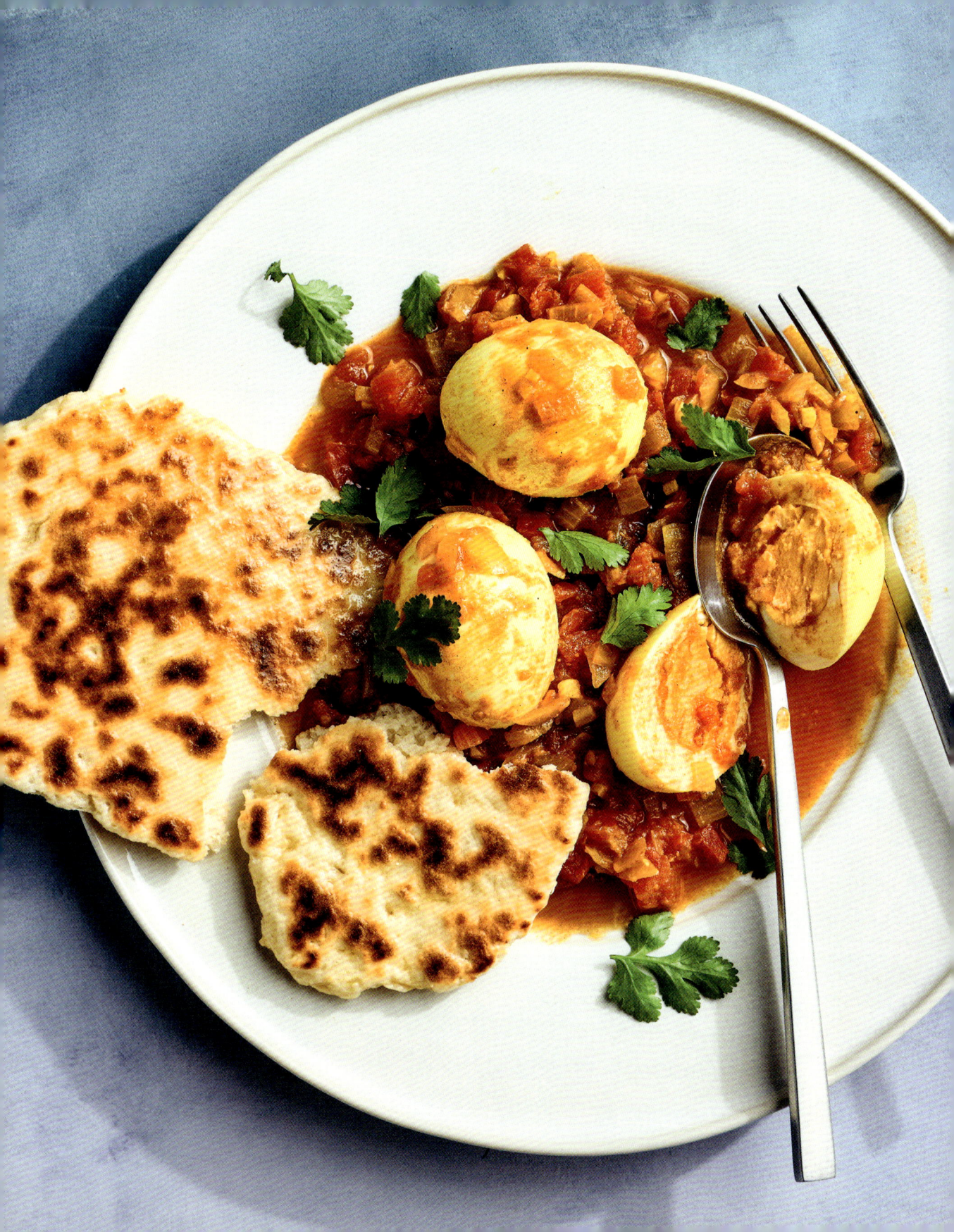

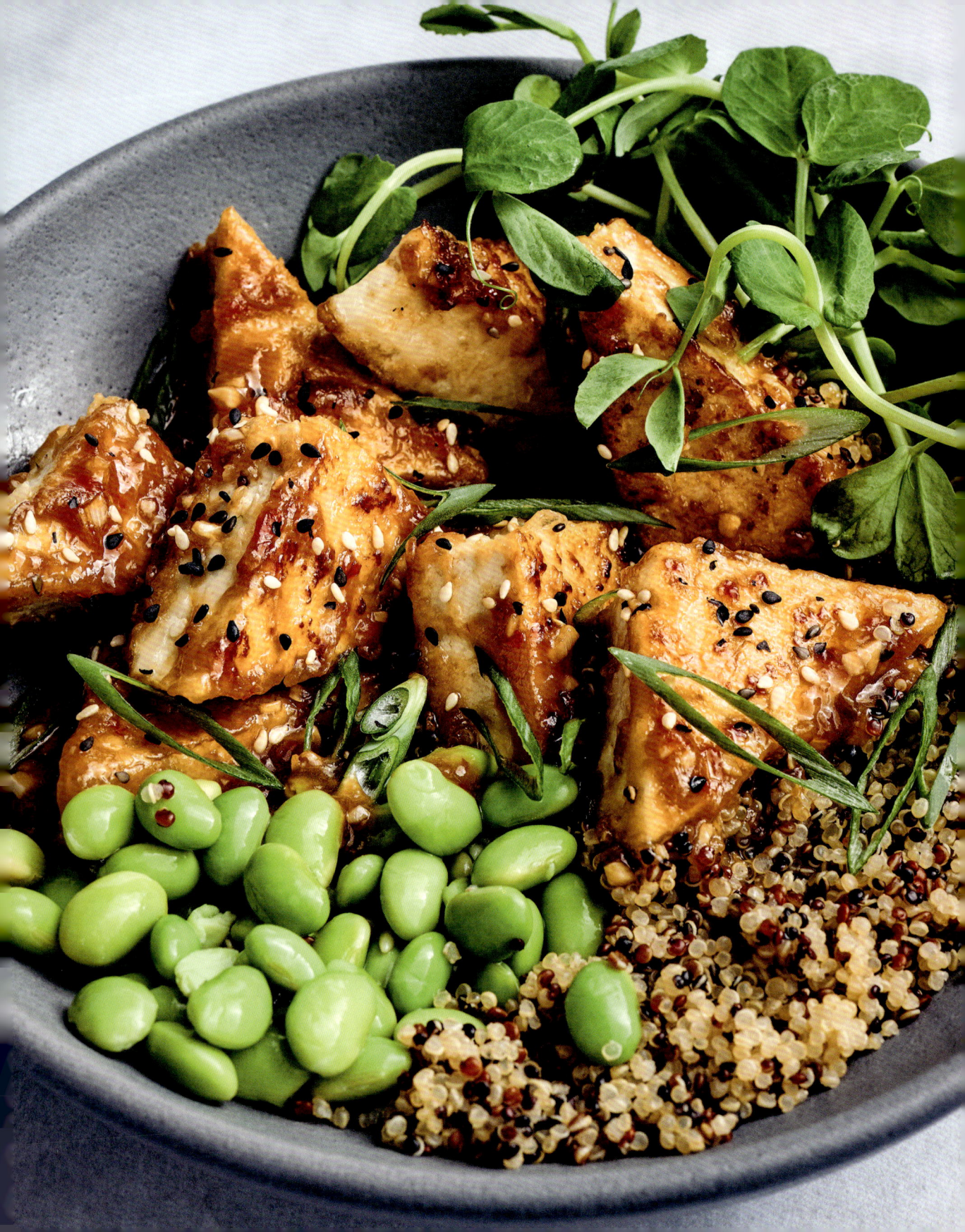

STICKY GLAZED TOFU QUINOA BOWLS

The savory-sweet glaze transforms simple tofu into a crispy, flavorful dish with a chewy, sticky exterior and a tender, juicy interior. Extra-firm tofu works best for glazing, as it holds its shape and absorbs flavors more effectively than softer varieties. Pressing the tofu for 15 to 20 minutes before cooking removes excess moisture, ensuring it crisps up perfectly. For extra protein, I serve it over quinoa, but this can also be served over rice.

In a small pot, bring ⅔ cup water to a boil. Add the quinoa, reduce the heat to low, cover, and cook until the liquid is absorbed and the quinoa is fluffy, 15 to 18 minutes.

While the quinoa cooks, drain and press the tofu with either a tofu press or in between a clean kitchen towel with something heavy on top to remove the excess water, 15 to 20 minutes. Cut the tofu in half horizontally to make 2 thinner blocks and cut into 8 triangles total.

In a small bowl, combine the soy sauce, 1 teaspoon of the sesame oil, the vinegar, garlic, ginger, and sambal. Add 1 tablespoon of the cornstarch and ¼ cup water and stir or whisk to combine. Place the remaining 3 tablespoons cornstarch on a small plate and coat the tofu triangles on both sides.

Set out two bowls for serving (because the tofu cooks fast). Divide the quinoa between the two bowls (about ⅔ cup each) and top with edamame.

In a nonstick medium skillet, heat the remaining 1 tablespoon sesame oil over medium-high heat. Add the tofu in a single layer, making sure the pieces don't touch. Pan-fry until golden and crispy, 4 to 5 minutes on each side.

Once the tofu is crisp, pour the marinade into the pan and quickly flip all the tofu pieces so they are coated on both sides. Remove from the heat.

Divide the tofu between the two bowls of quinoa along with any sauce still in the pan. Garnish with the sesame seeds, scallion, and microgreens and serve.

Per Serving (1 bowl) | Calories 526 | **Protein 30 g** | Carbohydrate 51 g | Fiber 7.5 g | Sugars 7 g | Fat 23 g | Saturated Fat 3 g | Cholesterol 0 mg | Sodium 1,134 mg

SERVES 2

⅓ cup uncooked quinoa (red or tri-color), rinsed

1 (14-ounce) package extra-firm tofu

3 tablespoons reduced-sodium soy sauce or gluten-free tamari

1 tablespoon plus 1 teaspoon toasted sesame oil

1 tablespoon seasoned rice vinegar

2 garlic cloves, minced

1 teaspoon grated fresh ginger or ginger paste

1½ teaspoons sambal oelek

4 tablespoons cornstarch

¼ cup frozen shelled edamame, thawed

1 teaspoon sesame seeds, for garnish

1 scallion, chopped, for garnish

½ cup microgreens or pea shoots, for garnish

LENTIL CHILI

The beauty of this dish lies in its simplicity—just one pot, a few basic ingredients, and a blend of spices that turn ordinary lentils into a flavor-packed chili. Here I used a poblano pepper and yellow squash, but jalapeños could also be used for more kick, and you can play around with different vegetables, like zucchini, carrots, or eggplant. It's a perfect weeknight dinner that only gets better as leftovers for lunch, and it freezes beautifully for make-ahead meals, too. Bonus: It's also a high-fiber meal that's loaded with nutrients. I had to get creative to get this to 30 grams of protein, but it turns out that crushing up some Quest protein chips on top really makes the dish!

Heat a large pot over medium-low heat and add the oil. Once hot, add the onion and poblano pepper and cook until softened, about 5 minutes. Add the garlic and cook until fragrant, 1 minute more.

Add the yellow squash, diced tomatoes, lentils, vegetable broth, 1½ cups water, the chili powder, onion powder, salt, cumin, garlic powder, and smoked paprika. Bring to a boil over high heat. Reduce the heat to medium-low and cook, stirring occasionally, until the lentils are tender, 40 to 50 minutes.

To serve: Pour into bowls and top each with 2 tablespoons yogurt, 2 tablespoons cheddar, 2 tablespoons red onion, and some cilantro. Crush the tortilla chips on top and enjoy.

TO FREEZE: Divide into 6 freezer-safe meal-prep containers. Freeze for up to 3 months. To reheat, transfer to the refrigerator overnight to thaw or reheat from frozen in 30-second intervals until heated through.

Perfect Pairings
Top this with whatever you like on your chili, such as sliced avocado, scallions, or chopped tomatoes.

Per Serving (1½ cups) | Calories 503 | **Protein 35 g** | Carbohydrate 67 g | Fiber 12 g | Sugars 12 g | Fat 13 g | Saturated Fat 4.5 g | Cholesterol 21 mg | Sodium 1,035 mg

SERVES 6

1½ tablespoons extra-virgin olive oil

1 medium yellow onion, diced (about 1 cup)

1 poblano pepper, seeded and diced

3 garlic cloves, chopped

2 small yellow squash (10 ounces total), chopped

1 (10-ounce) can diced tomatoes and green chilies (I like Rotel)

1 pound uncooked green lentils

1 (32-ounce) carton low-sodium vegetable broth*

2 tablespoons chili powder

2 teaspoons onion powder

2 teaspoons kosher salt

1 teaspoon ground cumin

½ teaspoon garlic powder

½ teaspoon smoked paprika

FOR SERVING

¾ cup whole-milk yogurt or nondairy yogurt

¾ cup shredded cheddar cheese or vegan cheddar, such as Violife

1 small red onion, diced

Chopped fresh cilantro

3 (1.1-ounce) bags Quest Loaded Taco Tortilla-Style Protein Chips

*Read the label to be sure this product is gluten-free.

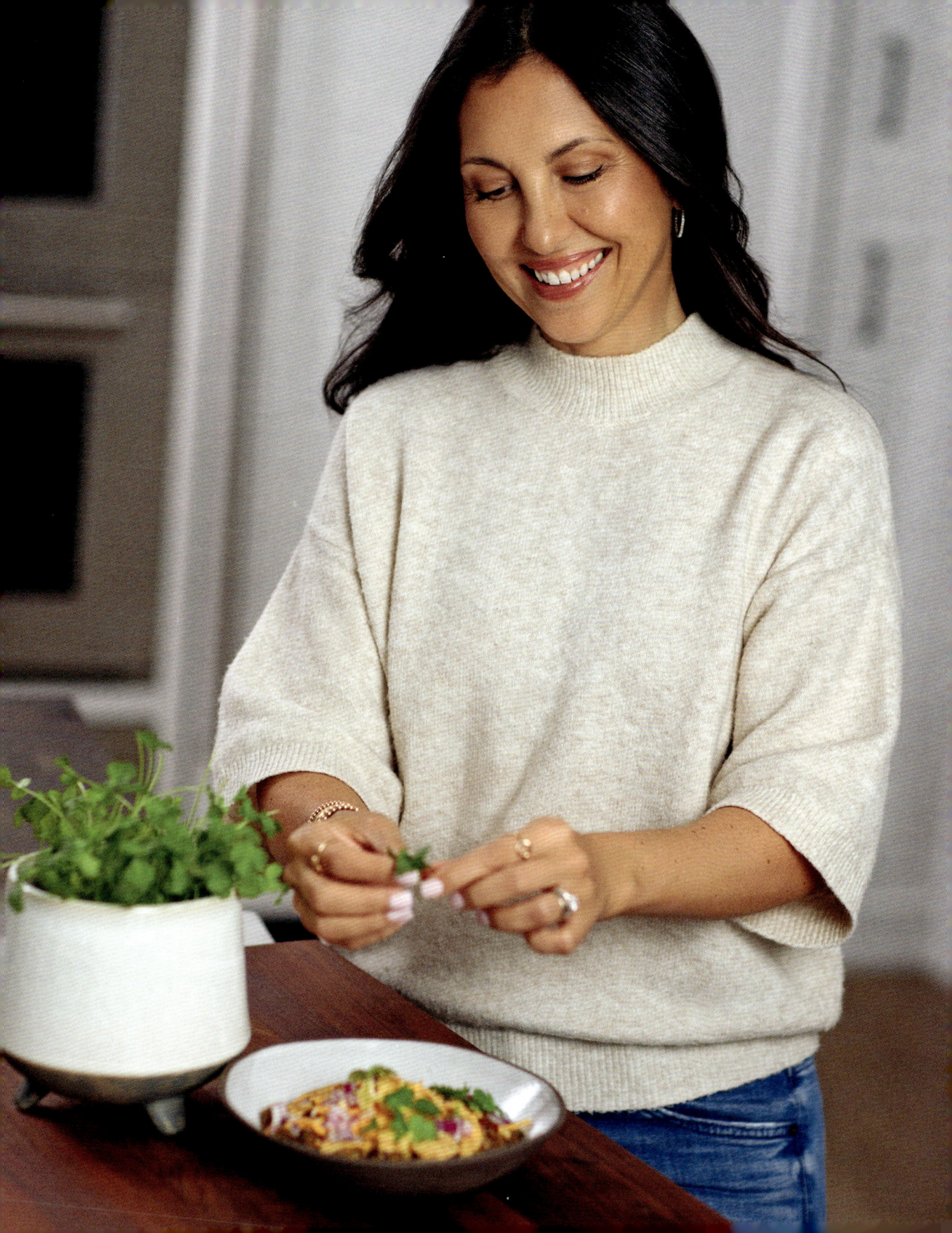

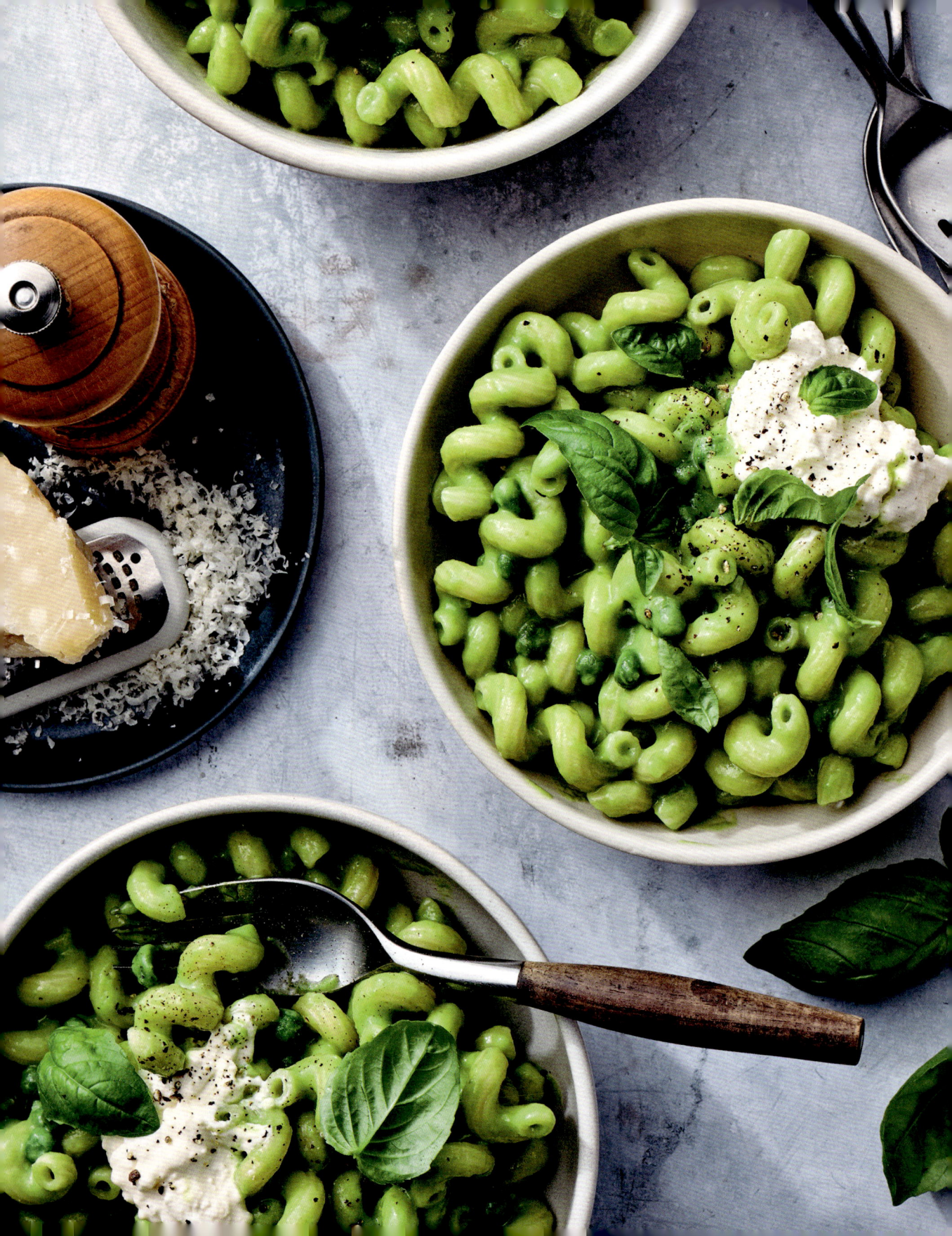

CREAMY PARMESAN & PEAS PASTA

I really hated peas growing up, but over time I've learned to love them—especially when they're pureed into a creamy and flavorful sauce. This dish takes the simplicity of sweet peas and pasta to the next level with a velvety Parmesan sauce that's pure comfort in a bowl. It's quick to make and it will give you a protein boost to keep you full and satisfied. My aunt absolutely loves this dish, and it's become one of her favorites.

Bring a large pot of generously salted water to boil over high heat. Add the pasta and cook to al dente according to the package directions. Reserving 1 cup of the pasta water, drain the pasta.

Meanwhile, in a large deep nonstick skillet, heat the olive oil over medium heat. Add the shallot and gently sauté, stirring often, until soft, 5 to 6 minutes.

Toss in the peas with a splash of hot pasta water and season with ¼ teaspoon kosher salt. Cook, stirring occasionally, until soft, about 5 minutes.

Remove three-quarters of the cooked peas with a slotted spoon (leaving the rest in the pan) and place in a blender with ½ cup of the pasta water. Puree until smooth.

In a small bowl, whisk together the eggs and Parmesan.

Pour the blended peas into the skillet and add the drained pasta. Stir to combine and cook over medium heat until warmed through, 1 to 2 minutes. Remove from the heat and add the egg/cheese mixture. Mix well to create a smooth and creamy sauce.

Divide the pasta among four large pasta bowls. Top with a dollop of ricotta and garnish with basil, black pepper to taste, and more grated Parmesan cheese, if desired.

SERVES 4

Kosher salt

12 ounces high-protein short pasta, such as bow ties or cavatappi, or whole wheat or gluten-free pasta

1 tablespoon extra-virgin olive oil

1 large shallot, finely chopped

12 ounces fresh or frozen petit peas

2 large eggs

2½ ounces good-quality Parmesan cheese, grated, plus more (optional) for serving

¼ cup part-skim ricotta cheese, for serving

Fresh basil, for garnish

Freshly ground black pepper

Per Serving (2 generous cups) | Calories 521 | **Protein 32 g** | Carbohydrate 75 g | Fiber 11 g | Sugars 9 g | Fat 13 g | Saturated Fat 5 g | Cholesterol 110 mg | Sodium 616 mg

TOMATO-SCALLION LENTIL BOWLS
with Jammy Eggs

Making jammy eggs is a life skill everyone needs to know! They have runny, jam-like yolk centers with perfectly set egg whites. Serving them over steamed lentils with hogao, a Colombian sofrito made with tomatoes and scallions, is one of my favorite ways to eat them since I'm always trying to get more fiber in my diet. This delicious dish is simple, hearty, and loaded with protein and fiber. And for me, a meal becomes complete when you put an egg on it!

In a medium skillet, heat the oil over medium-low heat. Add the tomatoes, scallions, garlic, and cumin and cook gently, stirring, until softened, 6 to 8 minutes. Reduce the heat to low, add the salt, and cook, stirring, until the tomatoes have broken down slightly and become saucy, about 3 more minutes. Add the lentils and cook until heated through, about 1 minute. If needed, add a few tablespoons of water or broth to loosen if dry.

Meanwhile, set up a bowl of ice and water and have near the stove. Bring a medium saucepan of water to a boil over medium-high heat. Using a slotted spoon, carefully lower the eggs into the water one at a time. Cook for 6 minutes, adjusting the heat to maintain a gentle boil. Transfer the cooked eggs to the ice bath and chill until just slightly warm, about 2 minutes.

Gently crack the eggs all over, peel, and rinse under warm water to remove any stubborn bits of shell.

Divide the lentils between two shallow bowls. Cut each egg in half and divide among the bowls along with the avocado and some cilantro. Season with a pinch of salt and pepper. Top with hot sauce, if you like it spicy, and enjoy!

TIP: Many brands offer precooked lentils such as Melissa's, Trader Joe's, or Nature's Promise, to name a few. Some come seasoned; others you will need to add your own seasonings to, so adjust to your taste.

SERVES 2

1½ teaspoons extra-virgin olive oil

1 cup diced tomato (2 medium tomatoes)

½ cup chopped scallions

2 garlic cloves, minced

¾ teaspoon ground cumin

¼ teaspoon kosher salt, plus more to taste

2 cups cooked lentils, canned or from 2 (5.3-ounce) packets

4 large eggs

2 ounces sliced avocado (about ½ small Hass)

Chopped fresh cilantro, for garnish

Freshly ground black pepper

Hot sauce (optional)

Per Serving (1 bowl) | Calories 470 | **Protein 32 g** | Carbohydrate 48 g | Fiber 19 g | Sugars 7 g | Fat 18 g | Saturated Fat 4.5 g | Cholesterol 372 mg | Sodium 775 mg

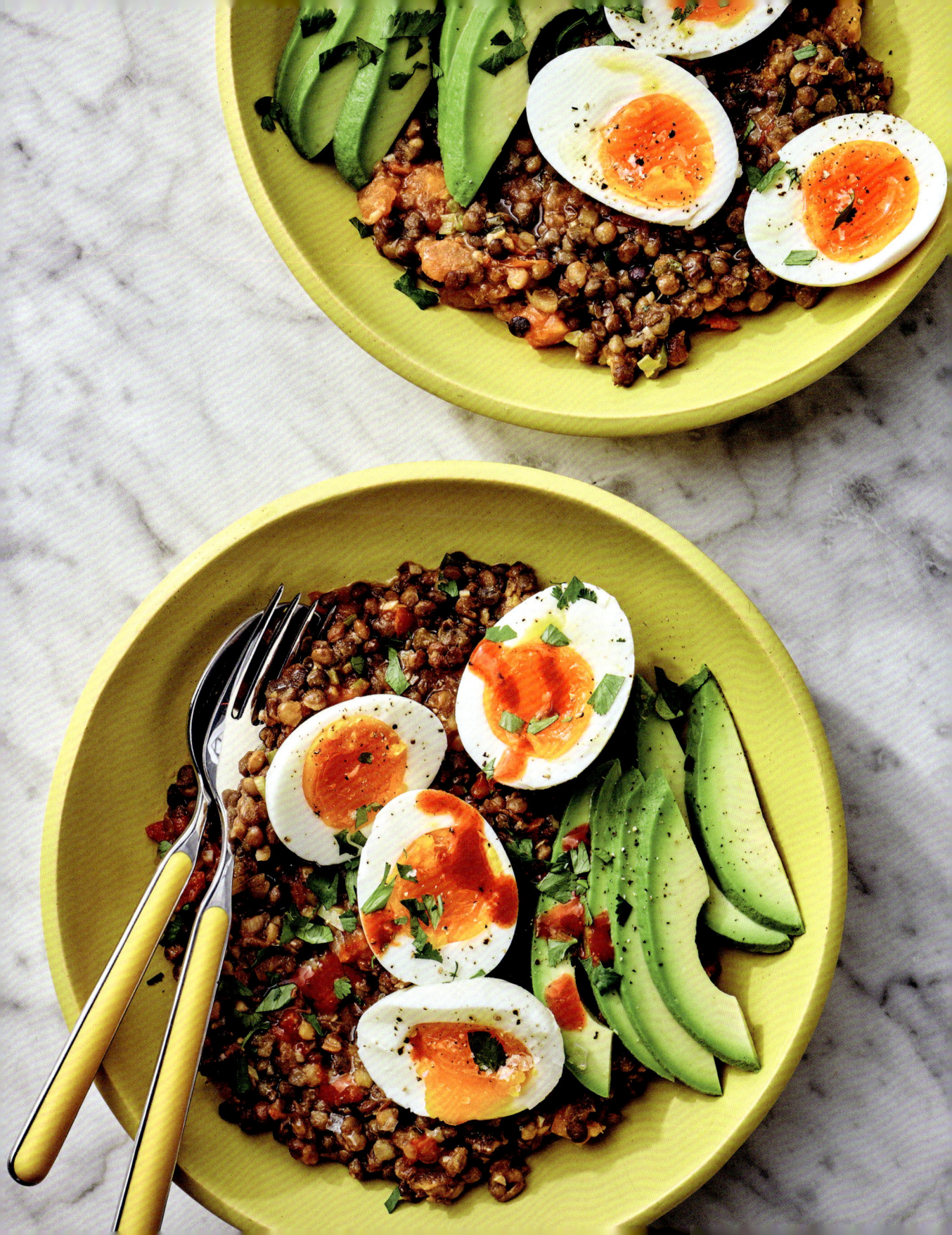

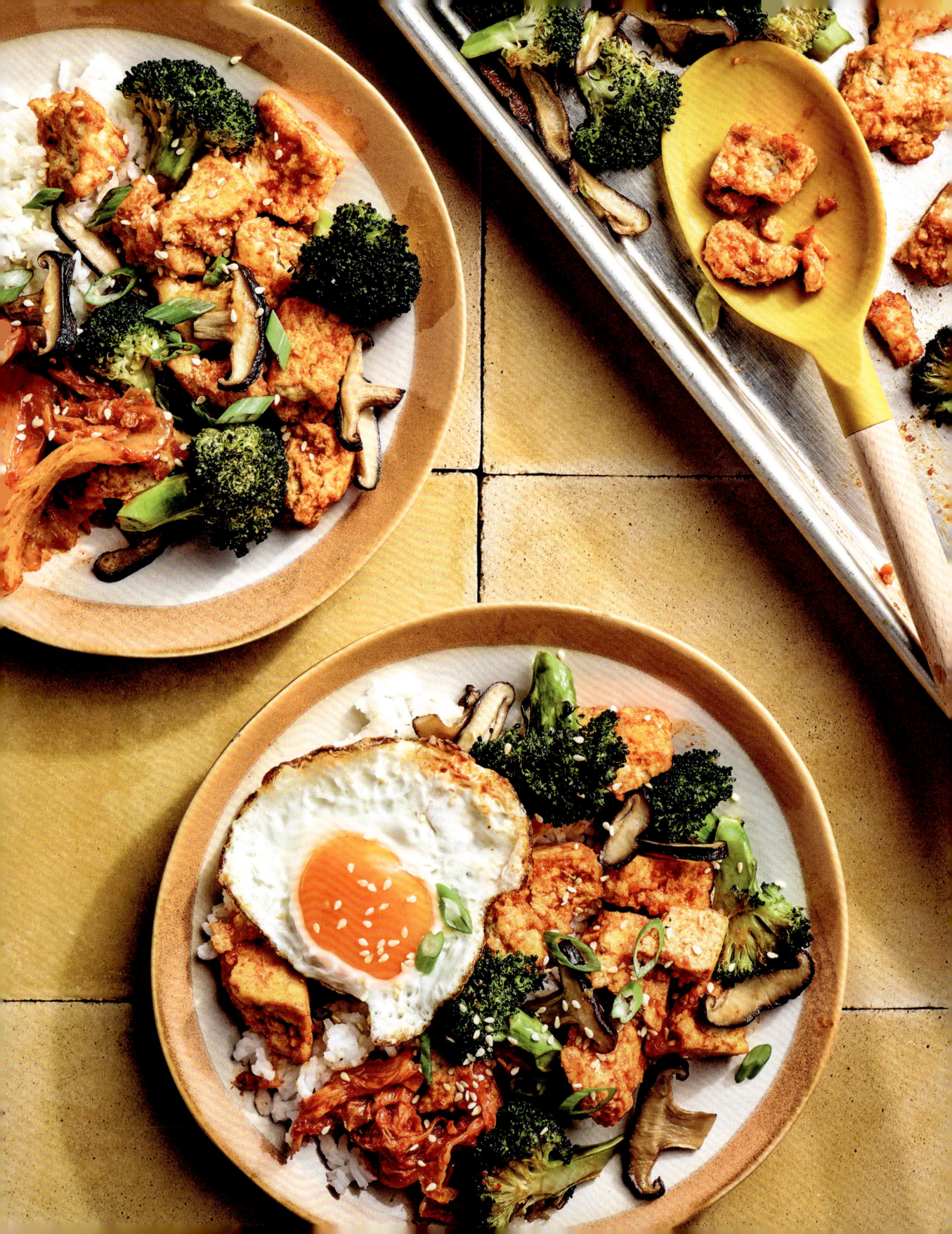

SHEET PAN GOCHUJANG TOFU with Vegetables

I love making this Korean-inspired tofu with gochujang (a sweet and spicy chile paste) and roasting the veggies right alongside the tofu on the same sheet pan. Tearing the tofu by hand into bite-size pieces and baking it with a little oil creates lots of nooks and crevices for the gochujang glaze to coat. The whole meal is ready in just 20 minutes, and it's delicious served over fluffy white rice. For a quick vegetarian bibimbap-inspired variation (a Korean rice bowl), crisp up the rice in a skillet with a little oil and top it with a fried egg!

ROAST THE TOFU AND VEGETABLES: Preheat the oven to 425°F. Spray a sheet pan with oil.

Place the tofu on a clean kitchen towel or paper towels. Cover with another towel and set a heavy object on top to remove as much excess moisture as possible. After pressing for 1 to 2 minutes, break the tofu up with your hands into ½- to 1-inch pieces.

Place the tofu pieces on one side of the oiled sheet pan in an even layer and toss with 1 teaspoon of the sesame oil. Place the broccoli, mushrooms, and scallion whites and light-green parts on the other side of the sheet pan and toss with the salt and the remaining 2 teaspoons sesame oil.

Roast until the tofu is lightly browned and the broccoli and mushrooms are tender, about 20 minutes, flipping the tofu and veggies halfway through.

MEANWHILE, MAKE THE GOCHUJANG GLAZE: In a small bowl, whisk together the gochujang, soy sauce, mirin, sesame oil, ginger, garlic, and agave.

When the tofu is ready, spoon the gochujang glaze over the tofu and toss well to coat, then bake for 2 more minutes to heat through.

TO SERVE: Spoon the rice into two bowls and top with the gochujang tofu and vegetables. Garnish with the scallion greens and sesame seeds. If desired, add a side of kimchi and top with a fried egg.

Per Serving (¾ cup rice + 2½ cups tofu and veggies) | Calories 574 | **Protein 30 g** | Carbohydrate 67 g | Fiber 6 g | Sugars 12 g | Fat 21 g | Saturated Fat 3 g | Cholesterol 0 mg | Sodium 625 mg

SERVES 2

TOFU AND VEGETABLES

Olive oil spray

1 (15.5-ounce) package extra-firm tofu

3 teaspoons toasted sesame oil

3 cups broccoli florets

4 ounces sliced fresh shiitake mushrooms

2 scallions, sliced, white and green parts kept separate

¼ teaspoon kosher salt

GOCHUJANG GLAZE

1 tablespoon gochujang paste, regular or gluten-free*

2 teaspoons soy sauce or gluten-free tamari

2 teaspoons mirin

1 teaspoon toasted sesame oil

½ teaspoon grated ginger

1 small garlic clove, minced

1 teaspoon agave or honey

FOR SERVING

1½ cups steamed white rice

¼ teaspoon sesame seeds

Kimchi (optional)

Fried eggs (optional)

*Read the label to ensure this product is gluten-free.

LASAGNA ROLL-UPS
with Cottage Cheese

I swapped out the ricotta for cottage cheese in these lasagna roll-ups, and no one in my family even noticed! In fact, my daughter Madison told me she liked them even better than when I use ricotta. I used to turn up my nose whenever someone mentioned using cottage cheese instead of ricotta in lasagna, but cottage cheese has come a long way. Brands like Nancy's and Good Culture taste amazing and they have completely won me over!

Preheat the oven to 350°F.

Bring a large pot of salted water to a boil. Add the noodles and cook to al dente according to the package directions. Drain the pasta. Place a piece of wax paper on the counter and lay out the lasagna noodles so they don't stick together.

Meanwhile, in a large bowl, combine the cottage cheese, Parmesan, parsley, pesto, egg, ¼ teaspoon kosher salt, and black pepper to taste and mix.

Ladle about 1 cup marinara on the bottom of a 9 × 13-inch or large oval baking dish.

Make sure the noodles are dry, then take ⅓ cup of the cheese mixture and spread evenly over the length of a noodle. Roll carefully and place seam side down into the baking dish. Repeat with the remaining noodles, placing one snugly against the next.

Ladle the remaining marinara over the noodles and top each one with 1 tablespoon mozzarella cheese. Cover the baking dish with foil, being careful not to touch the cheese, and transfer to the oven.

Bake until heated through and the cheese melts, about 40 minutes.

Serve hot, garnished with fresh basil or parsley.

SERVES 4

Kosher salt

8 lasagna noodles, wheat or gluten-free

16 ounces 2% cottage cheese, drained (I like Good Culture)

½ cup grated Parmesan cheese

¼ cup chopped fresh parsley

2 tablespoons prepared pesto

1 large egg

Freshly ground black pepper

2 cups marinara, plus more for serving

½ cup shredded part-skim mozzarella cheese (about 2 ounces)

Chopped fresh basil or parsley, for garnish

Perfect Pairings
Since I try to get a cup of vegetables with every meal, I serve this with a green salad and roasted vegetables like broccolini.

Per Serving (2 rolls) | Calories 443 | Protein 31 g | Carbohydrate 51 g | Fiber 3.5 g | Sugars 9 g | Fat 15 g | Saturated Fat 6 g | Cholesterol 79 mg | Sodium 1,045 mg

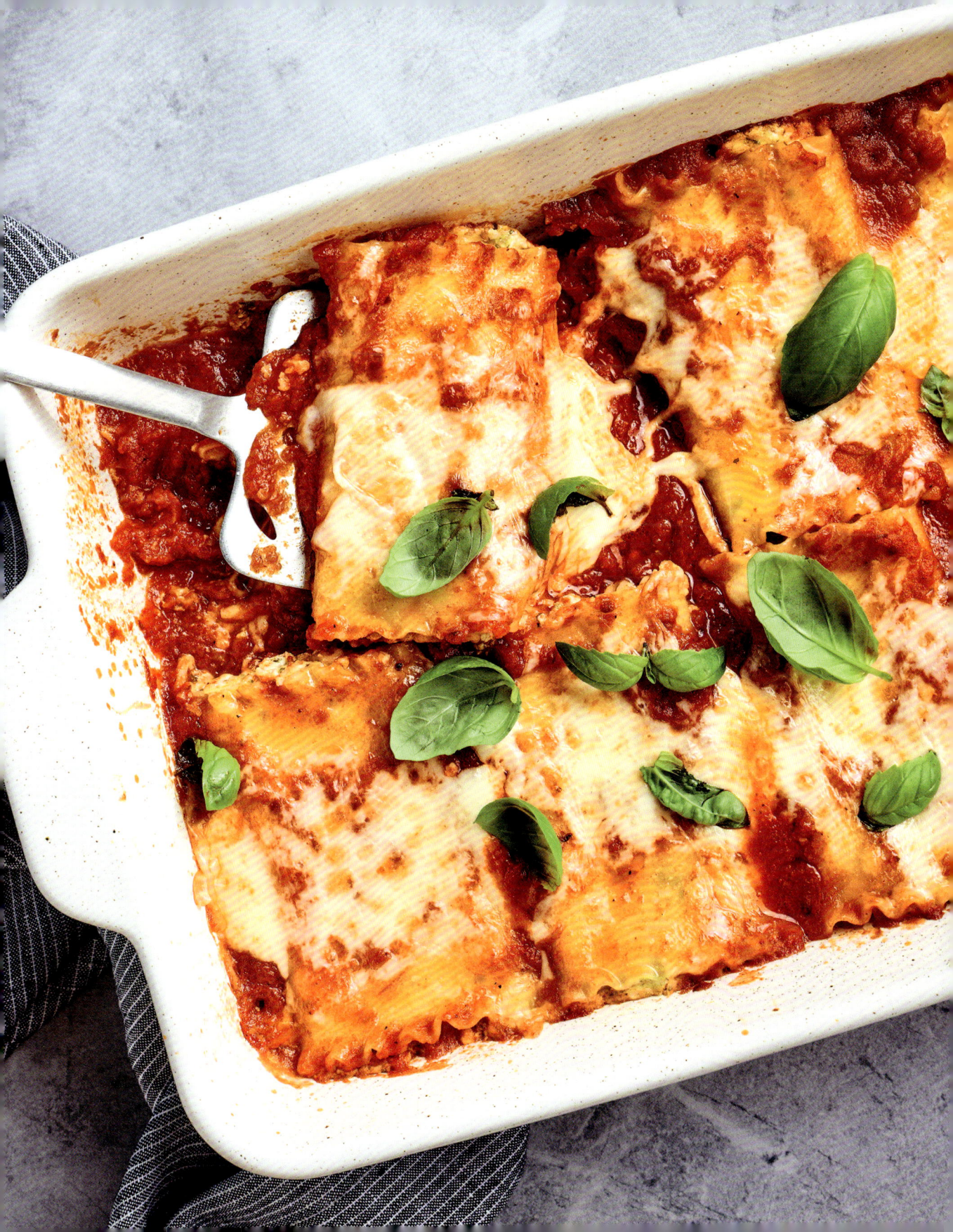

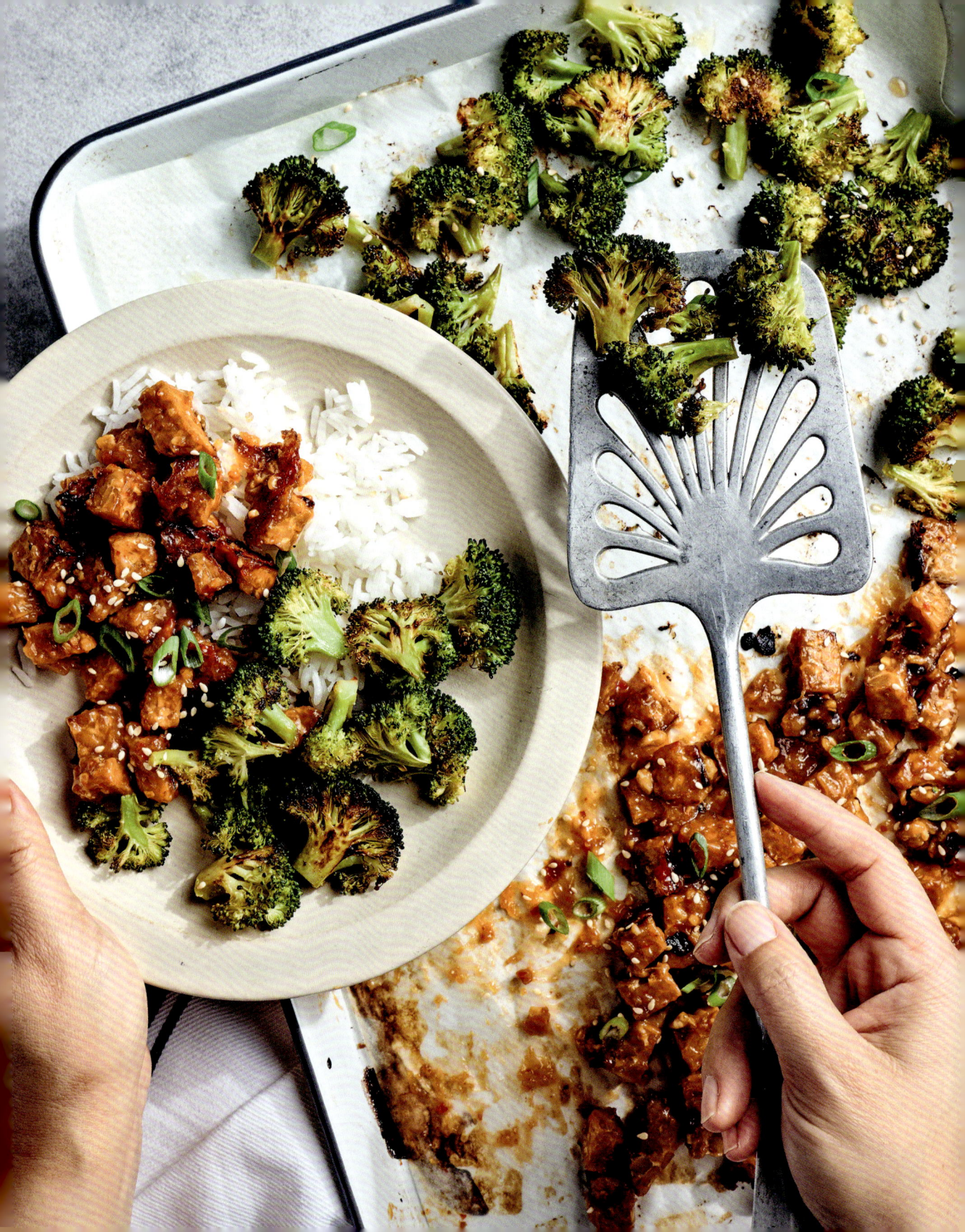

SHEET PAN TEMPEH & BROCCOLI

I've been experimenting with tempeh a lot this year—a plant-based protein made from fermented soybeans. The soybeans are formed into a firm, dense block and has a slightly nutty, earthy flavor with a hearty texture. It's a nutritional powerhouse, and unlike tofu, tempeh retains the whole soybean, which provides more fiber and a meatier consistency. After much trial and error, I personally find that cutting the tempeh into small cubes and marinating it at least 2 hours before roasting really helps the flavor soak in. In this dish, the marinade is spicy and savory, which I thought was great alongside rice, but I can also see myself enjoying this tempeh in summer rolls, salads, and more.

In a small shallow dish, whisk together the soy sauce, 1 tablespoon of the sesame oil, the garlic, ginger, vinegar, sweet chili sauce, Sriracha, cornstarch, and 1 tablespoon water. Add the tempeh and marinate in the fridge for at least 2 hours, tossing halfway through.

When ready to cook, preheat the oven to 400°F. Line a large sheet pan with parchment paper.

Spread the broccoli out on the prepared pan and toss with the remaining ½ tablespoon sesame oil and the salt. Push to one side of the pan. Use a slotted spoon to remove the tempeh, saving the marinade. Place the tempeh on the sheet pan and transfer to the oven.

Roast until the tempeh is golden and the broccoli is tender, about 30 minutes, tossing halfway through.

Meanwhile, stir 2 tablespoons water into the reserved marinade. When the tempeh is ready, pour the reserved marinade into a medium skillet over medium heat. Simmer until the sauce thickens, 30 to 60 seconds. Add the roasted tempeh and toss to coat.

Serve with the broccoli and rice, garnished with sesame seeds and sliced scallions.

SERVES 2

3 tablespoons reduced-sodium soy sauce or gluten-free tamari

1½ tablespoons toasted sesame oil

1 garlic clove, minced

1 teaspoon minced fresh ginger

1 tablespoon seasoned rice vinegar

2 tablespoons Thai sweet chili sauce

1 teaspoon Sriracha sauce

2 tablespoons cornstarch

1 (8-ounce) block tempeh, cut into ¼-inch dice

4 cups chopped broccoli florets

Pinch of kosher salt

1½ cups cooked sticky rice or basmati rice

Sesame seeds, for garnish

Sliced scallions, for garnish

Per Serving (generous ¾ cup tempeh + 1¼ cups broccoli + ¾ cup rice) |
Calories 599 | **Protein 32 g** | Carbohydrate 71 g | Fiber 6.5 g | Sugars 14 g |
Fat 24 g | Saturated Fat 4.5 g | Cholesterol 0 mg | Sodium 1,443 mg

ROASTED AUTUMN VEGGIE FRITTATA

This dinner frittata is a hearty, satisfying meatless meal that's incredibly versatile and ideal for using up leftovers or highlighting fresh, in-season ingredients. Here, butternut squash and cauliflower are roasted directly in the skillet, letting the edges get beautifully charred and caramelized. The eggs are combined with creamy whole-milk Greek yogurt, giving the frittata an irresistibly smooth texture, plus an extra boost of protein.

Preheat the oven to 450°F.

In a large bowl, whisk together the whole eggs, egg whites, Pecorino, ¾ cup of the yogurt, 1 teaspoon kosher salt, and ¼ teaspoon black pepper until incorporated. Set aside.

Set a 12-inch ovenproof skillet over medium-high heat. Add 2 tablespoons of the olive oil and heat until it starts to shimmer. Add the cauliflower and butternut squash, stir to coat in the oil, and let cook undisturbed until it starts to brown, about 4 minutes. Stir in the shallots and ¼ teaspoon salt and cook until everything is browned, about 5 more minutes. Give it one last stir and transfer the pan to the oven.

Roast until the veggies are tender and browned all over, about 10 minutes. Remove the skillet from the oven—carefully, as it will be hot!—and decrease the oven temperature to 300°F.

Measure out 1 cup of the roasted veggies and set aside. Set the skillet with the remaining vegetables over medium-high heat. Pour in the egg mixture and let cook undisturbed until the edges are just beginning to set, 30 seconds to 1 minute. Carefully return the pan to the oven, and bake the frittata until the top-center is just set, 25 to 30 minutes.

In a small bowl, stir the lemon zest and the remaining ½ cup yogurt.

Slice the frittata in 4 pieces. Just before serving, in a medium bowl, toss the arugula with the remaining 1 teaspoon olive oil and a pinch of salt. Top each slice of frittata with the arugula, the reserved roasted veggies, and 2 tablespoons lemony yogurt. Finish with black pepper.

SERVES 4

8 large eggs

¾ cup egg whites

¾ cup freshly grated Pecorino Romano cheese

1¼ cups whole-milk Greek yogurt

Kosher salt and freshly ground black pepper

2 tablespoons plus 1 teaspoon extra-virgin olive oil

1 pound cauliflower florets, chopped in small pieces

1 pound butternut squash, peeled and cut into ½-inch pieces

¾ cup roughly chopped shallots

Grated zest of ½ lemon

3 cups baby arugula

TIP: Swap the butternut squash for any variety of winter squash or even sweet potatoes for a seasonal twist.

Per Serving (1 wedge + 1 cup salad + 2 tablespoons yogurt) | Calories 489 | **Protein 36 g** | Carbohydrate 29 g | Fiber 6.5 g | Sugars 11 g | Fat 27 g | Saturated Fat 10 g | Cholesterol 401 mg | Sodium 943 mg

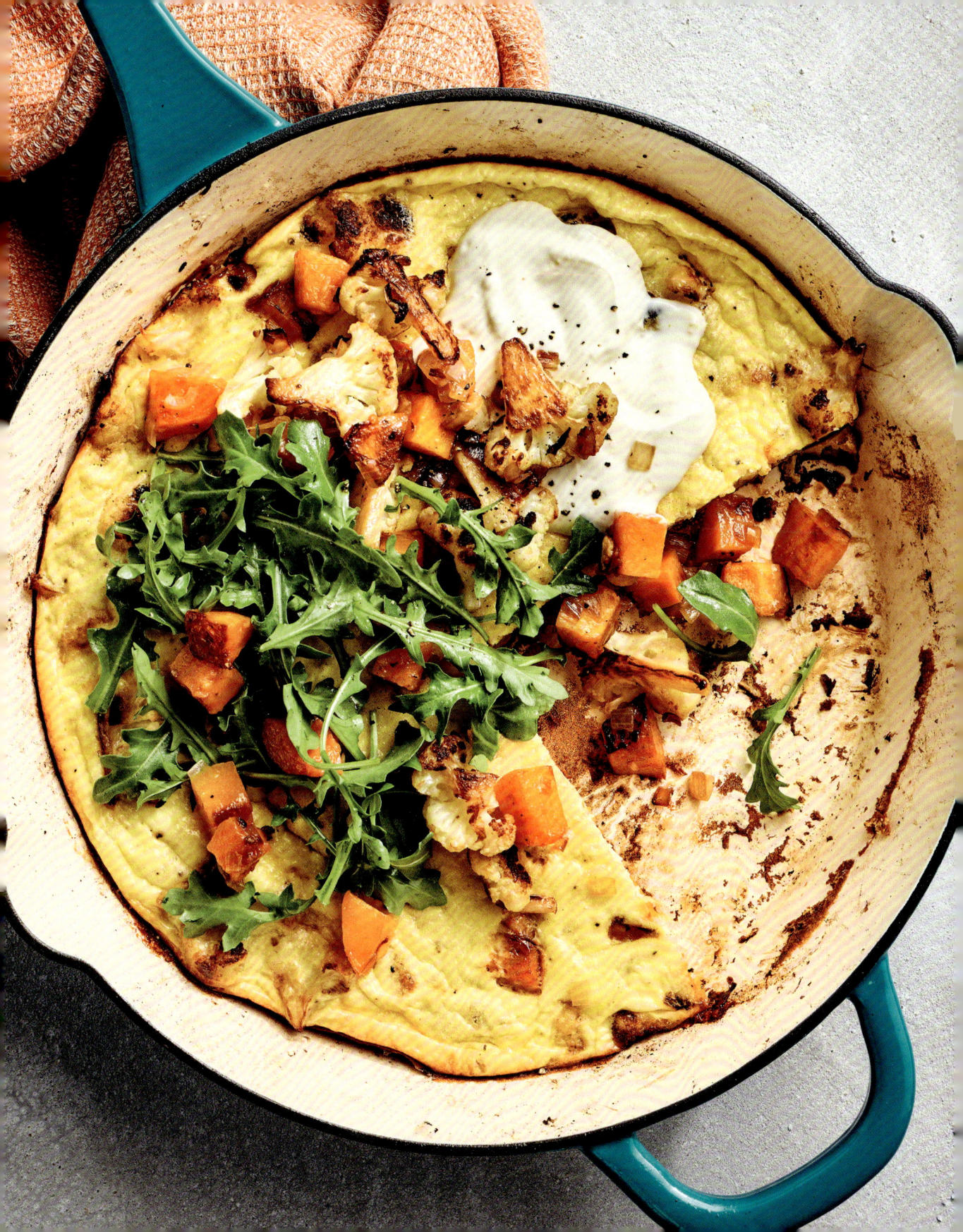

POULTRY
PERFECTION

Crispy, juicy, and incredibly versatile, chicken and turkey dinners are some of the most popular recipes on my website and in my home—and it's no surprise why! Poultry is affordable, naturally high in protein, and easy to cook, making it a go-to for busy weeknights and beyond.

But let's be honest: Chicken made the same way week after week can get a little boring. That's where Poultry Perfection comes in. The recipes in this chapter are packed with fresh ideas and bold flavors—these recipes will inspire you to take poultry to the next level.

In this chapter, you'll find a variety of dishes to suit every mood and craving. From hearty soups like Shortcut Turkey Meatball Minestrone (page 169) and one-pot meals like Sheet Pan Soy-Glazed Meatloaf & Veggies (page 149), to quick air-fryer meals like Air Fryer Chicken Schnitzel with Cabbage-Kale Slaw (page 154), to satisfying bowls like Air Fryer Chicken Satay Bowls with Spicy Peanut Sauce & Mango Slaw (page 166) and more, these recipes show just how versatile and exciting poultry can be. Whether you're cooking for the family, meal-prepping for the week, or just trying something new, these dishes are here to keep things easy, delicious, and anything but boring!

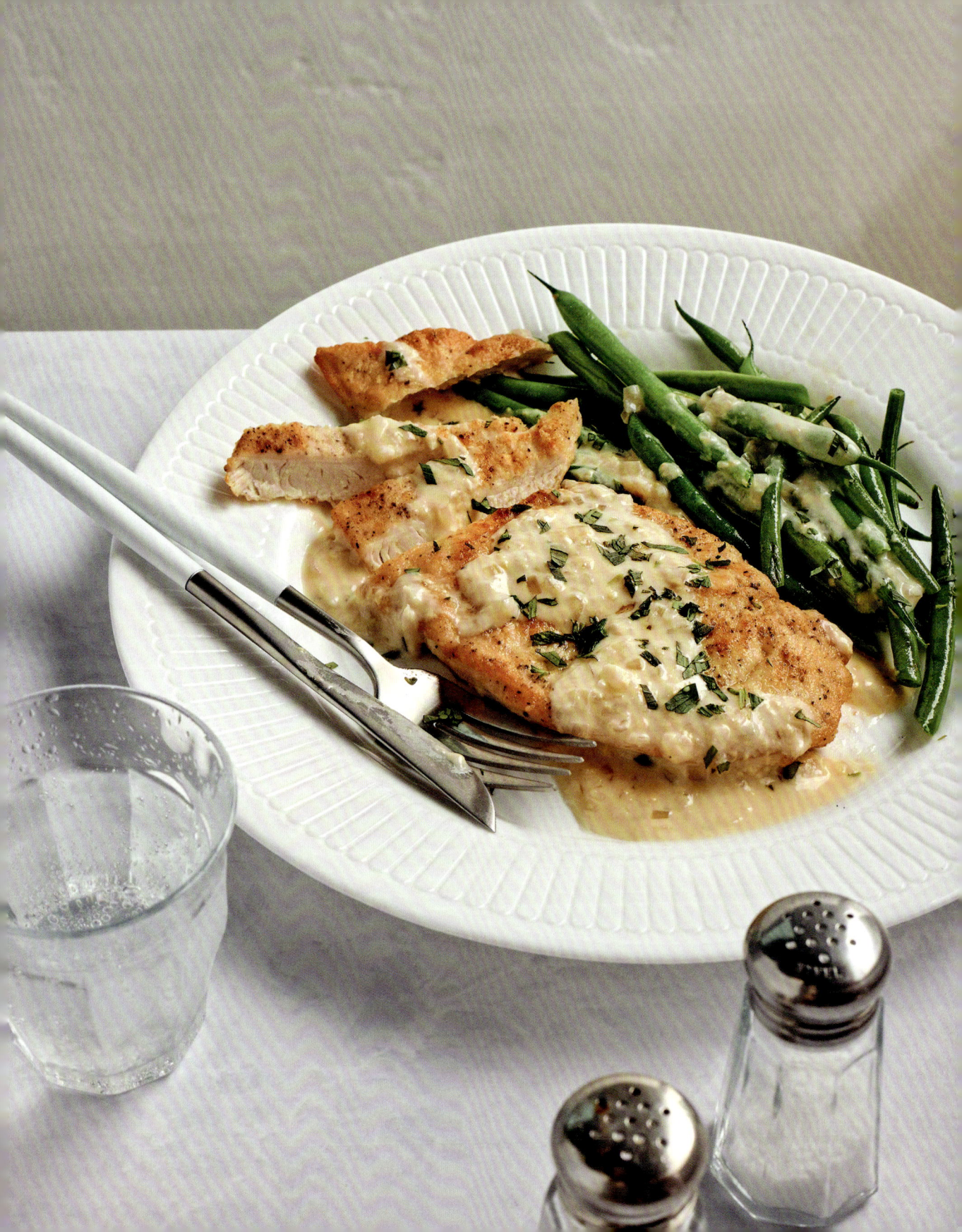

CREAMY MUSTARD CHICKEN

This simple and flavorful chicken dish is a real winner in my home! The creamy mustard sauce takes just a few minutes to make, and it transforms boring chicken breasts into something incredibly delicious. This recipe will come to the rescue on nights when you're staring at a package of chicken breasts and feeling totally uninspired.

In a large skillet, heat ½ teaspoon of the olive oil over medium-high heat. Add the green beans and toss to coat. Cover the pan and cook until crisp-tender, 2 to 4 minutes. Transfer to a plate and reserve the skillet.

Between two pieces of plastic wrap, pound the halved chicken breasts to an even thickness (about ½ inch). Season all over with the salt and pepper. Place the flour in a shallow bowl. Dredge each piece of chicken in the flour and shake off any excess. Set aside on a plate.

In the reserved skillet, heat 1 tablespoon of the olive oil over medium-high heat. Add the chicken and cook, flipping halfway, until cooked through and golden brown, 4 to 5 minutes per side. Remove and set aside.

Reduce the heat to medium and add the remaining 1 teaspoon olive oil. Add the minced shallot and garlic and sauté until the shallot is translucent, 1 to 2 minutes.

Add the wine and scrape up any browned bits from the bottom of the pan. When the wine has reduced by about half, add the chicken bone broth, cream cheese, and half-and-half. Use a whisk to mix until the cream cheese is fully melted and the sauce is smooth.

Whisk in the Dijon mustard and tarragon, then increase the heat slightly to bring to a simmer. Nestle the cooked chicken and green beans into the sauce and simmer for a few minutes to heat through.

Serve immediately, sprinkled with some chopped tarragon.

SERVES 4

1 tablespoon plus 1½ teaspoons extra-virgin olive oil

8 ounces haricots verts or green beans, trimmed

2 boneless, skinless chicken breasts (8 ounces each), halved horizontally to make 4 thin cutlets total

1 teaspoon kosher salt

¼ teaspoon freshly ground black pepper

¼ cup all-purpose flour or gluten-free flour

1 shallot, minced

2 garlic cloves, minced

½ cup low-calorie dry white wine, such as Kim Crawford Illuminate Sauvignon Blanc, a 70-calorie wine

1 cup chicken bone broth*

3 tablespoons (1½ ounces) ⅓-less-fat cream cheese (I like Philadelphia)

3 tablespoons half-and-half

2 tablespoons Dijon mustard

2 teaspoons minced fresh tarragon, plus more for serving

*Read the label to be sure this product is gluten-free.

Per Serving (1 piece chicken with sauce + 2 ounces green beans) | Calories 325 | **Protein 31 g** | Carbohydrate 14 g | Fiber 2.5 g | Sugars 2 g | Fat 13 g | Saturated Fat 3.5 g | Cholesterol 94 mg | Sodium 666 mg

ONE-POT FIESTA CHICKEN & RICE

Craving a hearty and flavorful meal that's easy on prep and cleanup? This recipe has you covered! It's a perfect weeknight meal—it's quick to prepare, high in fiber, requires minimal cleanup, AND it's guaranteed to satisfy everyone at my table. Plus, it's easily customizable. Don't like corn? Swap it for diced tomatoes or green chiles. Love cheese? Top it with Monterey Jack for a gooey, delicious finish. In my house, we love it with hot sauce and some avocado on the side.

In a medium bowl, combine the chicken, ½ teaspoon of the salt, half of the minced garlic, the paprika, onion powder, garlic powder, cumin, and pepper and toss to coat.

Spray a large skillet with a tight-fitting lid with oil and place over medium-high heat. When hot, add the chicken and sear until browned on both sides, 1 to 2 minutes per side. Transfer the chicken to a plate.

Reduce the heat to low and add the 1 teaspoon oil. Add the remaining minced garlic and cook until fragrant, about 30 seconds. Add the rice, then return the chicken and any of its juices to the pan along with the corn, black beans, 2 cups water, and 1½ teaspoons salt. Stir to combine. Bring to a boil and let it simmer on medium-high heat until the liquid is absorbed and just skimming the top of the rice, 6 to 8 minutes.

Cover, reduce the heat to low, and cook for 15 minutes, undisturbed. Remove the pan from the heat and, without lifting the lid, let it finish steaming, 5 more minutes.

Uncover and fold in the cilantro and lime juice. Serve right away and top with hot sauce, if desired.

SERVES 4

1¼ pounds boneless, skinless chicken thighs, cut into ½-inch pieces

2 teaspoons kosher salt

6 garlic cloves, minced

1 teaspoon sweet paprika

½ teaspoon onion powder

½ teaspoon garlic powder

¼ teaspoon ground cumin

¼ teaspoon freshly ground black pepper

Olive oil spray

1 teaspoon extra-virgin olive oil

1¼ cups uncooked long-grain white rice, rinsed

½ cup frozen corn kernels

½ cup canned black beans,* rinsed and drained

¼ cup finely chopped fresh cilantro

Juice of 1 lime

Hot sauce (optional), for serving

*Read the label to be sure this product is gluten-free.

Per Serving (1¾ cups) | Calories 449 | **Protein 35 g** | Carbohydrate 58 g | Fiber 4 g | Sugars 1 g | Fat 8 g | Saturated Fat 2 g | Cholesterol 133 mg | Sodium 796 mg

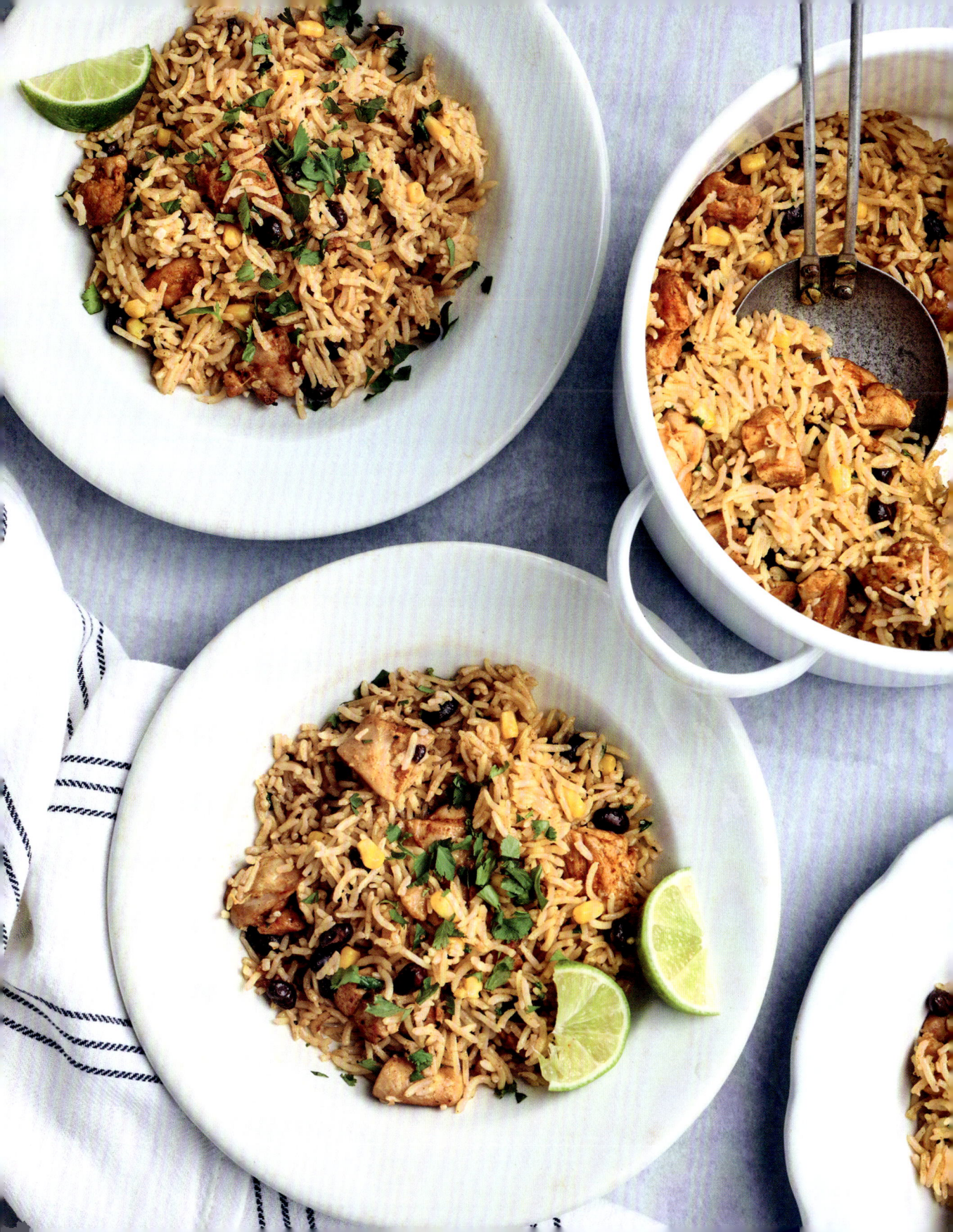

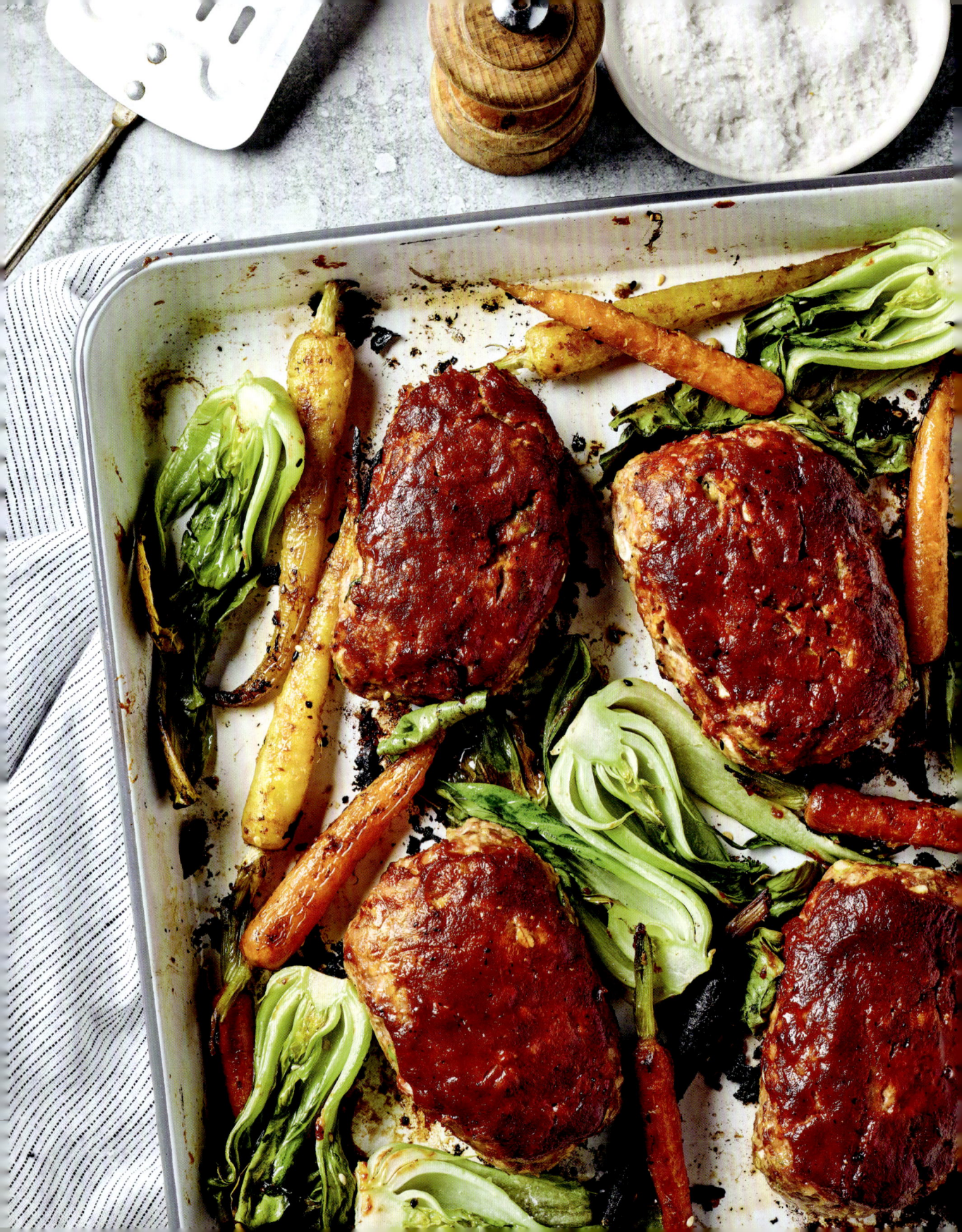

SHEET PAN SOY-GLAZED MEATLOAF & VEGGIES

Forget the typical ketchup glaze for your meatloaf—this soy-glazed turkey version bursts with sweet, savory, and warm gingery flavors. I love ginger, so for me the more the better, but if you're not a fan, feel free to reduce the amount. Individual-size loaves (they cook quicker than one large loaf) are baked alongside some delicious Asian-inspired veggies. One pan with minimal cleanup—it's a perfect one-and-done recipe for those busy weeknights.

Preheat the oven to 425°F. Line a sheet pan with parchment paper.

In a small bowl, combine the soy sauce, tomato paste, honey, sesame oil, and pepper. Set the soy glaze aside.

MAKE THE MEATLOAVES: In a large bowl, combine the garlic, ginger, scallion, egg, oats, and salt and mix to a paste with a fork. Add the turkey and mix thoroughly.

Divide the turkey mixture into 4 equal portions. Shape each portion into a 4½ × 2½–inch loaf and place on the prepared sheet pan, leaving room for the vegetables. Spoon the soy glaze on top of the loaves and spread to coat.

PREPARE THE VEGETABLES: In a medium bowl, combine the carrots with a spritz of olive oil spray, the ginger, sesame seeds, and ⅛ teaspoon of the salt. Add the carrots to the sheet pan around the loaves, spreading them out in a single layer, and reserve the bowl.

Transfer the sheet pan to the oven and roast for 12 minutes.

While the meatloaves and carrots bake, wet the bok choy in the sink and place in the reserved bowl. Add the sesame oil and remaining ⅛ teaspoon salt and toss to coat.

Remove the sheet pan from the oven. Flip the carrots over and add the bok choy around the loaves with the carrots. Return to the oven.

Bake until the vegetables are tender and the meatloaves are cooked through, an additional 15 minutes. Serve immediately.

Per Serving (1 small loaf + 1 cup veggies) | Calories 368 | **Protein 33 g** | Carbohydrate 25 g | Fiber 5 g | Sugars 11 g | Fat 17 g | Saturated Fat 4 g | Cholesterol 151 mg | Sodium 865 mg

SERVES 4

2 tablespoons reduced-sodium soy sauce or gluten-free tamari

2 tablespoons tomato paste

1 tablespoon honey

1 teaspoon toasted sesame oil

¼ teaspoon black pepper

TURKEY MEATLOAVES

3 garlic cloves, finely chopped

1 tablespoon grated ginger

¼ cup finely chopped scallion

1 large egg

½ cup quick-cooking oats*

1 teaspoon kosher salt

1¼ pounds ground turkey (93% lean)

VEGETABLES

10 ounces small heirloom rainbow carrots, trimmed, halved lengthwise if thick

Olive oil spray

1½ teaspoons grated ginger

½ teaspoon black and white sesame seeds

¼ teaspoon kosher salt

4 baby bok choy, halved

1 teaspoon toasted sesame oil

*Read the label to be sure this product is gluten-free.

MARRY ME CHICKEN & GNOCCHI

The Skinnytaste fan-favorite recipe "Marry Me Chicken" is made even better with the addition of tender gnocchi. This popular dish features chicken cooked in a creamy sauce with sun-dried tomatoes, garlic, Parmesan, and herbs and is said to be so impressive that it could inspire a marriage proposal! The gnocchi pairs really well with the creamy sauce (it makes Tommy want to marry me twice), taking this dish to yet another level. It's not only the way to my husband's heart, it's also family-friendly and a real crowd-pleaser.

Bring a large pot of salted water to a boil over high heat.

Cut the chicken into ½-inch cubes. Season with 1 teaspoon kosher salt and the pepper.

Heat a large skillet over medium-high heat and spray with oil. Add the chicken and cook, flipping halfway, until golden brown and cooked through, about 5 minutes. Remove the chicken from the skillet and set it aside. Reserve the skillet.

Add the gnocchi to the boiling water and cook according to the package directions. Drain well.

Meanwhile, in the same skillet, heat the sun-dried tomato oil over medium-low heat. Add the shallot and garlic and sauté until they become fragrant and translucent, 1 to 2 minutes.

Stir in the tomato paste and cook until heated through, another 1 to 2 minutes.

Add the chopped sun-dried tomatoes and baby spinach to the skillet. Cook until the spinach wilts, 3 to 5 minutes.

Reduce the heat to low and add the cream cheese, chicken broth, half-and-half, and oregano. Stir until the cream cheese is fully melted and the sauce is well combined.

Return the cooked chicken along with the gnocchi to the skillet and let it simmer over low heat in the sauce for a few minutes until heated through. Sprinkle with the Parmesan, if using, and serve.

Per Serving (1⅓ cups) | Calories 392 | **Protein 32 g** | Carbohydrate 26 g | Fiber 3 g | Sugars 3 g | Fat 17 g | Saturated Fat 8 g | Cholesterol 115 mg | Sodium 827 mg

SERVES 4

Kosher salt

16 ounces boneless, skinless chicken breast, preferably organic

¼ teaspoon freshly ground black pepper

Olive oil spray

1 (1-pound) package refrigerated or shelf-stable gnocchi*

1½ teaspoons oil from the sun-dried tomatoes

1 small shallot, minced

2 garlic cloves, minced

1 teaspoon tomato paste

¼ cup oil-packed sun-dried tomatoes, drained and chopped

4 cups packed baby spinach, roughly chopped

3 tablespoons ⅓-less-fat cream cheese (1½ ounces) (I like Philadelphia)

1 cup low-sodium chicken broth*

3 tablespoons half-and-half

¼ teaspoon dried oregano

2 tablespoons freshly grated Parmesan cheese, plus more (optional) for serving

*Read the label to be sure this product is gluten-free.

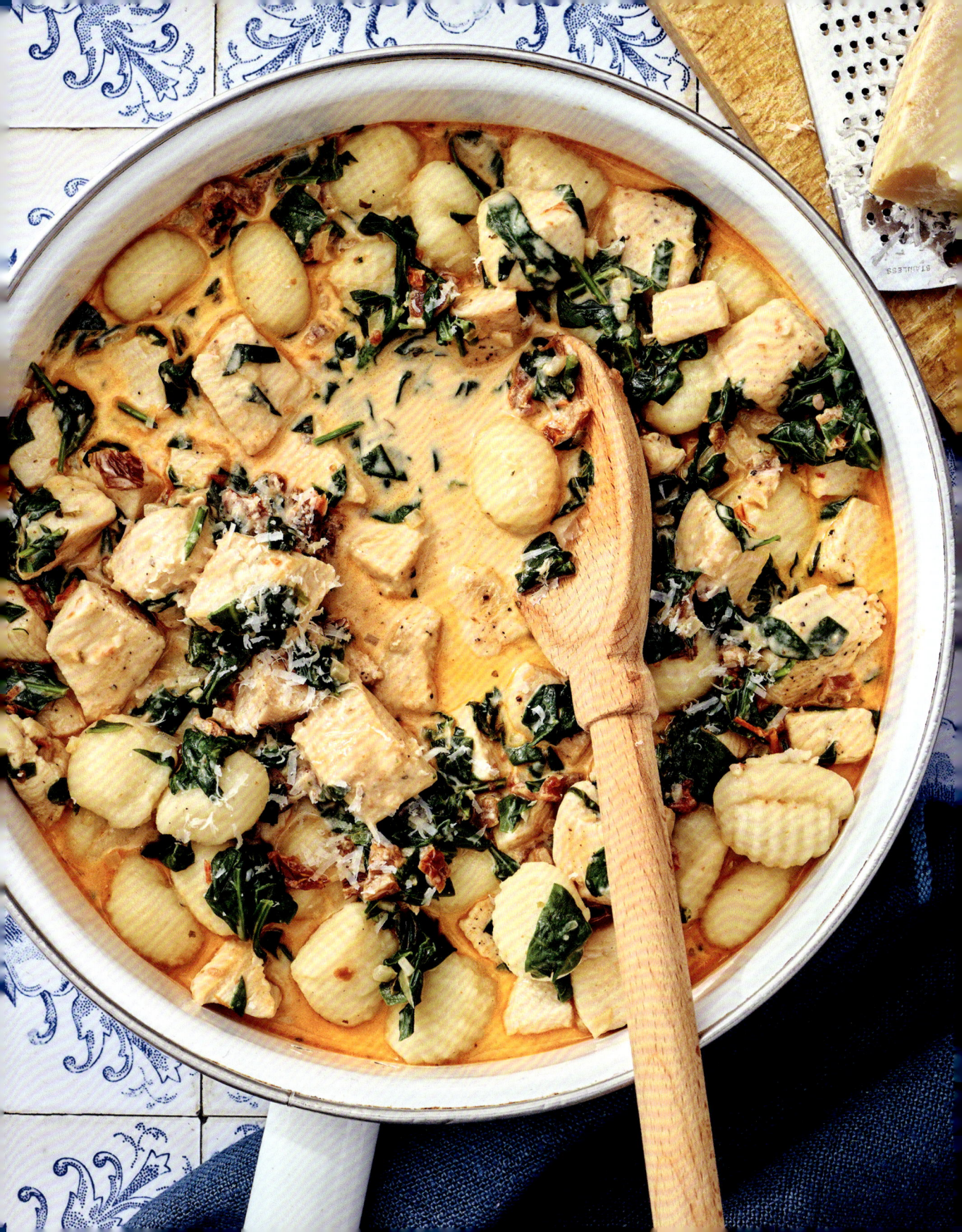

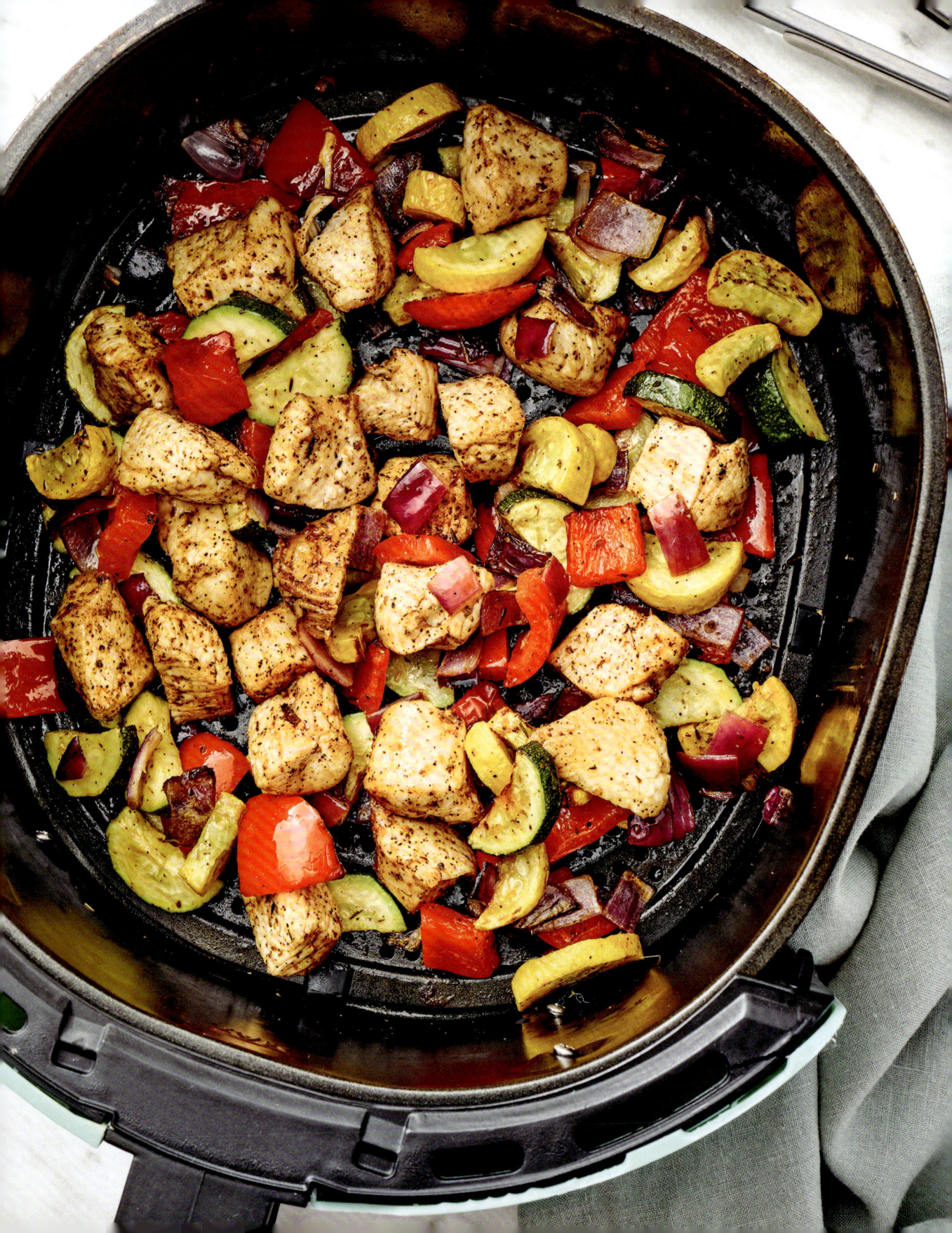

AIR FRYER CAJUN CHICKEN & VEGGIES

I love the simplicity of this low-carb, vegetable-rich dish—it's easy to whip up for a quick dinner and it's also ideal for meal-prepping! The first time I made this, I put the seasoning on the chicken and then had to run an unexpected errand outside the house, so I left it in the fridge a few hours before cooking. Well, it turned out so flavorful that now it's the only way I make it! For best results I highly recommend using organic chicken, since I find that nonorganic chicken breasts have an unpleasant woody texture.

In a large bowl, combine the chicken and Creole seasoning and toss to coat. If you have time, refrigerate for a few hours. If you don't, no worries.

Add the zucchini, yellow squash, bell pepper, onion, garlic, and salt to the bowl with the chicken and toss everything with the olive oil.

Cooking in two batches as needed (for smaller baskets), arrange the chicken and vegetables in the air fryer basket in a single layer and cook at 400°F for 10 minutes, shaking the basket two or three times, until the chicken is browned and the vegetables are tender.

Set aside and repeat with the remaining chicken and veggies.

Once both batches are cooked, return the first batch to the air fryer and cook for 1 minute, until everything is heated through. Serve immediately.

No Air Fryer? No Problem!

Cook this in a large skillet over high heat in two batches for 7 minutes until cooked through.

SERVES 4

1¼ pounds chicken breast, preferably organic, cut into ½-inch pieces

1 tablespoon Cajun or Creole seasoning (I like Zatarain's)*

1 medium zucchini (8 ounces), sliced into ¼-inch-thick half-moons

1 medium yellow squash (8 ounces), sliced into ¼-inch-thick half-moons

1 large red bell pepper, cut into thin 1-inch square pieces

½ medium red onion, cut into ½-inch chunks

3 garlic cloves, minced

¼ teaspoon kosher salt

2 tablespoons extra-virgin olive oil

*Read the label to be sure this product is gluten-free.

Per Serving (1½ cups) | Calories 265 | **Protein 34 g** | Carbohydrate 7 g | Fiber 2 g | Sugars 4 g | Fat 11 g | Saturated Fat 2 g | Cholesterol 104 mg | Sodium 1,042 mg

AIR FRYER CHICKEN SCHNITZEL
with Cabbage-Kale Slaw

Air frying is the absolute best way to get crispy chicken cutlets without all the extra oil that comes from frying. These cutlets are delicious on their own, but topping them with a tangy slaw adds a refreshing crunch that's super tasty! Enjoy this on its own for a light and satisfying lunch or dinner, or serve it with your favorite grain or vegetables.

MAKE THE SALAD: In a large bowl, whisk together the olive oil, vinegar, mustard, salt, and pepper to taste. Add the onion, cabbage, kale, and radishes and toss to combine. Cover and refrigerate while you cook the chicken.

COAT THE CHICKEN: Set up a dredging station in two shallow bowls. In one bowl, beat the eggs with 1 tablespoon water. In a second bowl, combine the panko and Parmesan. Season the cutlets on both sides with the salt. Coat them first in the egg mixture, letting the excess drip off, and then coat with the panko mixture. Transfer to a work surface and spray both sides generously with oil.

Cooking in two batches as needed (for smaller baskets), air fry the chicken at 400°F for 7 minutes. Flip and cook until the crumbs are golden brown and the center is no longer pink, 2 to 3 more minutes.

Set 2 cutlets on each of four plates and top with 1 cup slaw. Serve immediately.

TIP: If you can't find thin-sliced chicken cutlets, buy 4 chicken breasts (about 2 pounds total) and cut your chicken breasts in half horizontally. Place them between two sheets of plastic wrap and use a meat mallet or rolling pin to pound them to a thickness of about ¼ inch.

No Air Fryer? No Problem!

Bake on a sheet pan in a preheated 425°F oven for 12 to 14 minutes, flipping halfway, until golden and cooked through.

Per Serving (2 cutlets + 1 cup slaw) | Calories 460 | **Protein 59 g** | Carbohydrate 17 g | Fiber 2 g | Sugars 2 g | Fat 16 g | Saturated Fat 3.5 g | Cholesterol 262 mg | Sodium 948 mg

SERVES 4

SALAD

1½ tablespoons extra-virgin olive oil

4 teaspoons red wine vinegar

2 teaspoons Dijon mustard

¼ teaspoon kosher salt

Freshly ground black pepper

½ small red onion, thinly sliced

2 cups thinly sliced green cabbage

2 cups thinly sliced kale, stems and ribs removed

2 radishes, thinly sliced

CHICKEN

2 large eggs

1½ cups seasoned panko bread crumbs, regular or gluten-free

⅓ cup finely grated Parmesan cheese

8 thin-sliced chicken breast cutlets (about 4 ounces each and ¼ inch thick), preferably organic

1 teaspoon kosher salt

Olive oil spray

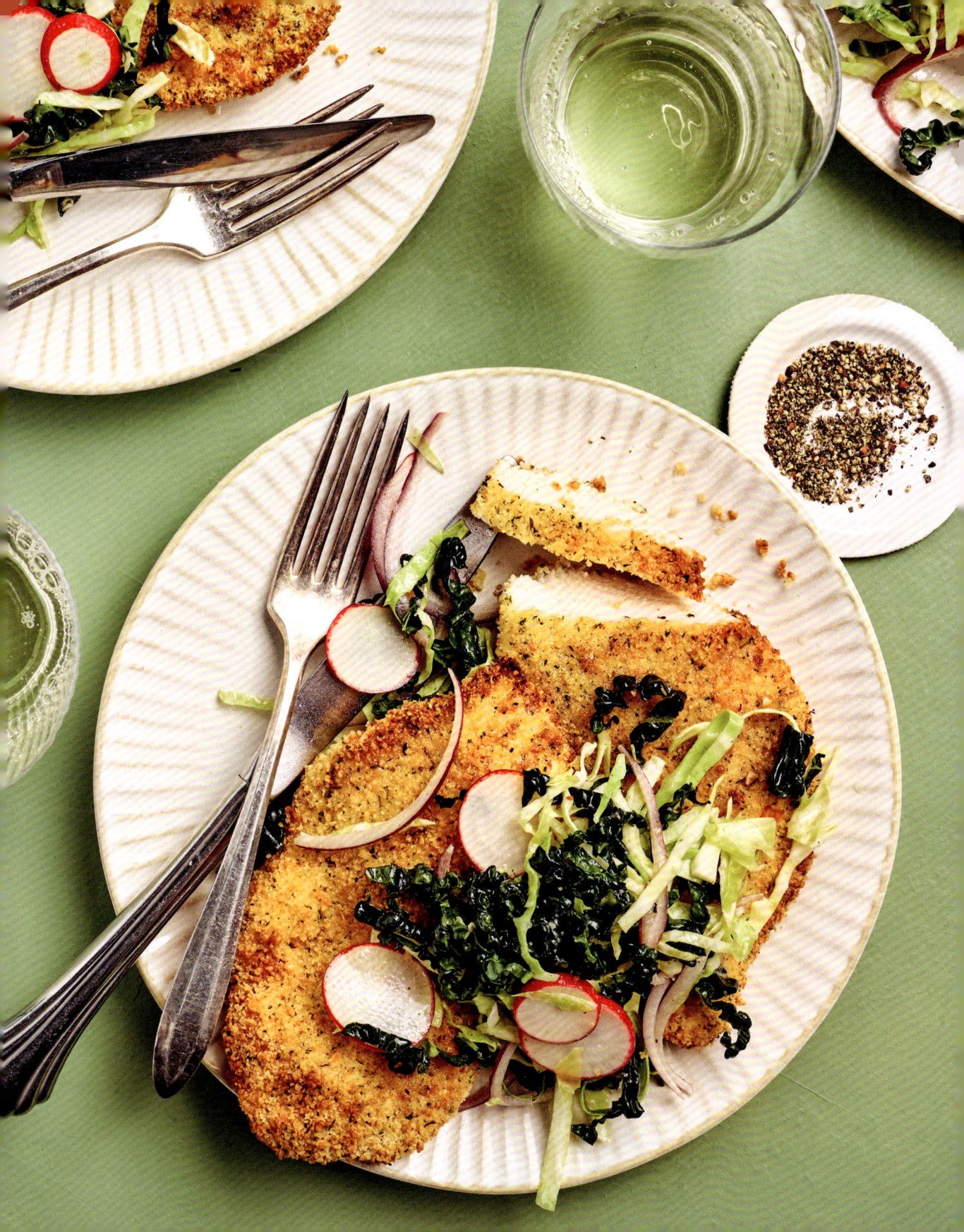

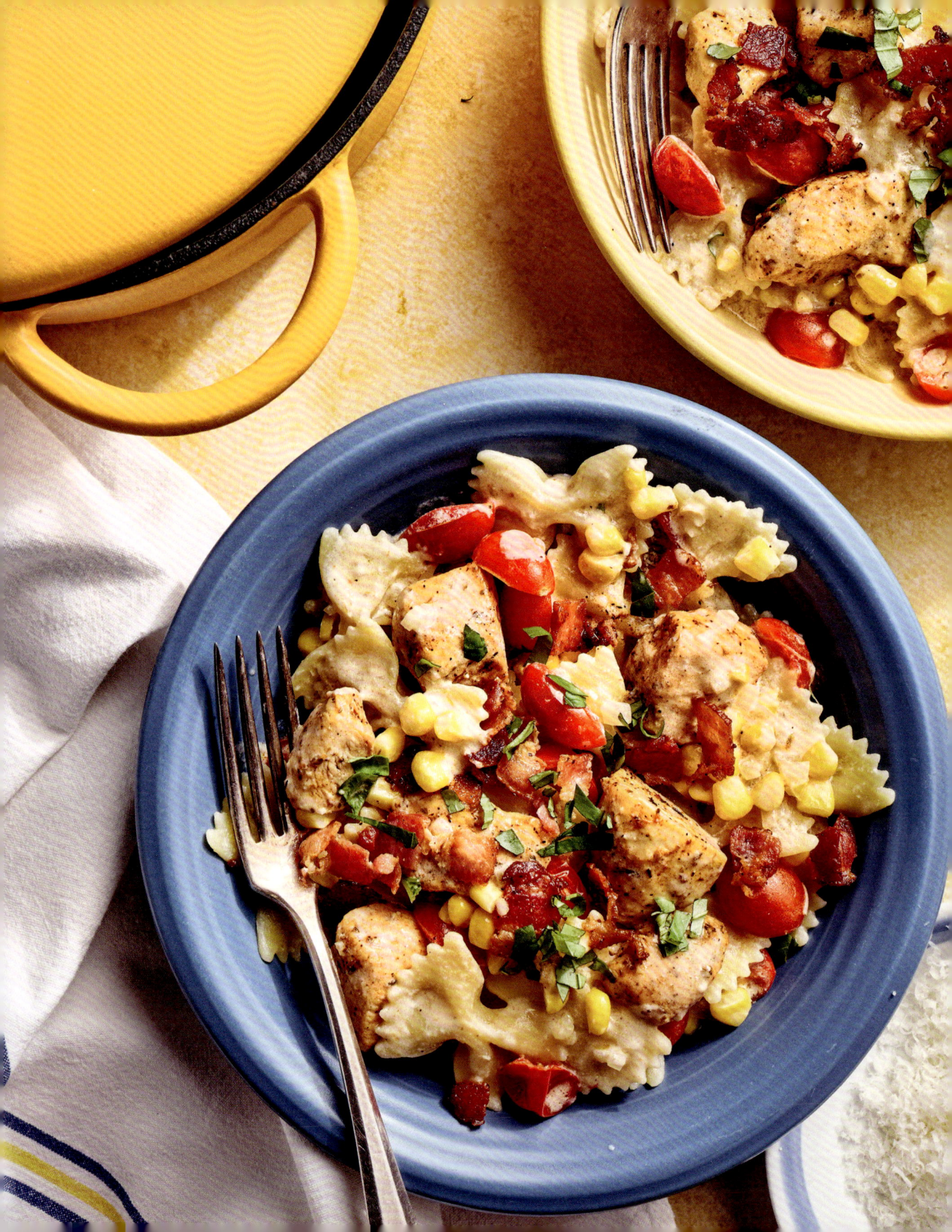

ONE-POT SUMMER PASTA with Chicken, Corn & Bacon

This pasta dish combines the savory flavors of bacon and chicken with the sweetness of corn, all tied together with a creamy yet light sauce. I streamlined this dish so everything cooks in a single pot. It gets plenty of protein from the chicken, milk, cheese, and high-protein pasta, but if you want to increase it a little more, you can swap the chicken broth for chicken bone broth.

In a small blender, combine the milk, Pecorino, and cream cheese and blend until smooth. Set aside.

Season the chicken all over with the Cajun seasoning.

Heat a large pot or Dutch oven over high heat. When the pot is very hot, spray it with oil and add the chicken in a single layer. Cook, undisturbed, until the bottom browns, about 3 minutes. Flip and cook the other side until the chicken is browned on all sides and cooked through, 2 to 3 minutes. Transfer to a plate.

Line a plate with paper towels and set it near the stove. Reduce the heat under the pot to medium, add the bacon, and cook until browned, 3 to 4 minutes. Remove with a slotted spoon and place on the paper towels, leaving the fat in the pot. Add the garlic and shallot and cook until golden and fragrant, about 1 minute.

Add a splash of the broth and scrape any browned bits from the bottom of the pot. Add the remaining broth, the cream cheese mixture, and the pasta. Stir to combine and bring to a boil. Reduce the heat to medium-low, cover, and simmer, stirring occasionally to help the pasta cook evenly, until the pasta is almost cooked, about 15 minutes.

Gently stir in the tomatoes and corn and cover again. Cook until the corn is crisp-tender, the pasta is tender, and the liquid is mostly absorbed, about 3 minutes. (If it seems dry before it's all cooked, you can add a little more broth.)

Uncover and add the chicken and any juices that have accumulated and stir to combine. Cook just for about 30 seconds to warm the chicken through.

Remove from the heat and serve topped with the bacon and basil.

Per Serving (2¼ cups) | Calories 556 | **Protein 54 g** | Carbohydrate 53 g | Fiber 6 g | Sugars 9 g | Fat 15 g | Saturated Fat 6 g | Cholesterol 132 mg | Sodium 756 mg

SERVES 4

1 cup fat-free milk

⅓ cup freshly grated Pecorino Romano or Parmesan cheese

⅓ cup ⅓-less-fat cream cheese (I like Philadelphia)

1¼ pounds boneless, skinless chicken breast, preferably organic, cut into ½-inch pieces

1 tablespoon Cajun seasoning

Olive oil spray

5 slices center-cut bacon, chopped

3 garlic cloves, minced

1 large shallot, minced

2 cups low-sodium chicken broth, plus more as needed

8 ounces high-protein bow tie pasta, such as Barilla, or gluten-free pasta

1½ cups cherry or grape tomatoes, halved

1 ear corn, kernels sliced off from cob (about 1 cup)

¼ cup finely chopped fresh basil

GRILLED CHICKEN THIGHS & CHARRED CORN SUMMER SALAD

News flash: Resting hot-off-the-grill chicken over raw summer tomatoes and red onions creates a simple salad that doesn't require any dressing! I fell in love with this technique from a recipe I saw in *The New York Times,* and I was blown away when I tested this out for myself. The raw onions mellow out from the heat of the chicken, and the juices mix with the tomatoes and fresh thyme to create a warm sauce that's ridiculously good, especially for its simplicity! The addition of charred corn at the end really ties the entire dish together. So simple, so delicious.

In a medium bowl, season the chicken with 1½ teaspoons of the oil, ¾ teaspoon of the salt, the onion powder, garlic powder, paprika, and oregano and toss to coat well.

Preheat an outdoor grill to medium-high heat.

On a large platter, layer the tomatoes followed by the red onion. Drizzle with the remaining 1½ teaspoons olive oil and ½ teaspoon salt. This will be the base of the salad.

When ready to grill, clean and oil the grates. Add the corn to one side of the grill and the chicken thighs to the other side. Cook until charred, turning every few minutes, about 10 minutes total. Cook the chicken until browned on both sides and cooked through, 6 to 7 minutes per side.

Transfer the chicken to the platter over the onions and top with the thyme leaves. Let the chicken rest for 5 to 10 minutes before serving, letting the drippings from the chicken create a warm dressing.

Meanwhile, place the corn on a cutting board, cut the kernels off the cob and add to the platter, scattered around the chicken. Serve immediately.

SERVES 4

8 boneless, skinless chicken thighs, fat trimmed (about 4 ounces each trimmed)

3 teaspoons extra-virgin olive oil

1¼ teaspoons kosher salt

1 teaspoon onion powder

1 teaspoon garlic powder

½ teaspoon sweet paprika

½ teaspoon dried oregano

3 large heirloom tomatoes, thinly sliced

1 small red onion, thinly sliced

1 large ear corn, husked

Leaves from 1 sprig of thyme

Per Serving (2 thighs + 1½ cups salad) | Calories 373 | **Protein 47 g** | Carbohydrate 15 g | Fiber 3 g | Sugars 6 g | Fat 14 g | Saturated Fat 3 g | Cholesterol 213 mg | Sodium 580 mg

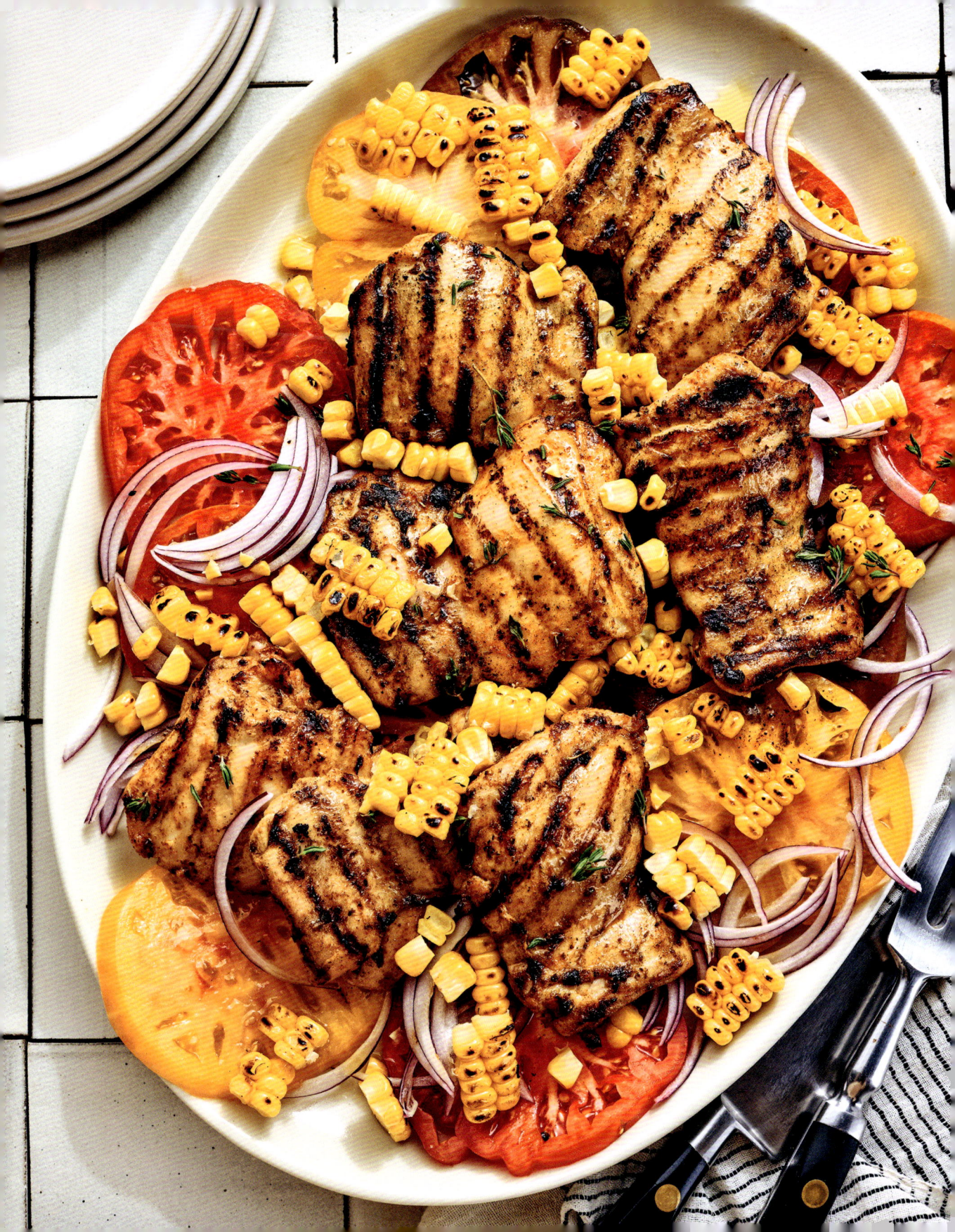

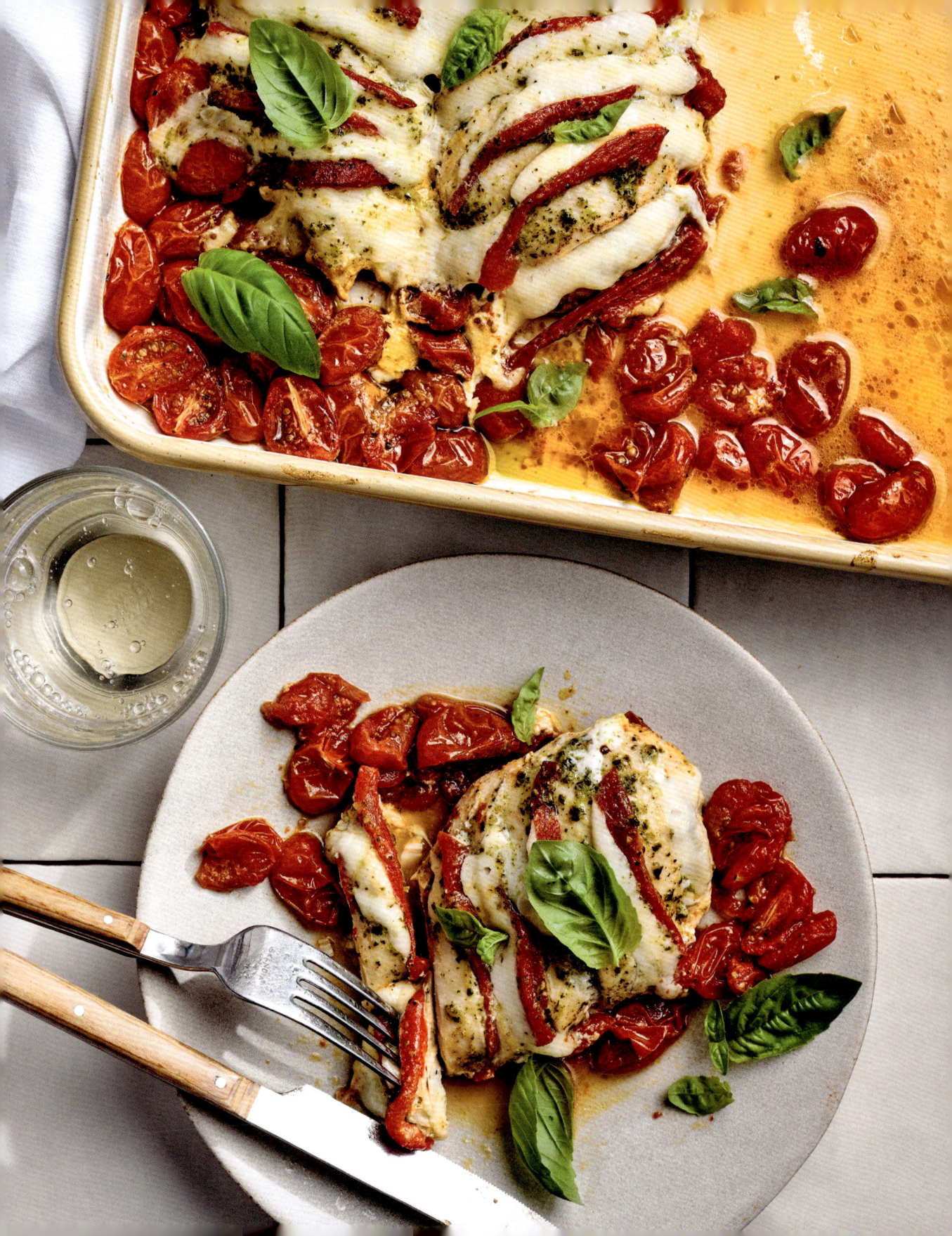

PESTO PIZZA CHICKEN BAKE

I called this dish "Pizza Chicken," because that's what my first delicious bite tasted like! This Hasselback chicken recipe takes its inspiration from the famous Hasselback potatoes, where thin, accordion-style cuts are made in the vegetable for even cooking and to create spaces to infuse flavor. Here, I fill the chicken with fresh mozzarella cheese, pesto, and roasted peppers, then bake them alongside cherry tomatoes, which creates a tasty sauce.

Preheat the oven to 400°F. Spray a 9 × 13-inch baking dish with oil.

Add the tomatoes to the baking dish, drizzle with the olive oil, and season with ¼ teaspoon of the salt and pepper to taste.

Bake until just partially cooked, about 10 minutes.

Meanwhile, cut 8 slits into the tops of each chicken breast, ½ inch apart and about 75 percent of the way down, being careful not to cut all the way through.

Season the chicken with the remaining ½ teaspoon kosher salt and pepper to taste.

Rub 2 tablespoons of the pesto over the top of the chicken and into the slits. Place a roasted pepper strip and mozzarella strip into each slit. Top with the remaining pesto.

Remove the tomatoes from the oven and stir, then nestle the chicken in the center of the baking dish.

Bake until the cheese has melted, the tomatoes are tender, and the chicken is cooked through, about 25 minutes.

Garnish with fresh basil leaves and serve immediately.

SERVES 4

Olive oil spray

20 ounces cherry tomatoes, halved

2 teaspoons extra-virgin olive oil

¾ teaspoon kosher salt

Freshly ground black pepper

4 boneless, skinless chicken breasts (about 8 ounces each), preferably organic

3 tablespoons prepared pesto

8 ounces fresh mozzarella, cut into 32 strips (2 × ¼-inch)

1 (12-ounce) jar roasted red peppers, cut into 32 strips (2 × ¼-inch)

Small fresh basil leaves, for garnish

Perfect Pairings

This can be served over spaghetti, orzo, or quinoa, with some garlic bread, or with a garden salad to keep it light.

Per Serving (1 chicken breast + ¼ cup tomatoes) | Calories 557 | **Protein 66 g** | Carbohydrate 10 g | Fiber 2 g | Sugars 7 g | Fat 27 g | Saturated Fat 10 g | Cholesterol 212 mg | Sodium 1,117 mg

ONE-POT CHICKEN ORZO CAPRESE

One-pot meals are ideal for busy weeknights, and this one features the flavors of a caprese salad—juicy tomatoes, creamy mozzarella, and fresh basil—all cooked together with orzo and chicken breasts. This is a meal the whole family will love, but perhaps the best part is that it's an easy way to make dinner extra special in under 30 minutes and with little cleanup!

In a medium bowl, season the chicken with 1 teaspoon of the olive oil, 1 teaspoon of the salt, 1 clove of minced garlic, the Italian seasoning, and black pepper to taste.

Heat a large deep skillet over high heat. When hot, spray with oil and add the chicken. Cook for about 5 minutes, turning, until browned on all sides and no longer pink in the center. Remove the chicken and set aside.

Add the remaining 1 tablespoon olive oil to the skillet. When hot, add the remaining garlic and sauté until golden, about 30 seconds. Add the tomatoes and ¼ teaspoon of the salt and cook until the tomatoes begin to soften, 2 to 3 minutes.

Add 2 cups water and bring to a boil over high heat. Add the orzo and season with the remaining ½ teaspoon salt. Reduce the heat to low, cover, and cook, stirring occasionally, until the liquid is absorbed and the pasta is tender, 12 to 14 minutes. Uncover and stir in the chicken. Cook until the chicken is warmed through, 1 more minute.

Remove from the heat and stir in the mozzarella cheese and half of the fresh basil. To serve, divide the orzo among four pasta bowls and top with the remaining basil.

SERVES 4

1 pound boneless, skinless chicken breast, preferably organic, cut into ½-inch cubes

1 tablespoon plus 1 teaspoon extra-virgin olive oil

1¾ teaspoons kosher salt

5 garlic cloves, minced

½ teaspoon Italian seasoning

Freshly ground black pepper

Olive oil spray

2 cups cherry tomatoes, halved

8 ounces uncooked orzo (1⅓ cups) or gluten-free pasta

3 ounces mini fresh mozzarella balls, halved if larger than ½ inch (about ⅔ cup)

¼ cup thinly sliced fresh basil

Perfect Pairings

Serve this with a big green salad on the side if you want to add more veggies to your meal.

Per Serving (1½ cups) | Calories 452 | **Protein 37 g** | Carbohydrate 44 g | Fiber 3 g | Sugars 3 g | Fat 13 g | Saturated Fat 4 g | Cholesterol 100 mg | Sodium 679 mg

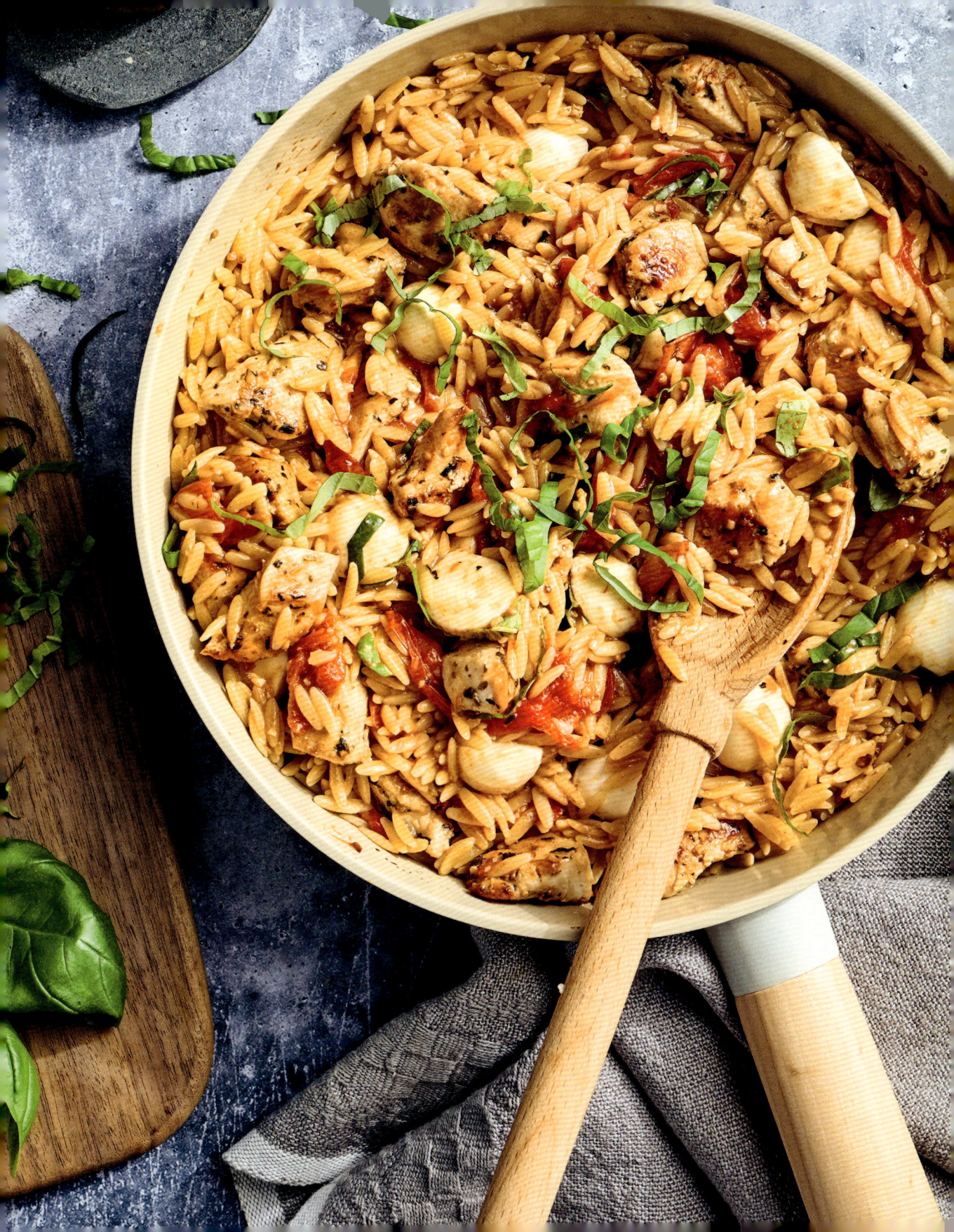

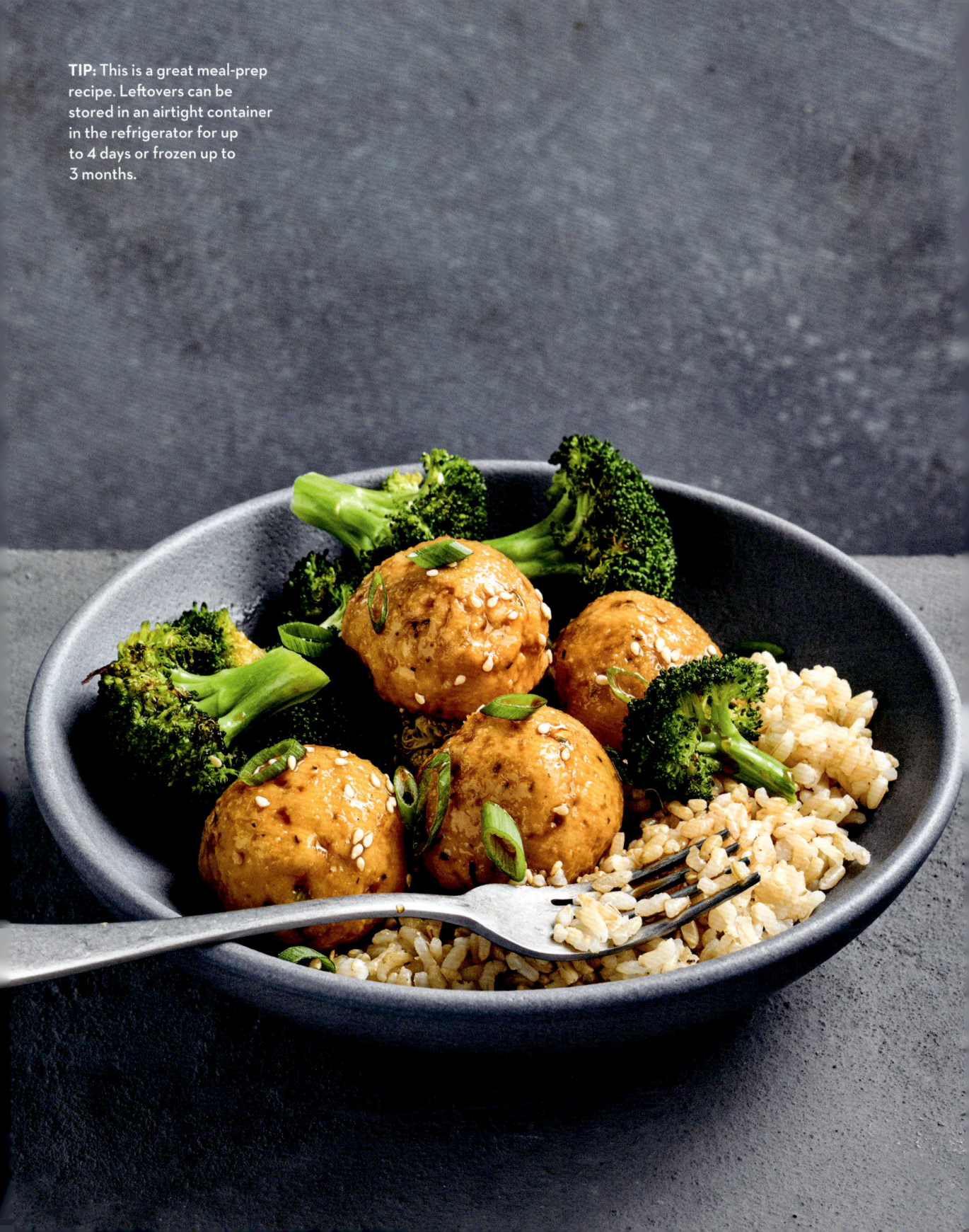

TIP: This is a great meal-prep recipe. Leftovers can be stored in an airtight container in the refrigerator for up to 4 days or frozen up to 3 months.

BAKED TERIYAKI CHICKEN MEATBALLS

Italian meatballs (polpette), Swedish meatballs (köttbullar), Turkish meatballs (köfte) . . . I've never met a meatball I didn't like! And tsukune, savory Japanese-style ground chicken meatballs, are no exception. Inspired by that version, this dish is a fun way to experience a taste of Japanese bar food at home, without a grill.

Position racks in the center and top third of the oven and preheat the oven to 400°F. Line two large sheet pans with foil or parchment paper and spray with oil.

MAKE THE MEATBALLS: In a large bowl, combine the ground chicken, panko, scallion whites, ginger, soy sauce, mirin, egg, and sesame oil. Mix with a fork until combined. Be careful not to overmix, which can make the meatballs tough. Wet your hands to prevent sticking and form the mixture into 16 balls, then transfer to one of the sheet pans.

Transfer the pan of meatballs to the center rack and bake for 9 minutes.

MEANWHILE, PREPARE THE BROCCOLI: Place the broccoli on the second sheet pan and toss with the sesame oil and salt.

When the meatballs have been in for 9 minutes, flip them over and return to the oven. Add the broccoli to the bottom rack and bake both until almost cooked through, about 7 minutes.

MEANWHILE MAKE THE SAUCE: In a small saucepan, combine the soy sauce, mirin, sake, and honey. Bring to a simmer over medium heat, stirring occasionally, until the sauce thickens slightly, 1 to 2 minutes.

Brush the meatballs with half of the sauce and continue baking until cooked through, another 2 minutes.

TO SERVE: Divide the rice among four bowls, top each with 4 meatballs, some of the remaining sauce, and 1 cup broccoli. Garnish with scallion greens and sesame seeds, if using, and serve.

Per Serving (¾ cup rice + 4 meatballs + 1 cup broccoli) | Calories 450 | **Protein 30 g** | Carbohydrate 51 g | Fiber 5 g | Sugars 8 g | Fat 14 g | Saturated Fat 3 g | Cholesterol 130 mg | Sodium 708 mg

SERVES 4

MEATBALLS

Olive oil spray

1 pound ground chicken or ground turkey (92% lean)

⅓ cup panko bread crumbs, regular or gluten-free

¼ cup chopped scallions, white and green parts kept separate

1 tablespoon grated fresh ginger

1 tablespoon reduced-sodium soy sauce or gluten-free tamari

1 tablespoon mirin

1 large egg, beaten

1 teaspoon toasted sesame oil

ROASTED BROCCOLI

1 head broccoli (12 ounces), cut into florets

2 teaspoons toasted sesame oil

¼ teaspoon kosher salt

SAUCE

2 tablespoons reduced-sodium soy sauce or gluten-free tamari

2 tablespoons mirin

2 tablespoons sake

1 teaspoon honey

FOR SERVING

3 cups cooked brown rice

Sesame seeds (optional)

AIR FRYER CHICKEN SATAY BOWLS

with Spicy Peanut Sauce & Mango Slaw

If you like chicken satay, you're going to *love* this Southeast Asian–inspired rice bowl. Served over jasmine rice, the peanut sauce gives this bowl some heat, while the fresh mango cabbage slaw adds a touch of sweetness and the perfect crunch. The chicken does take a little time to marinate, but once that's done, this dish comes together pretty fast. It's also ideal for meal prep.

SERVES 4

CHICKEN

1½ pounds boneless, skinless chicken breast, preferably organic, cut into ¾-inch pieces

¾ cup canned light coconut milk

Juice of 1 lime

1 tablespoon minced fresh ginger or ginger paste

3 garlic cloves, minced

1 tablespoon curry powder

2 tablespoons reduced-sodium soy sauce or gluten-free tamari

1 tablespoon sambal oelek

2 tablespoons minced fresh cilantro

Olive oil spray

PEANUT SAUCE

1 teaspoon avocado oil or coconut oil

1 tablespoon minced fresh ginger or ginger paste

¾ cup canned light coconut milk

3 tablespoons unsweetened peanut butter

2 tablespoons reduced-sodium soy sauce or gluten-free tamari

1 tablespoon sambal oelek

1½ teaspoons curry powder

1 teaspoon sugar

MANGO SLAW

1 small head napa or Savoy cabbage (about 1½ pounds)

1 mango (I like Honey or Kent mangoes), sliced into thin strips

2 scallions, chopped

3 tablespoons minced fresh cilantro

3 tablespoons seasoned rice vinegar

1 tablespoon Thai sweet chili sauce

1 teaspoon toasted sesame oil

¼ teaspoon kosher salt

FOR SERVING

3 cups cooked jasmine rice, heated

Minced fresh cilantro, for garnish

1 tablespoon black sesame seeds

(recipe continues)

Per Serving (1 bowl) | Calories 619 | **Protein 49 g** | Carbohydrate 66 g | Fiber 9 g | Sugars 20 g | Fat 18 g | Saturated Fat 5.5 g | Cholesterol 124 mg | Sodium 1,055 mg

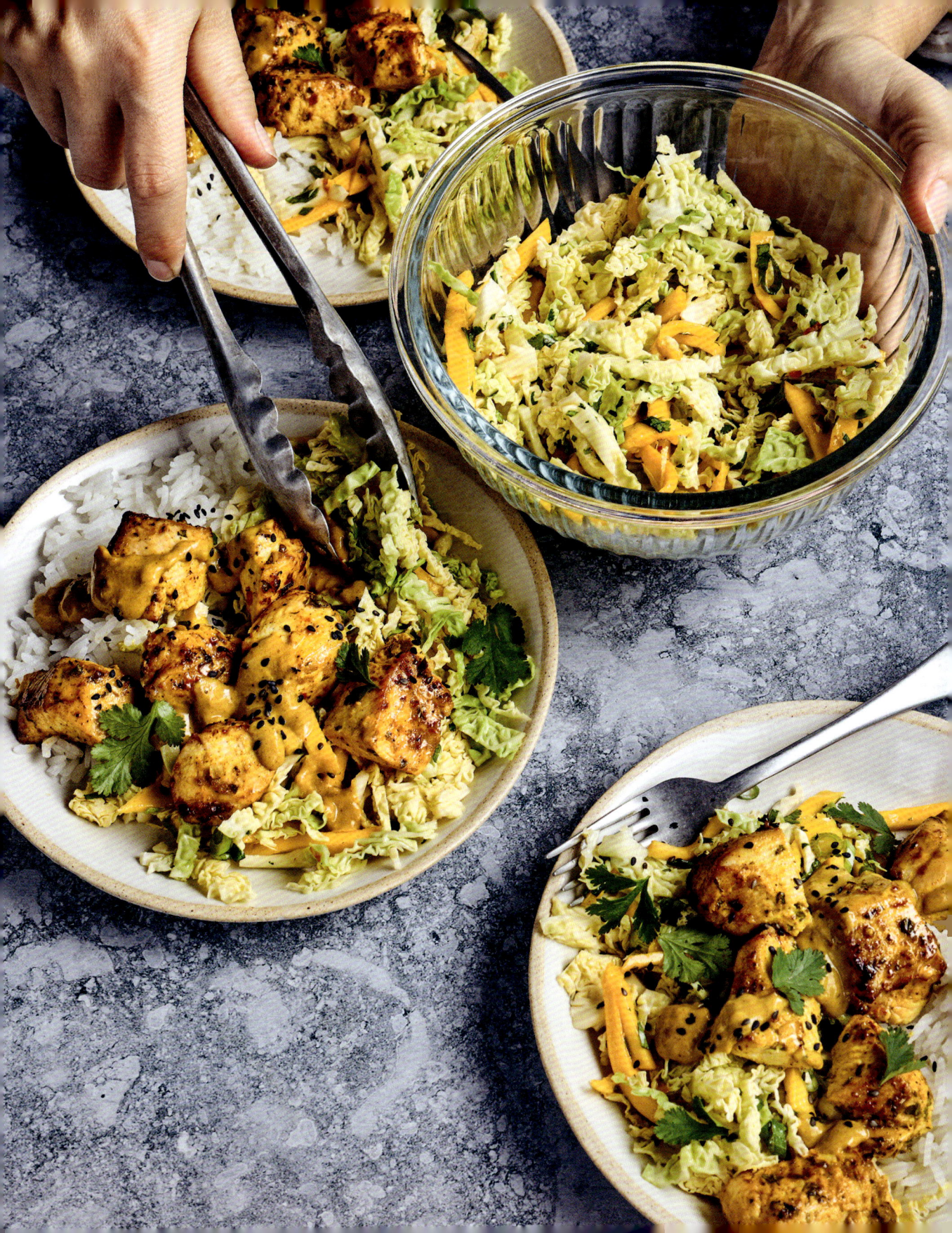

MARINATE THE CHICKEN: In a medium bowl, combine the chicken, coconut milk, lime juice, ginger, garlic, curry powder, soy sauce, sambal, and cilantro and mix well. Cover and refrigerate at least 1 to 2 hours or as long as overnight.

WHEN READY TO COOK, MAKE THE PEANUT SAUCE: In a small pot, heat the oil over medium-low heat and sauté the ginger until fragrant, about 1 minute. Add the coconut milk, peanut butter, soy sauce, 2 tablespoons water, the sambal, curry powder, and sugar. Mix until smooth and bring to a boil. Once it boils, remove from the heat and keep warm.

MAKE THE MANGO SLAW: Shred the cabbage into thin slices (about 8 cups). In a large bowl, combine the cabbage and mango with the scallions, cilantro, rice vinegar, sweet chili sauce, sesame oil, and salt and toss to mix. Keep chilled until ready to serve.

To make in an air fryer, spray the basket with oil. Cooking in batches as needed (for smaller baskets), arrange the chicken in a single layer (discard the marinade) in the air fryer basket and cook at 400°F for 9 to 10 minutes, shaking the basket halfway through, until the chicken is browned.

TO SERVE: Scoop ¾ cup rice into each of four bowls. Divide the chicken and slaw among the bowls, then top the chicken with 3 tablespoons peanut sauce and garnish with cilantro. Sprinkle the sesame seeds over the slaw and serve immediately.

No Air Fryer? No Problem!

In a skillet, spray with oil and cook the chicken in two batches over high heat for 3 to 4 minutes on each side.

SHORTCUT TURKEY MEATBALL MINESTRONE

My brother, who also loves to cook, often re-creates my recipes, and occasionally he puts his own spin on them! Recently, he took my classic minestrone soup and replaced the pasta with turkey meatballs. When he raved about how good it was, I knew I had to give it a try. He wasn't wrong—it's a warm, comforting soup that's made even better with tender turkey meatballs. To keep things simple, I skip rolling the meatballs and just sauté the meatball mixture in small pieces, creating flavorful bites in every spoonful.

SERVES 6

MEATBALL MIXTURE

¼ cup seasoned bread crumbs, regular or gluten-free

1 large egg

¼ cup chopped fresh Italian parsley

¼ cup grated Pecorino Romano cheese

2 garlic cloves, minced or grated

¾ teaspoon kosher salt

1 pound ground turkey (93% lean)

SOUP

1½ (15-ounce) cans no-salt-added white navy or cannellini beans,* rinsed and drained (2¼ cups)

1 (32-ounce) container chicken bone broth*

2 teaspoons extra-virgin olive oil

1 cup diced carrots

½ cup diced celery

½ cup chopped onion

2 garlic cloves, minced

1 (14.5-ounce) can no-salt-added petite diced tomatoes

Parmesan cheese rind (optional)

1 sprig of fresh rosemary

2 bay leaves

2 tablespoons chopped fresh basil

¼ cup chopped fresh Italian parsley

¼ teaspoon kosher salt, plus more to taste

Freshly ground black pepper

1 medium zucchini (about 8 ounces), diced

2 cups chopped Swiss chard or baby spinach

Parmesan cheese (optional), for serving

*Read the label to be sure this product is gluten-free.

(recipe continues)

Per Serving (1¾ cups) | Calories 378 | **Protein 40 g** | Carbohydrate 31 g | Fiber 9 g | Sugars 6 g | Fat 12 g | Saturated Fat 3 g | Cholesterol 91 mg | Sodium 986 mg

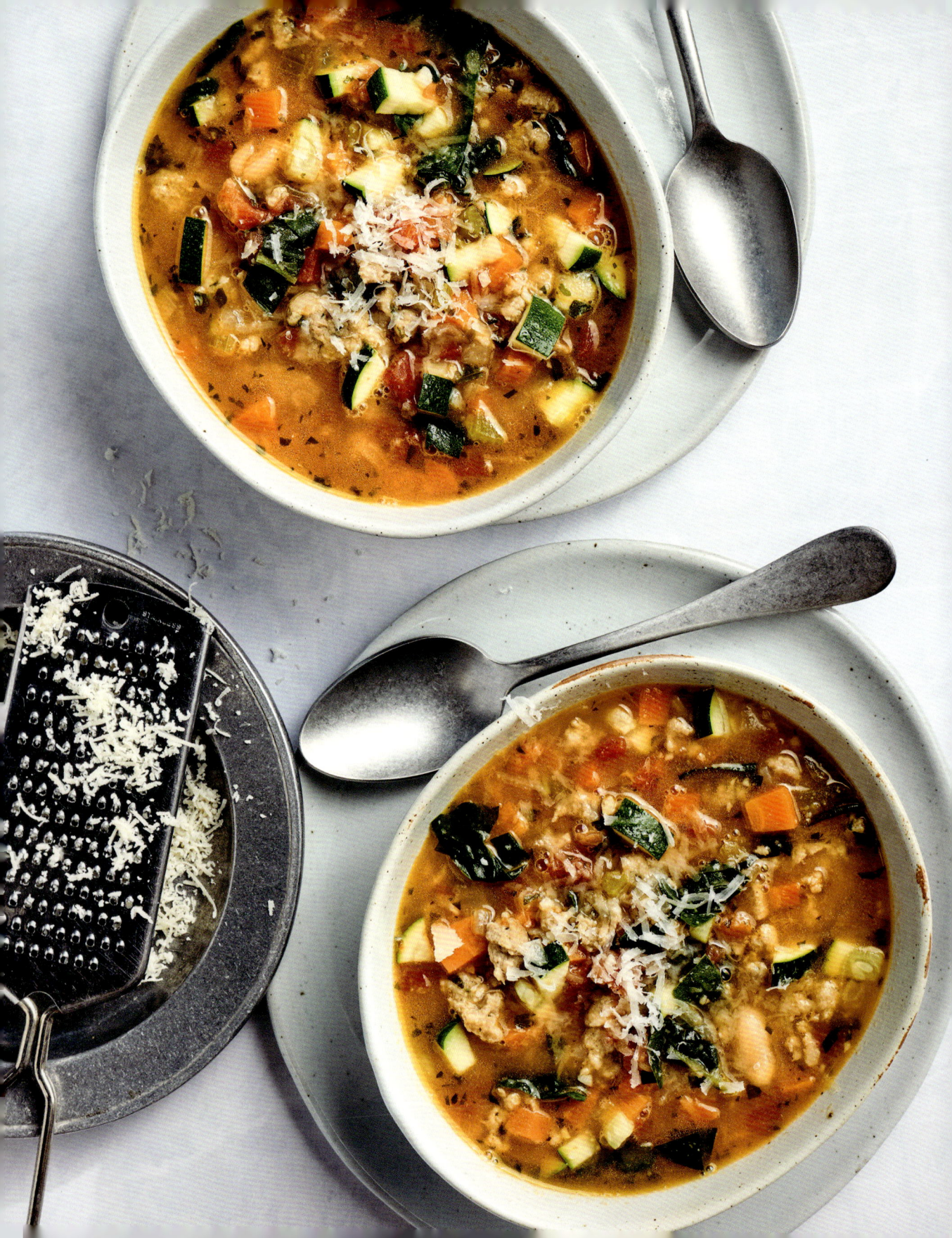

MAKE THE MEATBALL MIXTURE: In a large bowl, combine the bread crumbs, egg, parsley, grated cheese, garlic, and salt and mix well to combine. Add the turkey and mix using a fork to fully combine everything.

MAKE THE SOUP: In a blender, combine 1½ cups of the beans and 1 cup of the bone broth and puree until smooth.

Heat a large nonstick soup pot over medium-high heat. Add the meatball mixture and cook, breaking the meat up into smaller chunks, until browned, about 5 minutes. Transfer to a plate and set aside.

Add the olive oil to the pot and set over medium-high heat. Add the carrots, celery, onion, and garlic. Reduce the heat to low and sauté until tender and fragrant, about 15 minutes.

Return the meat to the pot. Add the remaining 3 cups bone broth, the tomatoes, pureed beans, remaining ¾ cup whole beans, the Parmesan cheese rind (if using), rosemary, bay leaves, basil, parsley, salt, and black pepper to taste. Bring to a boil over high heat. Reduce the heat to low, cover, and cook until the vegetables are tender and the flavors meld, about 40 minutes.

Add the zucchini and Swiss chard, cover again, and simmer until the zucchini is tender, about 6 minutes.

Discard the bay leaves, rosemary stem, and Parmesan rind (if used). Taste for salt and adjust as needed as this will vary depending on the broth you use.

Divide among six bowls and serve with extra Parmesan cheese, if desired.

TO STORE: Refrigerate up to 4 days or freeze up to 3 months in a freezer-safe container.

Perfect Pairings
This is a hearty soup, but if you want a side, you can serve it with crusty bread, garlic bread, or a simple salad.

CHICKEN SPAETZLE SOUP

If you're not familiar with spaetzle, it's a cross between an egg pasta and dumplings, but it's much quicker and easier to make. If you don't have a spaetzle maker, a colander with large holes or even the large holes of a cheese grater will work fine. My recipe uses more egg than most recipes I've seen, but that also means more protein, and I promise you, it's delicious.

MAKE THE SOUP: In a large pot or Dutch oven, heat the butter over medium heat. Add the onion, celery, and carrots and cook, stirring, until soft, 4 to 5 minutes. Reduce the heat to low. Add the garlic and cook, stirring, until fragrant, about 1 minute.

Add 6½ cups water, the chicken thighs, bouillon, bay leaves, and a generous amount of black pepper. Bring the broth to a boil, then reduce the heat to low so it bubbles gently. Cover and simmer until the chicken is tender and easily shreds with two forks, 35 to 40 minutes.

MEANWHILE, MAKE THE SPAETZLE: In a large bowl, whisk together the flour and salt. In a separate small bowl, beat together the eggs, milk, and herbs until thoroughly combined. Add the egg mixture to the flour and use a wooden spoon or spatula to gently stir together until you have a sticky dough. The dough shouldn't be too thin or too thick or it will be difficult to press the spaetzle through the holes of your spaetzle maker. If it's too thick add a tablespoon more liquid; if it's too thin, add a little more flour. Let the dough sit for at least 5 to 10 minutes while the soup simmers.

When the chicken is tender, remove and transfer to a bowl, leaving the lid on the soup. Shred the chicken with two forks and discard the bones. Discard the bay leaves and return the chicken to the soup. Increase the heat to medium-high and return to a rolling boil.

Working in about three batches, hold a spaetzle maker or colander with large holes over the pot and press the dough through the holes so the spaetzle drop into the boiling soup. Let the spaetzle cook until they float to the top, 2 to 3 minutes. Serve in bowls with more pepper and a sprinkle of parsley (if using).

Per Serving (1½ cups) | Calories 385 | **Protein 38 g** | Carbohydrate 29 g | Fiber 2.5 g | Sugars 6 g | Fat 12 g | Saturated Fat 4.5 g | Cholesterol 243 mg | Sodium 1,282 mg

SERVES 4

SOUP

1 tablespoon unsalted butter or nondairy butter

¾ cup diced onion

¾ cup diced celery

1 cup ¼-inch-thick half-moons peeled carrot

2 garlic cloves, minced

4 bone-in chicken thighs, skin removed

2 tablespoons chicken bouillon paste* (I like Better Than Bouillon)

2 bay leaves

Freshly ground black pepper

SPAETZLE

¾ cup all-purpose flour or gluten-free flour mix, such as Cup4Cup

⅛ teaspoon kosher salt

2 large eggs

⅓ cup whole milk (or water for dairy-free)

1 teaspoon chopped fresh herbs, such as thyme, parsley, or chives

Fresh parsley (optional), for garnish

*Read the label to be sure this product is gluten-free

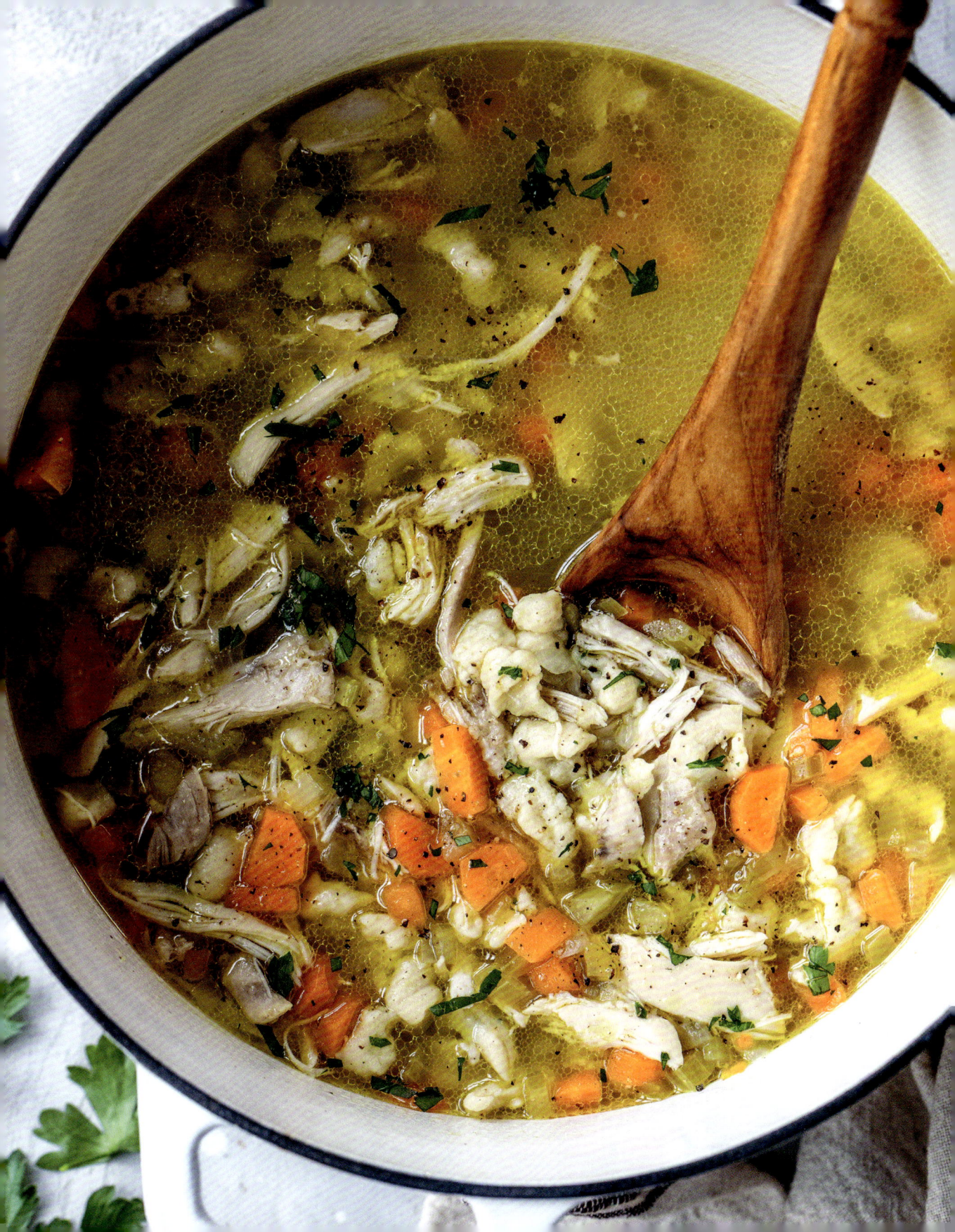

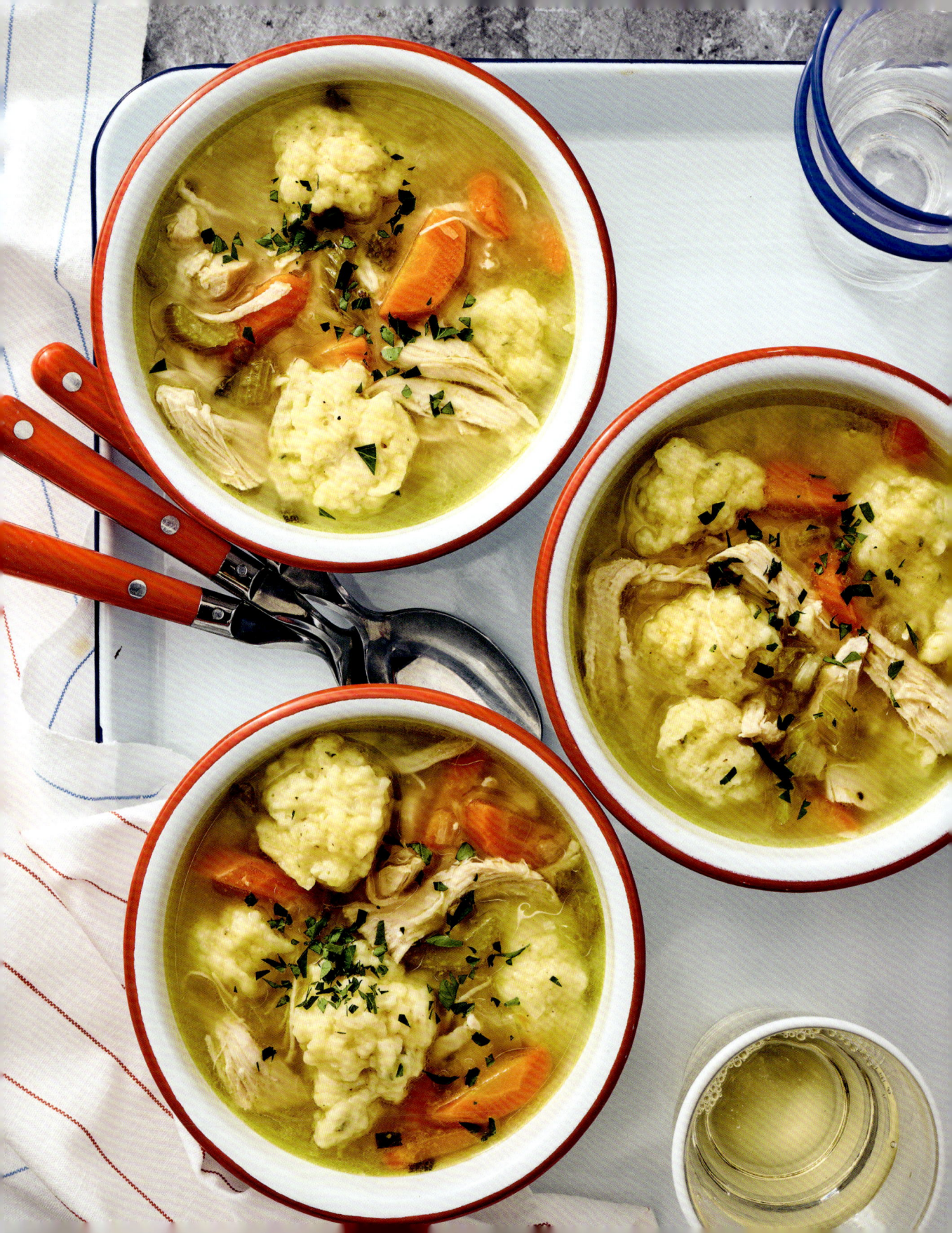

INSTANT POT TURKEY & SAGE DUMPLING SOUP

As the weather cools, my family and I crave hearty dishes that warm you up like a big hug, and nothing says comfort like a pot of soup! This turkey and dumpling soup is a satisfying meal in one, and it's a big hit with everyone in my house, from kids to adults. It's perfect for leftover Thanksgiving turkey and equally delicious with chicken breast. This is comfort food at its finest!

Press the sauté button on an electric pressure cooker and melt the butter. Add the onion, celery, carrots, and garlic and cook, stirring, until soft and fragrant, 5 to 8 minutes Sprinkle the flour over the vegetables and cook, stirring, until no longer raw, about 1 minute.

Add 7 cups water, the bouillon, turkey, sage, and bay leaves and season with black pepper to taste. Seal and cook on high pressure for 20 minutes. Quick or natural release, then open when the pressure subsides. Remove the turkey and shred or chop into bite-size pieces. Discard the bay leaves and return the turkey to the pot. Press sauté and bring to a boil.

MEANWHILE, MAKE THE DUMPLINGS: In a medium bowl, combine the flour, sage, baking powder, salt, and pepper. In a small bowl, whisk together the egg yolk and milk. Add the egg mixture to the flour mixture and mix until just blended (it will be thick).

When the soup comes to a boil, drop in scant teaspoons (they will expand a lot!). Seal and cook on high pressure for 5 minutes. Quick or natural release, then open when the pressure subsides.

Serve immediately, garnished with parsley.

No Instant Pot? No Problem!

You can simmer the soup in a large pot or Dutch oven until the turkey shreds easily, about 1 hour. Bring the soup to a boil before dropping in the dumplings and cook until they puff up and float to the top, about 2 to 4 minutes.

SERVES 6

1 tablespoon unsalted butter or nondairy butter

½ cup diced onion

1 cup chopped celery

1 cup chopped carrots

1 garlic clove, minced

2 tablespoons all-purpose flour

2 tablespoons turkey or chicken bouillon paste (I like Better Than Bouillon)

1½ pounds boneless, skinless turkey breast, cut into 4 pieces (turkey tenderloin or cutlets will also work)

2 fresh sage leaves, chopped

2 bay leaves

Freshly ground black pepper

DUMPLINGS

1 cup all-purpose flour

1 tablespoon minced fresh sage

1 teaspoon baking powder

½ teaspoon kosher salt

⅛ teaspoon freshly ground black pepper

1 large egg yolk, beaten

½ cup cold fat-free milk (or water for dairy-free)

Chopped fresh parsley, for garnish

Per Serving (1¾ generous cups) | Calories 277 | **Protein 32 g** | Carbohydrate 26 g | Fiber 2 g | Sugars 4 g | Fat 5 g | Saturated Fat 2 g | Cholesterol 105 mg | Sodium 1,025 mg

ONE-POT LEMONY ORZO with Chicken & Feta

My one-pot orzo recipes on the Skinnytaste website are some of my most popular—and I truly believe there can never be too many! This Mediterranean-inspired dish is packed with flavor: juicy chicken, zesty lemon, briny olives, and creamy feta all mingle with the tender orzo. The best part? It's quick, easy, and leftovers make a great lunch.

Season the chicken breasts on both sides with the paprika, 1 teaspoon of the oregano, ½ teaspoon of the salt, and the garlic powder.

Heat a large heavy-bottomed skillet over medium-low heat. When hot, add 1 teaspoon of the oil. Add the chicken and cook until browned on both sides and almost cooked through, about 5 minutes per side. Remove from the heat, leaving the juices in the pan, and tent with foil so the chicken continues cooking.

Add the remaining 1 teaspoon oil, the uncooked orzo, and garlic to the skillet. Toast the orzo for about 2 minutes over medium heat, stirring constantly.

Add the bone broth and remaining ¼ teaspoon salt and bring to a boil over high heat. Give the mixture a good stir, reduce the heat to low, cover, and cook until the liquid is absorbed and the orzo is tender, about 14 minutes.

Uncover and return the chicken breast to the skillet along with the lemon juice, cherry tomatoes, and olives. Stir to combine, then cover and cook for 2 minutes to heat through.

Meanwhile, in a medium bowl, combine the feta with the remaining ¼ teaspoon oregano, half of the basil, and black pepper to taste.

Sprinkle the feta mixture all over the skillet and cook for another minute to melt the feta. Garnish with the remaining basil and serve immediately.

SERVES 4

4 small boneless, skinless chicken breasts (about 6 ounces each), preferably organic

1 teaspoon sweet paprika

1¼ teaspoons dried oregano

¾ teaspoon kosher salt

½ teaspoon garlic powder

2 teaspoons extra-virgin olive oil

8 ounces orzo (1⅓ cups) or gluten-free orzo

3 garlic cloves, minced

2 cups unsalted chicken bone broth*

2 tablespoons fresh lemon juice

1 cup cherry or grape heirloom tomatoes, halved

⅓ cup pitted Castelvetrano olives, sliced into rounds

2 ounces feta cheese, crumbled (omit for dairy-free)

¼ cup chopped fresh basil

Freshly ground black pepper

*Read the label to be sure this product is gluten-free.

Perfect Pairings
This dish can be served as a standalone meal or paired with a simple side salad, such as a Greek cucumber-tomato version.

Per Serving (1 breast + 1 cup orzo) | Calories 511 | Protein 52 g | Carbohydrate 44 g | Fiber 3.5 g | Sugars 3 g | Fat 13 g | Saturated Fat 3.5 g | Cholesterol 139 mg | Sodium 665 mg

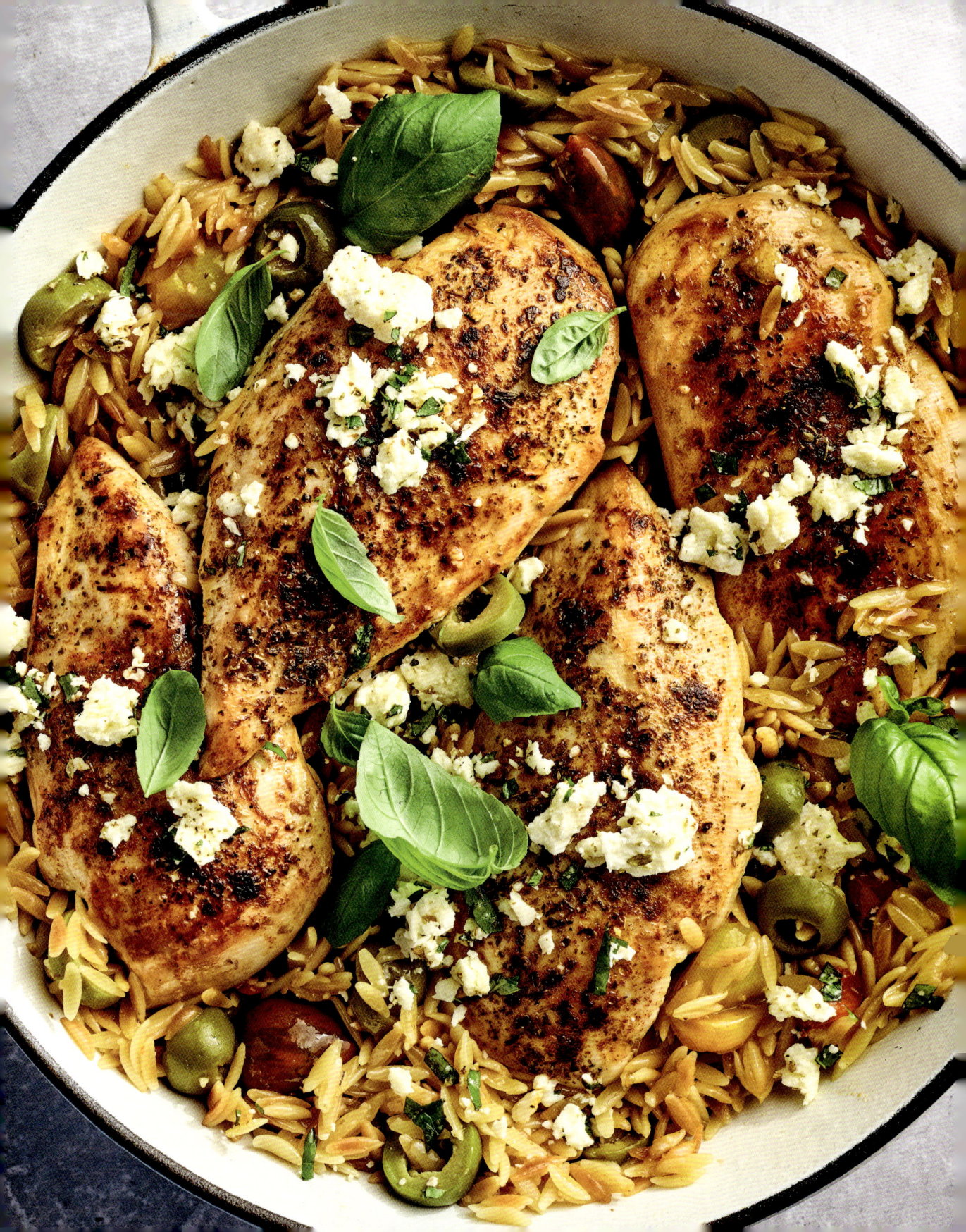

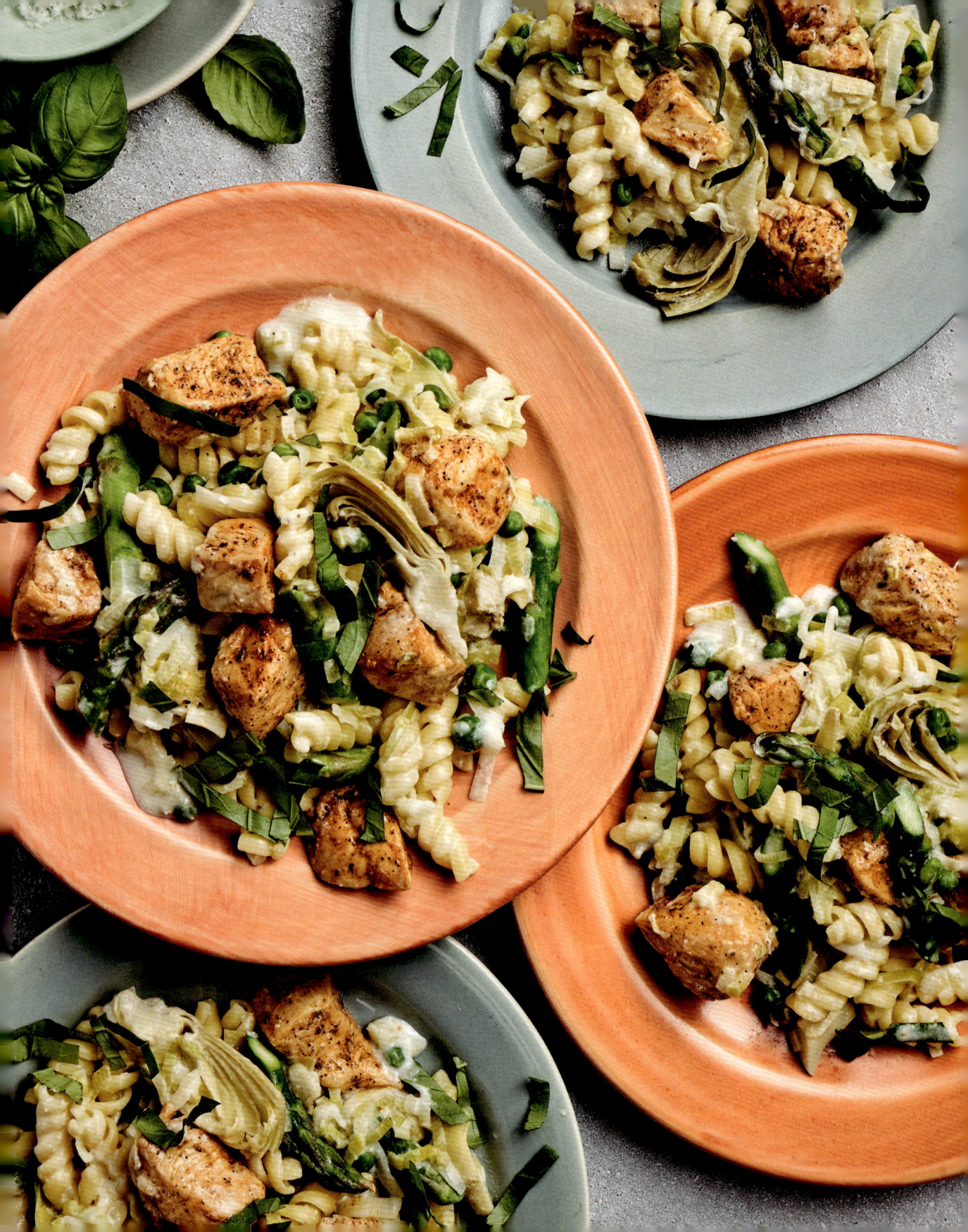

ONE-POT CHICKEN PASTA PRIMAVERA

Primavera means "spring" in Italian, so I thought the name for this one-pot pasta dish was fitting since it's made with springtime asparagus, leeks, artichokes, and peas. Each portion has a generous amount of veggies and Cajun-seasoned chicken, and who doesn't love a one-pot meal? It's light and flavorful, but it still hits all the cravings that a creamy Alfredo-type pasta would fulfill. The dish is loaded with protein, but if you want to add even more, simply swap the broth for bone broth and the regular pasta for high-protein pasta.

In a small blender, combine the milk, grated cheese, and cream cheese and blend until smooth. Set aside.

In a medium bowl, season the chicken with the Cajun seasoning.

Heat a large pot over high heat. When the pan is very hot, spray it with oil and add the chicken in a single layer. Cook, undisturbed, until the bottom browns, about 3 minutes. Flip and cook the other side until browned and cooked through, 2 to 3 minutes. Transfer to a plate and set aside.

Add a splash of the broth and scrape any browned bits from the bottom of the pot. Add the remaining broth, the cream cheese mixture, pasta, and leeks. Stir to combine and bring to a boil. Reduce the heat to medium-low, cover, and simmer, stirring occasionally to help the pasta cook evenly, for 15 minutes. Taste the pasta and if it's not al dente, or there is still a lot of liquid at the bottom of the pot, cover and cook for another minute and check again.

When the pasta is ready, gently stir in the asparagus and artichokes, cover, and cook until the asparagus is crisp-tender, the pasta is tender, and the liquid is mostly absorbed, about 3 minutes.

Uncover and stir in the chicken with any juices along with the peas. Cook just for about 30 seconds to warm the peas through.

Remove from the heat and stir in the basil. Serve with more Parmesan cheese for topping.

SERVES 4

1 cup fat-free milk

⅓ cup freshly grated Pecorino Romano or Parmesan cheese, plus more for serving

⅓ cup ⅓-less-fat cream cheese (I like Philadelphia)

1 pound boneless, skinless chicken breast, preferably organic, cut into ½-inch pieces

2 teaspoons Cajun seasoning

Olive oil spray

1½ cups low-sodium chicken broth*

8 ounces bow tie or other short pasta, whole wheat or gluten-free

2 medium leeks, white and light-green parts only, thinly sliced and rinsed well

6 ounces thin asparagus, tough ends trimmed, cut into 1-inch pieces

1 (14-ounce) can water-packed artichoke hearts, drained, rinsed, and quartered if necessary

1 cup frozen peas (no need to thaw)

¼ cup thinly sliced fresh basil

*Read the label to be sure this product is gluten-free.

Per Serving (1⅔ cups) | Calories 541 | **Protein 45 g** | Carbohydrate 66 g | Fiber 10 g | Sugars 9 g | Fat 10 g | Saturated Fat 4.5 g | Cholesterol 104 mg | Sodium 698 mg

HEARTY AUTUMN SALAD
with Chicken & Maple-Dijon Dressing

I eat salads all summer long, but when the weather cools, they get an autumn upgrade packed with the best fall produce. I swap in heartier greens like kale and shredded Brussels sprouts, giving the salad more texture and staying power. Roasted delicata squash is a favorite addition, not only for its sweet, nutty flavor, but also because there's no peeling required! To round this salad out, I toss in sweet, crunchy apples, juicy pomegranate seeds, toasted pecans, and some roasted chicken for protein. A maple-Dijon dressing ties it all together. It's perfect for meal prep—just store the dressing separately and mix when ready.

Preheat the oven to 425°F. Line a baking sheet with parchment paper.

MEANWHILE, MAKE THE VINAIGRETTE: In a small bowl, whisk together the vinegar, maple syrup, both mustards, the salt, and pepper. While whisking, gradually stream in the olive oil and whisk until incorporated.

PREPARE THE SALAD VEGETABLES: On the lined baking sheet, toss the delicata squash with 1 teaspoon of the olive oil, ¼ teaspoon of the kosher salt, and the pepper. Spread out and roast until caramelized and tender, about 20 minutes.

In a large bowl, combine the kale with the remaining 1 teaspoon olive oil. Massage the oil into the kale to help tenderize it, about 3 minutes. Add the Brussels sprouts and toss with the remaining ¼ teaspoon salt.

Just before serving, core and thinly slice the apple.

To assemble the salad, divide the prepped kale and Brussels among four bowls. Top with the roasted delicata, apples, pomegranate, pecans, cranberries, chicken, and cheese.

Drizzle the vinaigrette over top (about 1½ tablespoons each) and serve.

Per Serving (2 generous cups) | Calories 529 | **Protein 40 g** | Carbohydrate 37 g | Fiber 12 g | Sugars 15 g | Fat 27 g | Saturated Fat 6 g | Cholesterol 100 mg | Sodium 523 mg

SERVES 4

VINAIGRETTE

2 tablespoons cider vinegar

1 tablespoon pure maple syrup

1 teaspoon Dijon mustard

1 teaspoon whole-grain mustard

¼ teaspoon kosher salt

⅛ teaspoon black pepper

3 tablespoons extra-virgin olive oil

SALAD

1 delicata squash (about 14 ounces), seeded and cut into ¼-inch-thick half-rings

2 teaspoons olive oil

½ teaspoon kosher salt

⅛ teaspoon black pepper

2 cups shredded kale

2 cups shredded Brussels sprouts

1 medium apple

½ cup pomegranate seeds

⅓ cup roasted unsalted pecans, chopped

¼ cup unsweetened dried cranberries

3 cups chopped cooked chicken breast or turkey breast (from a rotisserie chicken or leftovers)

2 ounces blue cheese or Gorgonzola, crumbled (omit for dairy-free)

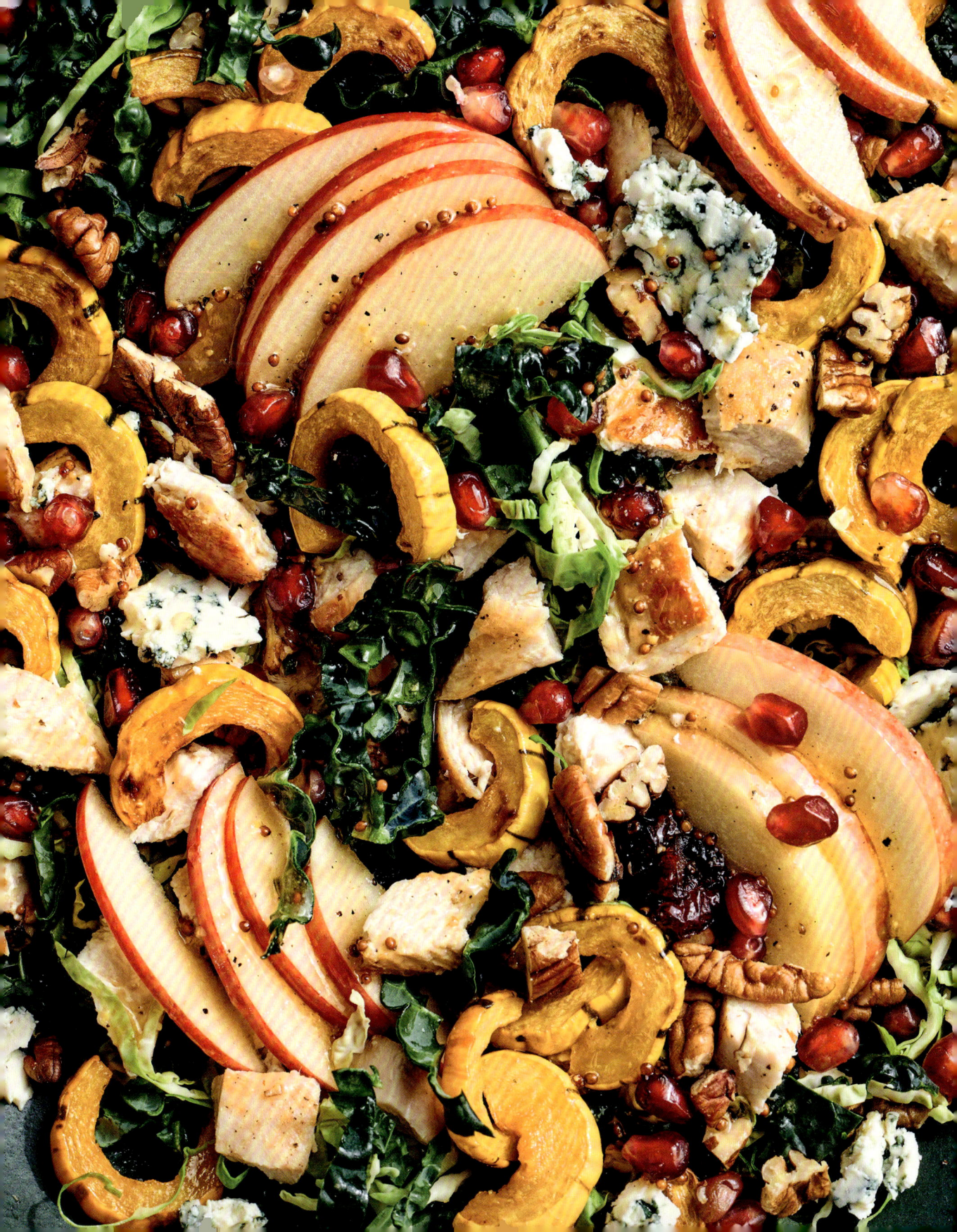

PRIME CUTS
& JUICY BITES

We are a family of meat lovers, so creating this chapter came naturally—it was definitely easier than tackling the meatless recipes! Beef, pork, lamb, and even bison are not only rich and flavorful, but also fantastic sources of protein, making them staples in many households, including mine.

This chapter is packed with recipes that highlight the bold, savory flavors of these prime cuts while keeping things healthy and light. Many of the dishes use leaner cuts, making them perfect for those looking to enjoy the richness of meat, while maintaining a balanced diet.

From tender roasts like my Sunday Pot Roast with Gravy (page 190) to slow cooker meals such as the Slow Cooker Chili con Carne (page 197), quick steaks like Colombian Thin-Cut Steaks with Fried Egg (page 212) to hearty soups like Instant Pot Mexican Beef Soup (page 203), and even creative ways to cook with bison like Sweet Potato Burger Bowls (page 194), these recipes are designed to showcase the flexibility of these proteins while helping you meet your goals in the most delicious way possible.

From quick and easy dinners to trying something new to elevate your weekly menu, this chapter has something for every meat lover who values great flavor and smart eating.

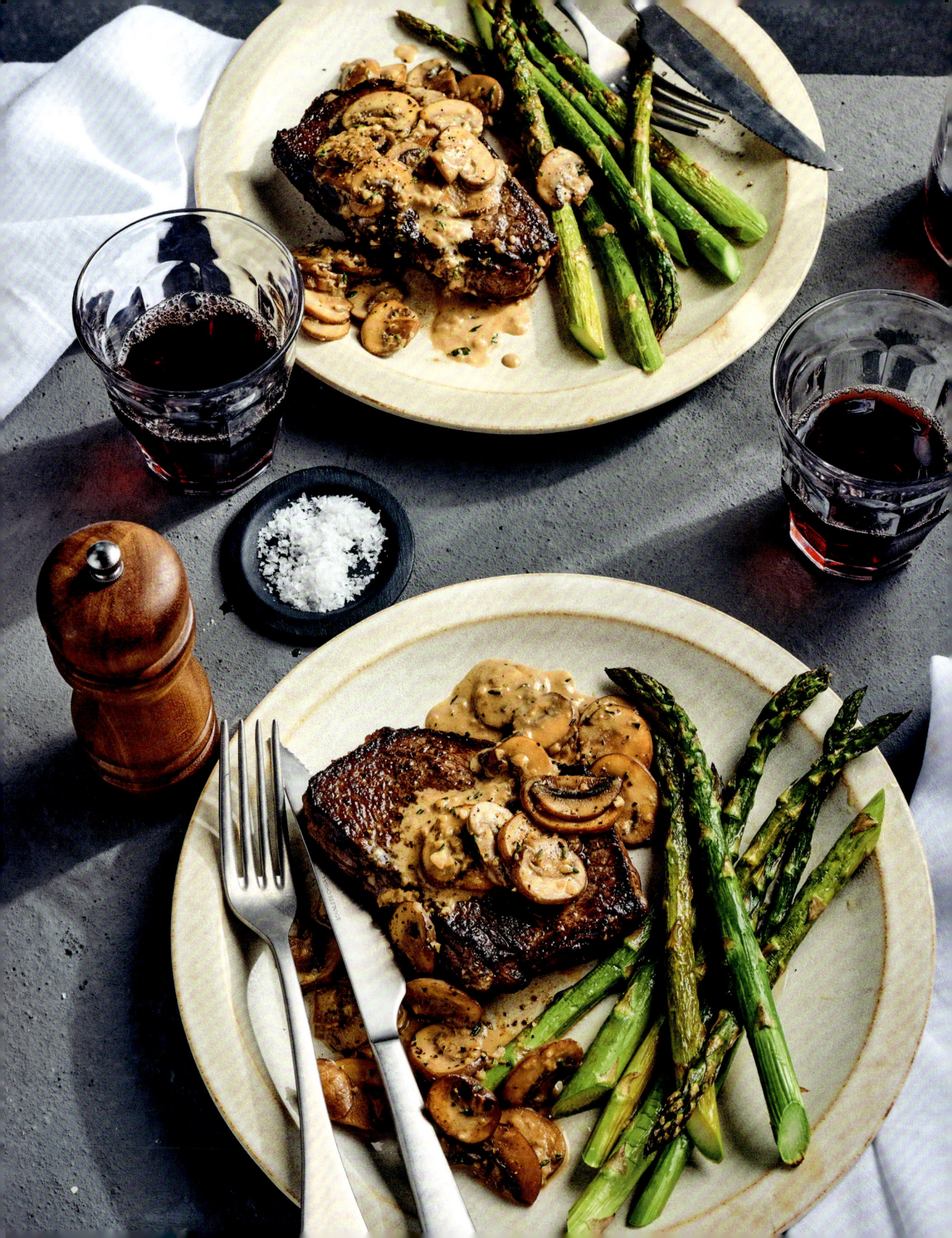

SEARED STEAKS

with Dijon-Mushroom Sauce & Roasted Asparagus

I love creating fancy steakhouse dinners at home! It's actually quite easy—just make sure you have everything prepped before you start. Also, to get a good sear on the steaks, let them come to room temperature while you prep the asparagus and sauce, and be sure to get your skillet very hot before adding the meat.

Season the steaks on both sides with ¾ teaspoon of the salt. Let them rest at room temperature for 30 minutes.

Preheat the oven to 400°F. Line a large sheet pan with foil and spray with olive oil.

Arrange the asparagus on the sheet pan in a single layer. Spritz with olive oil and season with the remaining ¼ teaspoon salt and pepper to taste. Roast until tender crisp, 12 to 14 minutes.

Meanwhile, heat a large cast-iron skillet over high heat. When hot, spray with oil.

Place the steaks in the pan in a single layer and cook for about 3 minutes. Flip and cook an additional 2 minutes for medium-rare (or longer if thicker), until the internal temperature reaches 125°F, or to your desired doneness.

Remove the steaks from the pan, transfer to a plate, tent with foil, and let them rest.

Meanwhile, return the skillet to medium heat and melt the butter. Add the garlic and sauté until fragrant, 30 to 60 seconds. Add the mustard, mushrooms, beef broth, and thyme, scraping any browned bits from the bottom of the pan. Cover and simmer until the mushrooms are soft, 2 to 3 minutes.

Stir in the half-and-half and simmer uncovered until the sauce slightly reduces, 1 to 2 minutes. Taste and adjust the salt and pepper if needed.

Spoon the mushroom sauce over the steaks and serve with asparagus.

Per Serving (1 steak + ⅓ cup mushroom sauce + asparagus) | Calories 329 | **Protein 42 g** | Carbohydrate 8 g | Fiber 3 g | Sugars 4 g | Fat 14 g | Saturated Fat 7 g | Cholesterol 121 mg | Sodium 499 mg

SERVES 4

4 top sirloin steaks (6 ounces each), about ¾ inch thick, trimmed

1 teaspoon kosher salt, plus more to taste

Olive oil spray

1 pound asparagus, tough ends trimmed

Freshly ground black pepper

2 tablespoons salted butter

2 garlic cloves, minced

1 teaspoon Dijon mustard

8 ounces Baby Bella mushrooms, thinly sliced (about 3 cups)

¼ cup beef broth*

1 teaspoon fresh thyme leaves, chopped

3 tablespoons half-and-half

*Read the label to be sure this product is gluten-free.

TIP: You can swap the asparagus for green beans or serve the steaks with your favorite steakhouse sides like baked potato or mashed potatoes.

ONE-POT PHILLY CHEESESTEAK PASTA

My husband, Tommy, loves this simple, one-pot dish that combines the flavors of a Philly cheesesteak with pasta. A package of lean ground beef (it's much quicker than chopping up steak!) is cooked with onion, bell peppers, and mushrooms, and then it's simmered with pasta in beef bone broth to absorb all the flavors and get super tender. Melted provolone adds a creamy finish, making it a hearty, family-friendly meal with minimal cleanup, so it's perfect for busy weeknights!

Heat a large deep skillet over medium heat. Add the beef and steak seasoning and cook, breaking the meat up into small pieces, until browned, 5 to 6 minutes. Add the onion and bell peppers and cook until tender, about 5 minutes.

Add the mushrooms and Worcestershire sauce and cook until tender, 2 to 3 minutes. Stir in the beef bone broth and pasta and bring to a boil. Reduce the heat to medium, cover, and cook, stirring halfway, until the pasta starts to become al dente and most of the liquid is absorbed, 8 to 10 minutes.

Reduce the heat to medium-low, stir in the milk, cover and cook, stirring every 5 minutes, until the pasta is al dente and most of the liquid is absorbed, 8 to 10 minutes.

Stir in the cheese and serve immediately.

TIP: I used provolone cheese here per Tommy's request, but mozzarella or cheddar would also be lovely. If your kids don't like a lot of spice, cut back on the steak seasoning, which has a lot of black pepper.

SERVES 4

¾ pound ground beef (96% lean)

2 teaspoons Montreal steak seasoning

½ cup chopped onion

1 green bell pepper, diced

1 red bell pepper, diced

4 ounces diced or sliced button mushrooms

1 tablespoon Worcestershire sauce*

2 cups beef bone broth (I like Dr. Kellyann Bone Broth)*

8 ounces rotini or shell pasta, regular or gluten-free

¾ cup fat-free milk

1 cup chopped provolone cheese, shredded mozzarella, or shredded cheddar (about 4 ounces)

*Read the label to be sure this product is gluten-free.

Per Serving (generous 1½ cups) | Calories 492 | **Protein 43 g** | Carbohydrate 53 g | Fiber 5 g | Sugars 7 g | Fat 12 g | Saturated Fat 6 g | Cholesterol 66 mg | Sodium 866 mg

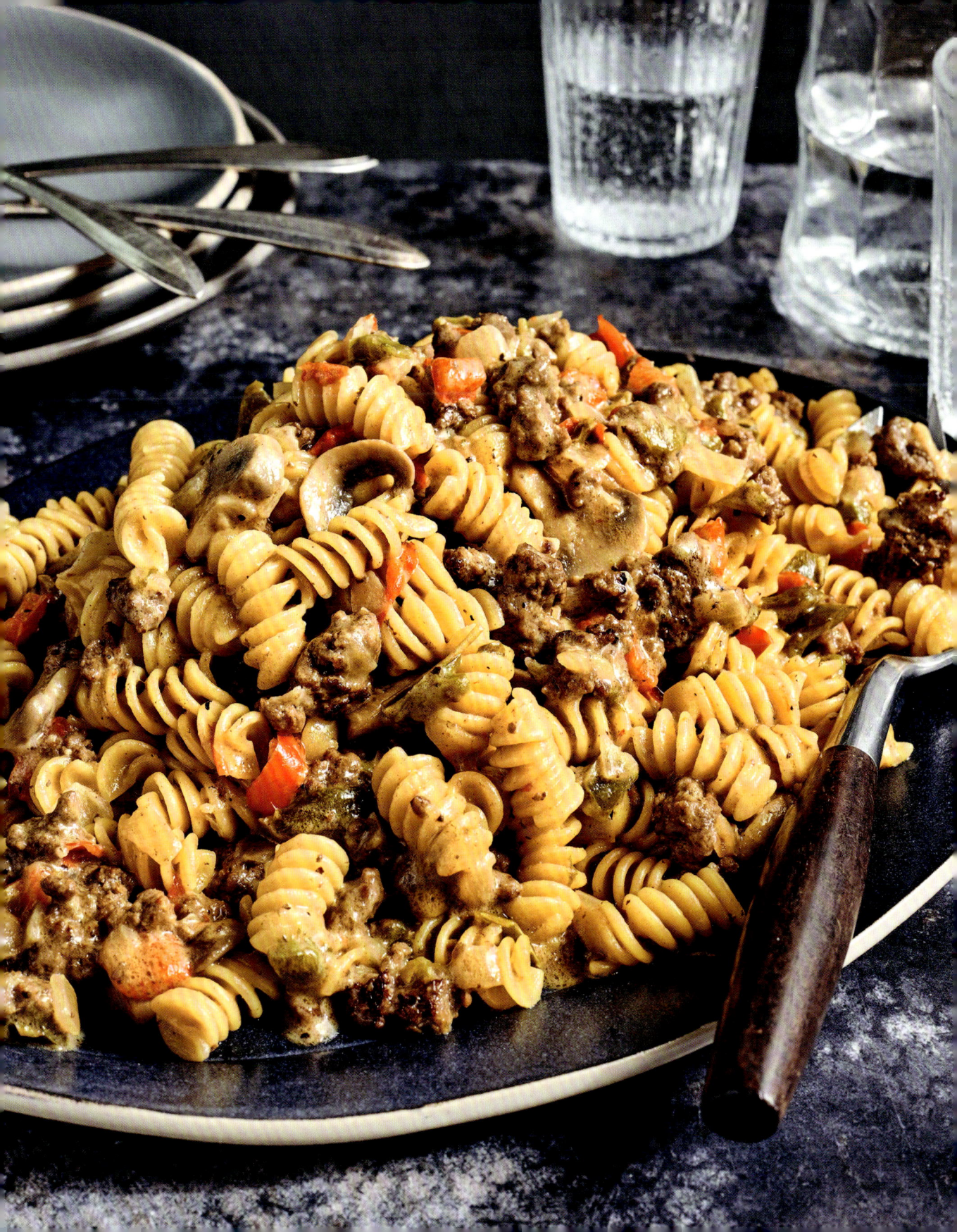

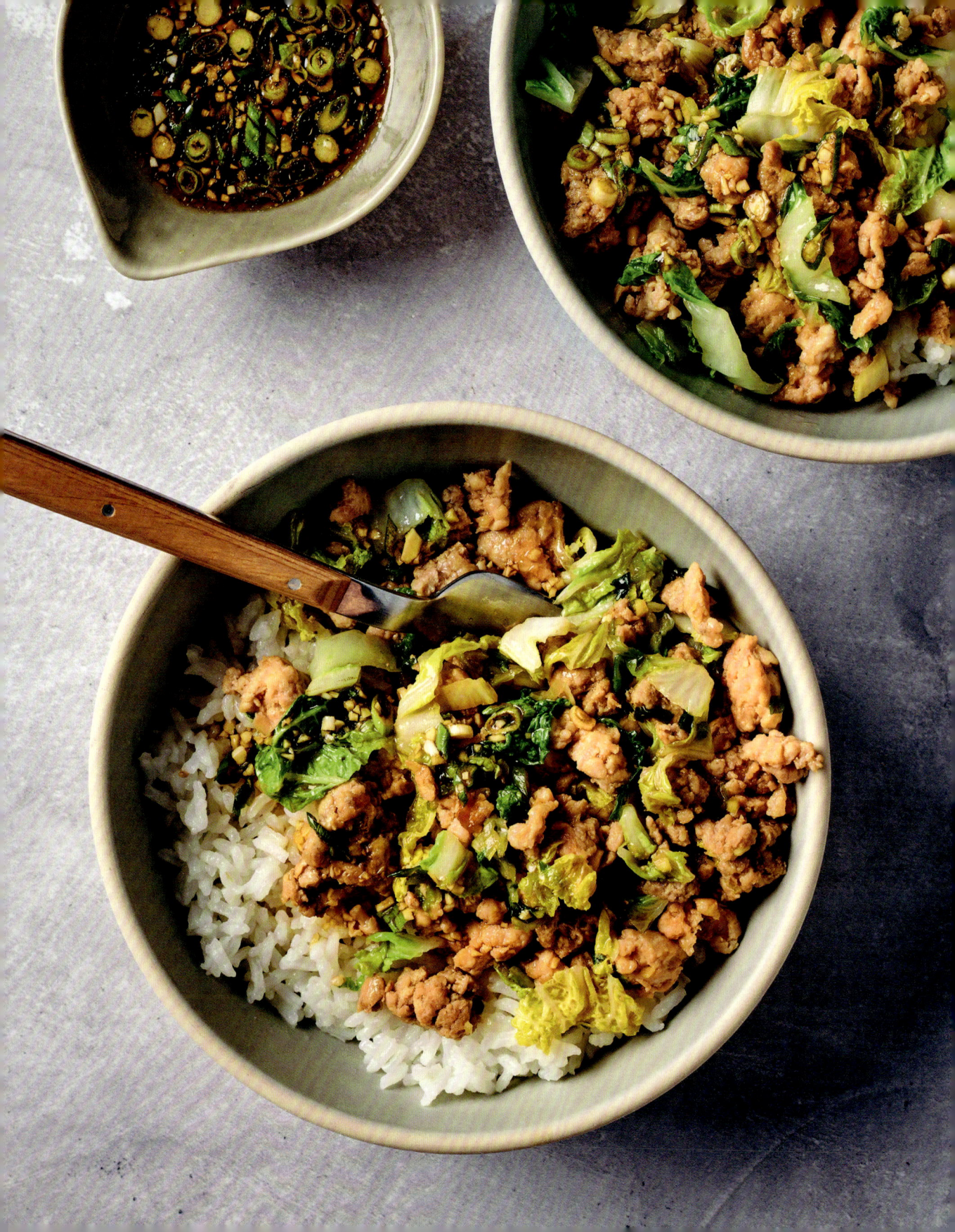

POTSTICKER RICE BOWLS

I'm so excited to share this simplified version of potstickers with you! Normally this delicious potsticker filling of meat, cabbage, ginger, sesame, and scallions would be wrapped in dumpling dough and pan-fried. But by serving this filling over rice instead, you get all those flavors, while turning dumplings into a main dish! Pork dumplings are my absolute favorite, but since ground pork tends to be pretty high in fat, I combined it with leaner chicken, which worked wonderfully. Tommy loves my dumpling sauce, and it's a must for drizzling on top of these bowls.

MAKE THE DUMPLING SAUCE: In a small bowl, combine the soy sauce, sweetener, vinegar, sesame oil, garlic, and scallion.

MAKE THE POTSTICKER "FILLING:" Heat a large deep skillet over medium heat. Add the sesame oil, ground pork, and ground chicken and cook, breaking the meat up into small pieces, until browned and cooked through, 5 to 6 minutes.

Add the ginger, scallions, soy sauce, and rice wine and mix well. Stir in the cabbage and cook until tender, 4 to 5 more minutes.

ASSEMBLE THE BOWLS: Spoon ¾ cup rice into each of four bowls and top with 1 cup of the pork filling. Drizzle with the dumpling sauce and serve.

Per Serving (1¾ cups) | Calories 504 | **Protein 32 g** | Carbohydrate 41 g | Fiber 2 g | Sugars 4 g | Fat 23 g | Saturated Fat 6.5 g | Cholesterol 121 mg | Sodium 1,330 mg

SERVES 4

DUMPLING SAUCE

2 tablespoons reduced-sodium soy sauce or gluten-free tamari

¾ teaspoon monk fruit sweetener or sugar

1½ tablespoons seasoned rice vinegar

1½ teaspoons toasted sesame oil

1 small garlic clove, grated

1 small scallion, finely chopped (about 2 tablespoons)

POTSTICKER "FILLING"

2 teaspoons toasted sesame oil

½ pound ground pork

¾ pound ground chicken (92% lean)

1½ tablespoons grated fresh ginger or ginger paste

⅓ cup chopped scallions

2 tablespoons reduced-sodium soy sauce or gluten-free tamari

1½ tablespoons rice wine or mirin

6 cups roughly chopped napa cabbage (8 ounces)

BOWLS

3 cups cooked white rice

SUNDAY POT ROAST with Gravy

As the weather cools, I always find myself craving my mom's pot roast. Slow-cooked to perfection, it's melt-in-your-mouth tender, with rich, savory gravy soaking into every bite. The meat practically falls apart at the touch of a fork. Her recipe is simple but takes time, so I usually save it for lazy Sundays when I'm home and can savor the process. While my mom traditionally served her pot roast with potato pancakes and applesauce, I like to lighten it up with mashed sweet potatoes and roasted vegetables like Brussels sprouts or broccoli.

Season the beef with the salt and black pepper to taste. Place the flour in a large dish and coat the beef on both sides. Set the beef aside and reserve the remaining flour.

In a liquid measuring cup or medium bowl, dissolve the beef bouillon in 2 cups water. Whisk in the reserved flour.

Heat a large Dutch oven or deep enamel skillet over medium-high heat and add the oil. Sear the beef until browned on both sides, about 5 minutes per side. Transfer to a plate and set aside.

Add the onion to the pot and reduce the heat to medium-low. Cook, stirring constantly, until soft and golden, 5 to 8 minutes.

Return the beef to the pot, nestling it in with the onions. Pour the beef bouillon liquid into the pot, add the thyme sprigs, and bring to a boil. Reduce the heat to low, cover tightly, and cook until the meat is very tender, about 3 hours, keeping an eye on the pot and adding more water if needed.

Remove the beef and transfer to a cutting board. Let it cool so it doesn't fall apart when slicing. Using a sharp knife, slice the meat across the grain into about ⅛-inch-thick slices. Return the sliced meat to the pot, submerging the meat under the gravy.

Cook over low heat to let the flavors meld and flavor the sliced meat, about 30 more minutes. Keep warm until ready to serve. Garnish with the parsley just before serving.

SERVES 6

3 pounds trimmed beef chuck roast

1½ teaspoons kosher salt

Freshly ground black pepper

⅓ cup all-purpose or gluten-free flour

1 beef bouillon cube, such as Knorr

2 tablespoons extra-virgin olive oil

1 large onion, diced

3 sprigs of fresh thyme

1 tablespoon chopped fresh parsley, for garnish

Per Serving (6 ounces meat + gravy) | Calories 489 | **Protein 45 g** | Carbohydrate 8 g | Fiber 0 g | Sugars 1 g | Fat 31 g | Saturated Fat 12 g | Cholesterol 157 mg | Sodium 832 mg

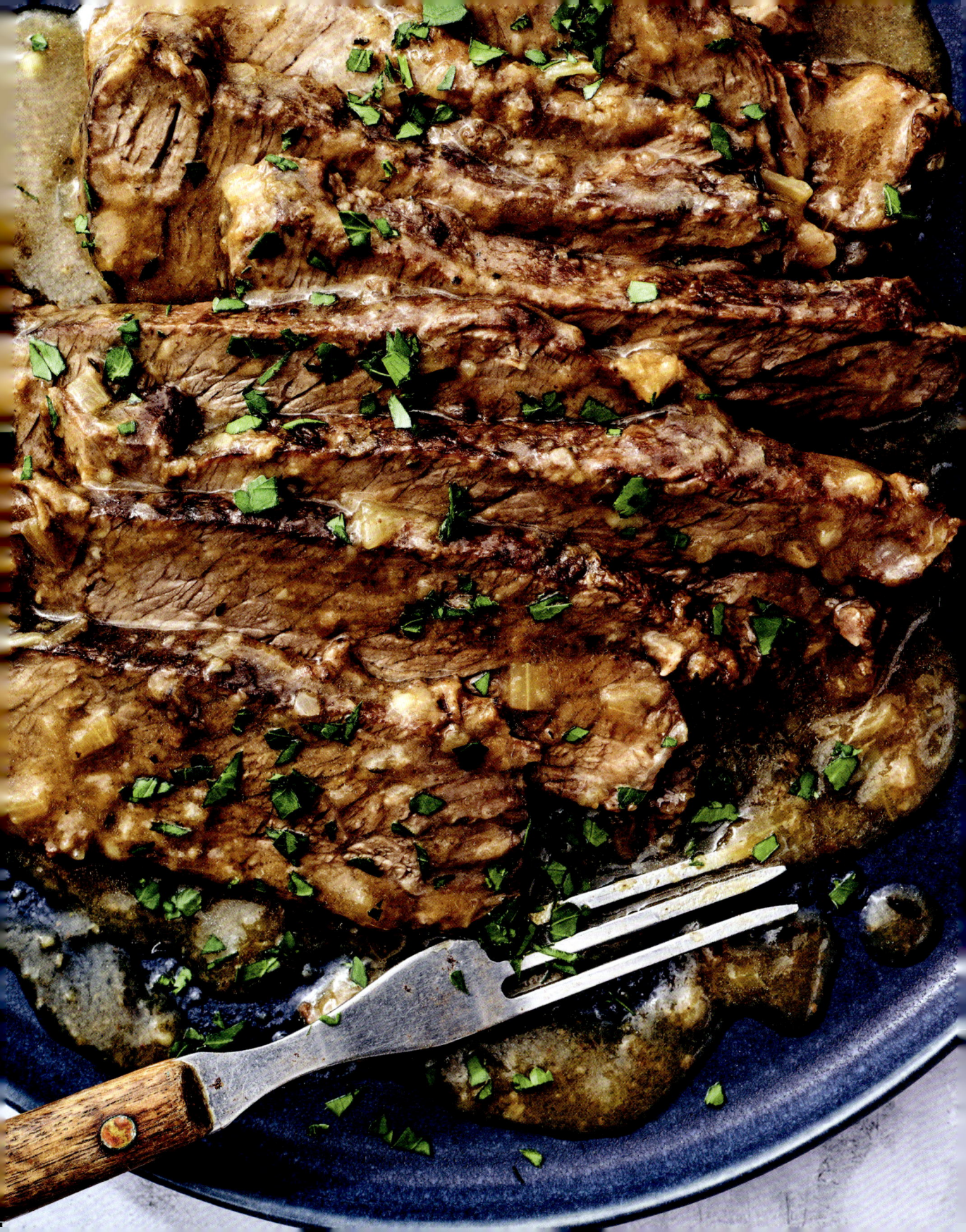

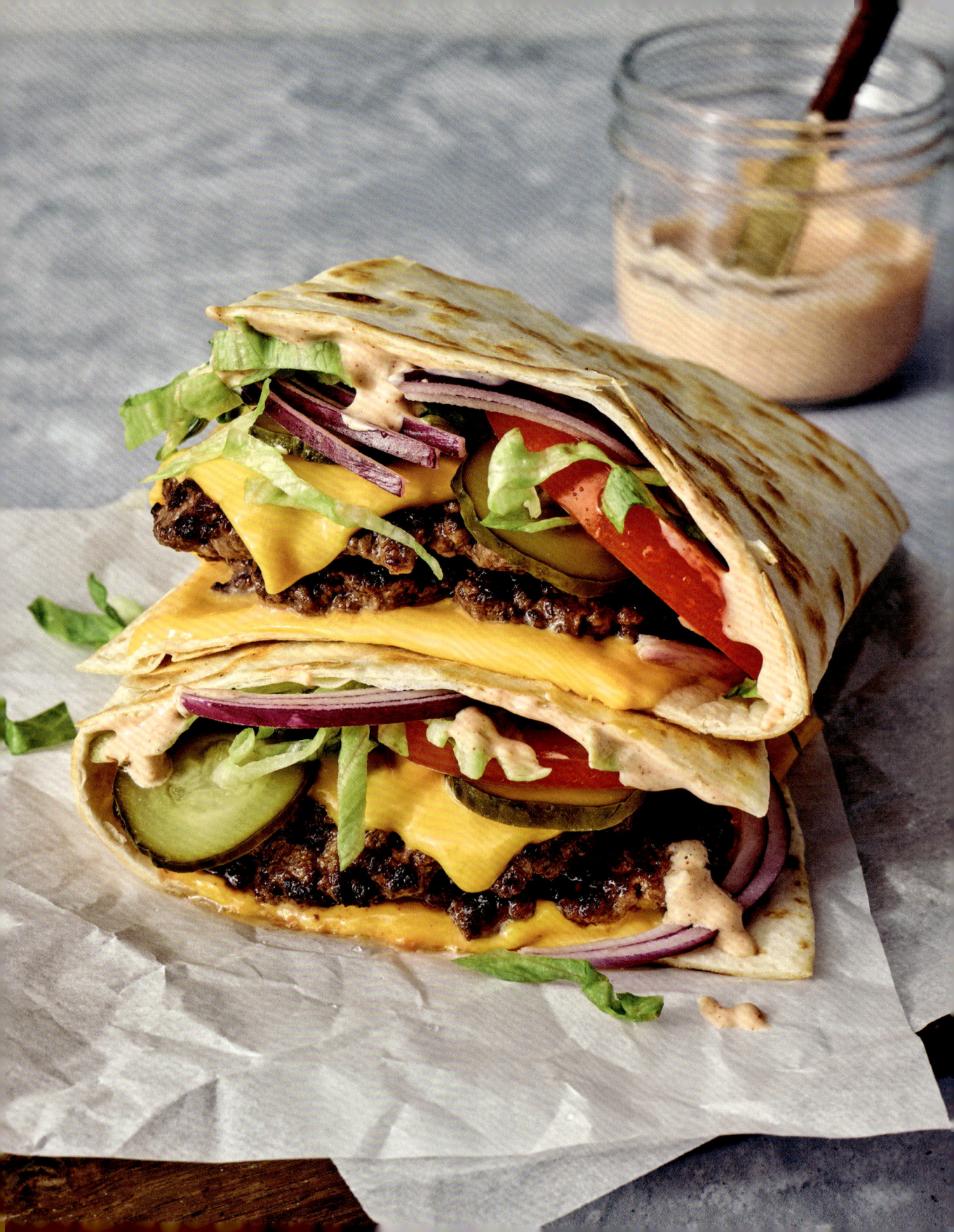

SMASH BURGERDILLA

We make smash burgers—burger patties that are literally smashed onto a hot griddle or skillet—all summer long on our Blackstone grill. One day I had the idea to serve the burgers on tortillas to lower the carbs, and the results are these delicious burger quesadillas! Burgerdillas are really fun to make and they can be customized with anything you typically put on your burger. I like topping mine with pickles, onions, ketchup, and a little mustard. Keep in mind that the meat spreads when you smash them.

Divide the beef into 8 equal portions and shape them into balls. Spray a burger press or large spatula with oil so it doesn't stick.

Heat a large skillet or griddle over medium-high heat until hot, then spray with oil. Place 4 balls of meat on the skillet, leaving plenty of space in between the balls for the meat to spread when smashed (if using a skillet, you may have to cook in smaller batches). Using the greased burger press or spatula, firmly smash each ball flat (about ¼ inch thick), then season each with half of the salt and some black pepper to taste. Cook, undisturbed, until the patties are browned and crisp on the bottom, 1 to 2 minutes. Flip and season each with the remaining salt.

On the other side of the griddle or in a large nonstick skillet, place the tortilla halves over medium-high heat (in batches as needed). Top each with 1 slice of cheese, 2 burger patties, and another slice of cheese, then fold in half to form a quesadilla. Cook until the tortilla is slightly browned and the cheese is melted, 30 to 60 seconds on each side.

Add the pickles, onions, and any toppings you desire and serve immediately.

SERVES 4

1 pound ground sirloin (90% lean) or ground meat of choice

Olive oil spray

1 teaspoon kosher salt

Freshly ground black pepper

2 (10-inch) low-carb flour tortillas or gluten-free tortillas, cut in half

8 slices cheddar or American cheese

1 dill pickle, sliced into thin rounds

½ small red onion, sliced

OPTIONAL TOPPINGS

Ketchup, mustard, special sauce (see recipe, page 194), sautéed onions, sautéed mushrooms, cooked bacon, shredded lettuce, thinly sliced tomatoes

Perfect Pairings
Serve with baked sweet potato wedges or baked fries, or skip the starchy vegetables and serve with a green salad.

Per Serving (1 burgerdilla) | Calories 388 | **Protein 35 g** | Carbohydrate 9 g | Fiber 5.5 g | Sugars 0 g | Fat 26 g | Saturated Fat 12 g | Cholesterol 114 mg | Sodium 905 mg

SWEET POTATO BURGER BOWLS
with Special Sauce

Building a deconstructed burger bowl is perfect if you're craving a burger but want to skip the bread. Plus, your family or friends can pick and choose their favorite burger toppings! I like using ground bison here because it's more tender than lean ground beef, and it tastes the same to me. But feel free to make this with any ground meat you prefer. Rather than a side of fries, roasted sweet potatoes are added to the bowl, creating the perfect balance of flavors and nutrients. The special sauce is what I love putting on my burgers at home, and it works great as a dressing.

ROAST THE SWEET POTATOES: Preheat the oven to 425°F. Lightly spray a sheet pan with oil.

In a medium bowl, toss the sweet potatoes with the olive oil, salt, garlic powder, and black pepper to taste. Spread out in an even layer on the prepared sheet pan and transfer to the oven.

Bake until tender, golden, and browned on the edges, 25 to 30 minutes, tossing every 10 to 15 minutes.

MEANWHILE, MAKE THE SPECIAL SAUCE: In a small bowl, combine the mayonnaise, yellow mustard, ketchup, barbecue sauce, onion powder, garlic powder, paprika, and dill pickle juice and mix well. (Makes about ½ cup.)

FOR THE BOWLS: Heat a large skillet over medium-high heat. When hot, spray with oil and add the ground bison, salt, garlic powder, and pepper to taste. Cook, undisturbed, until it starts to brown, 2 to 3 minutes. Continue cooking, breaking up the meat, for 5 to 6 minutes until cooked through.

Divide the lettuce among four large shallow bowls or plates. Top with the cooked bison, sweet potatoes, tomatoes, red onion, and pickles. Drizzle each with 2 tablespoons sauce and serve immediately.

Per Serving (1 bowl) | Calories 382 | **Protein 32 g** | Carbohydrate 30 g | Fiber 5 g | Sugars 11 g | Fat 16 g | Saturated Fat 5 g | Cholesterol 80 mg | Sodium 887 mg

SERVES 4

ROASTED SWEET POTATOES

Olive oil spray

2 medium sweet potatoes (14 ounces), peeled and cut into ¾-inch cubes

1½ teaspoons extra-virgin olive oil

¼ teaspoon kosher salt

½ teaspoon garlic powder

Freshly ground black pepper

SPECIAL SAUCE

¼ cup light mayonnaise

1 teaspoon yellow mustard

2 tablespoons ketchup

1½ teaspoons barbecue sauce

¼ teaspoon onion powder

¼ teaspoon garlic powder

¼ teaspoon sweet paprika

1 teaspoon dill pickle brine

BOWLS

1¼ pounds 90% lean ground grass-fed bison, beef, or turkey

1 teaspoon kosher salt

½ teaspoon garlic powder

Freshly ground black pepper

4 cups chopped iceberg or romaine lettuce

1 cup cherry tomatoes, halved

½ medium red onion, thinly sliced

1 dill pickle, chopped or sliced

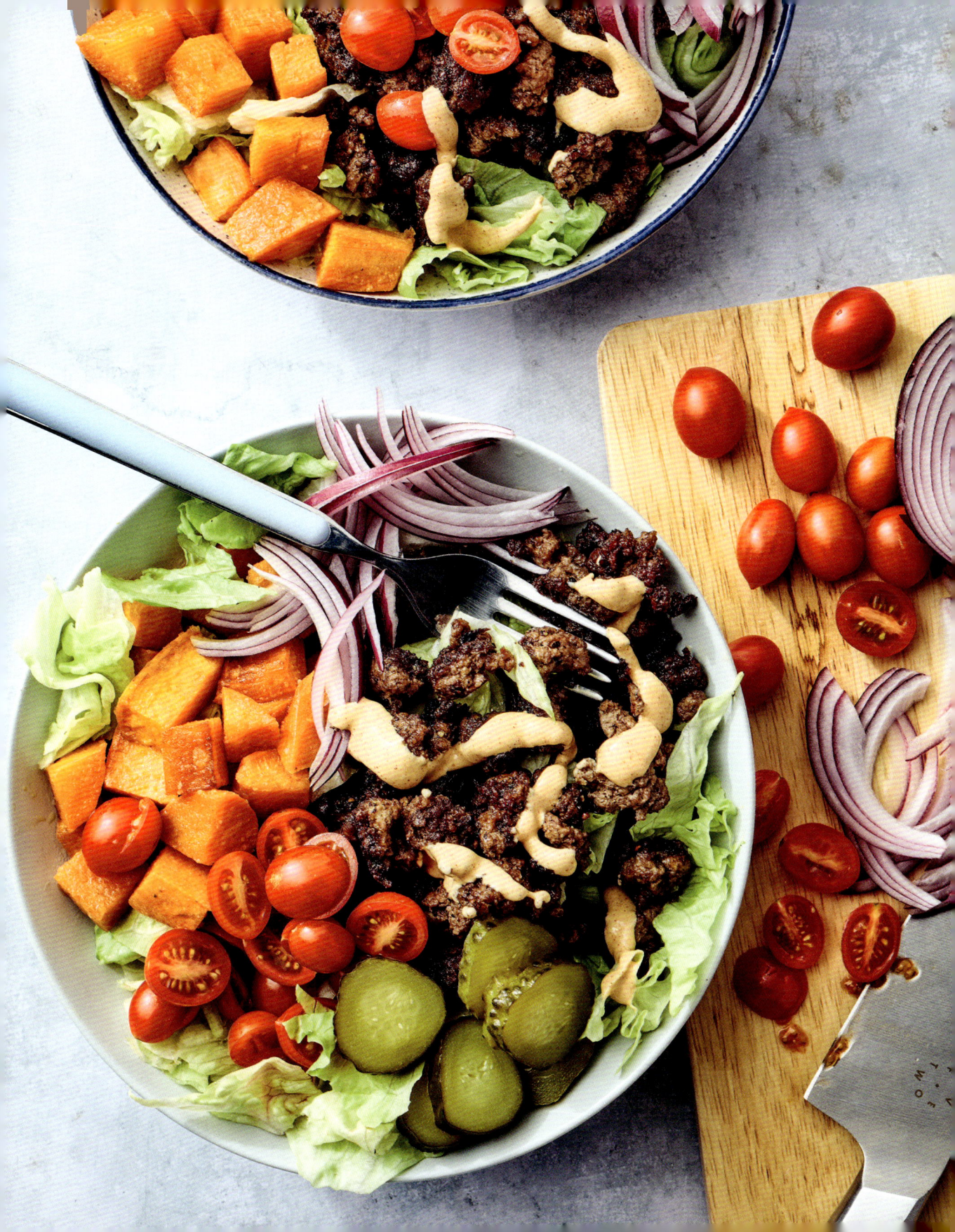

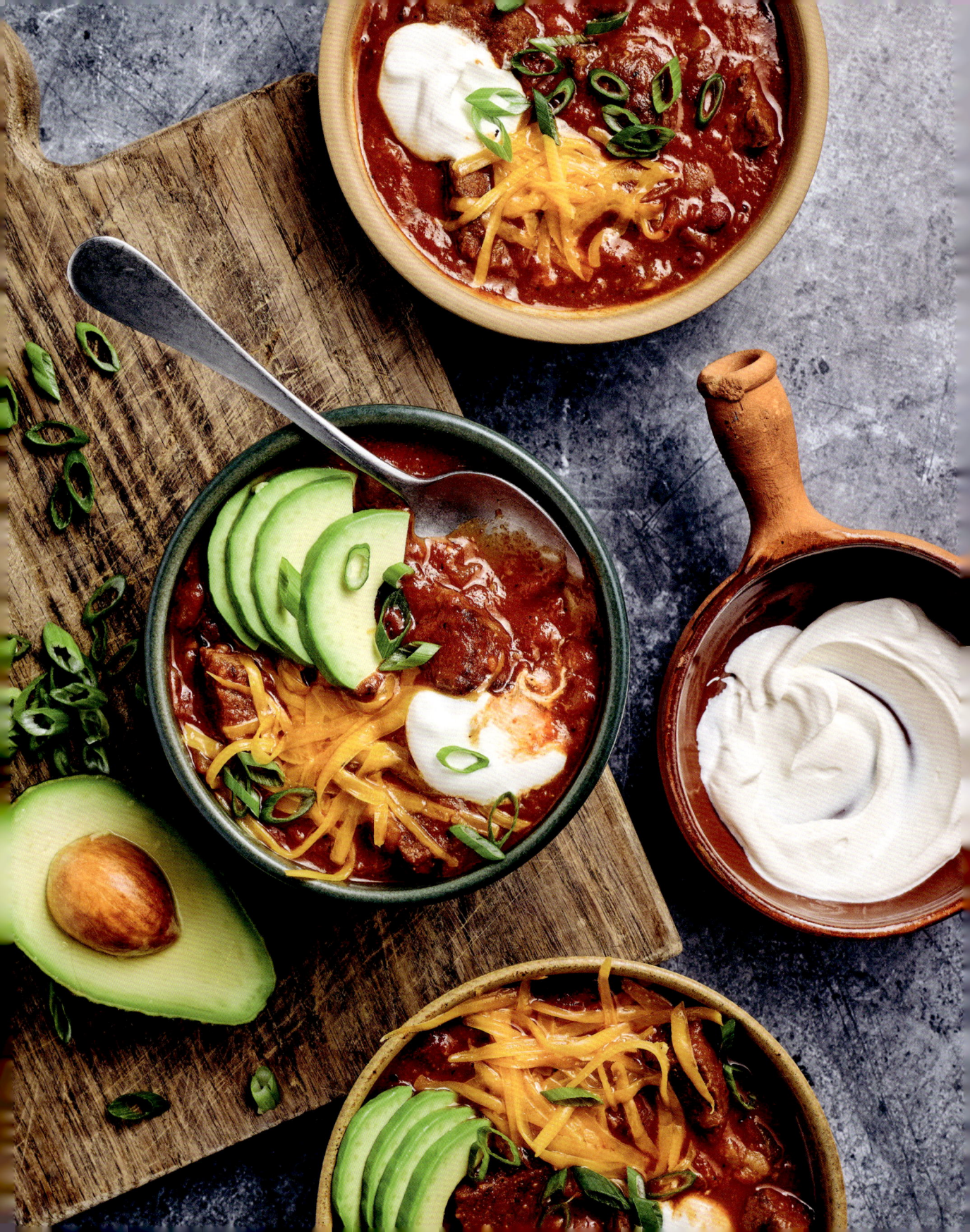

SLOW COOKER CHILI CON CARNE

Want to know the secret to the perfect chili? Low and slow cooking—and your slow cooker is the ideal tool for the job. This slow-cooked chili is sure to become your go-to, with each bite packing bold and savory flavors. The longer the chili simmers, the richer and deeper the flavors become, transforming the beef into melt-in-your-mouth tenderness. Be sure not to skip the essential step of browning the meat and veggies before adding them to the slow cooker—this small detail makes all the difference. For an extra layer of smokiness, I used fire-roasted tomatoes. This recipe makes a big batch of chili—perfect for leftovers the next day or to stash in the freezer for an easy, delicious meal down the road.

In a small bowl, combine the chili powder, cumin, smoked paprika, onion powder, and garlic powder.

In a large bowl, season the beef with the salt and toss to coat completely.

Heat a large skillet over medium-high heat. When hot, spray with oil. Working in two batches, brown the beef on all sides, 3 to 4 minutes per batch. Transfer the beef to a slow cooker and repeat with the remaining beef.

In the same skillet, add the olive oil and reduce the heat to medium. Add the onions, poblano pepper, and garlic and cook, stirring, until the vegetables are soft, about 5 minutes. Add 2 tablespoons of the spice mix and cook for 1 minute, until fragrant, being careful not to burn the spices. Add the tomato paste with the remaining spice mix and cook until caramelized, another 4 to 5 minutes.

Transfer the vegetables to the slow cooker. Stir in the crushed tomatoes, beef broth, and beans and add the bay leaves. Cover and cook on high for 6 hours, or on low for 8 to 9 hours, until the meat is fork-tender. Discard the bay leaves.

(recipe continues)

SERVES 8

1 tablespoon dark chili powder

1 tablespoon ground cumin

1 tablespoon smoked paprika

½ tablespoon onion powder

1 teaspoon garlic powder

2¼ pounds trimmed beef chuck roast, cut into ½-inch cubes

2 teaspoons kosher salt

Olive oil spray

1½ teaspoons extra-virgin olive oil

2 medium onions, chopped (about 2 cups)

1 large poblano pepper, seeded and chopped

3 garlic cloves, chopped

1 (6-ounce) can tomato paste

2 cups canned fire-roasted crushed tomatoes

3 cups low-sodium beef broth*

1 (15-ounce) can kidney beans,* rinsed and drained

3 bay leaves

¼ cup masa harina

Optional toppings: shredded cheddar cheese, sour cream, chopped fresh cilantro, sliced avocado, or scallions

*Read the label to be sure this product is gluten-free.

Per Serving (1¼ cups) | Calories 380 | **Protein 33 g** | Carbohydrate 28 g | Fiber 7 g | Sugars 6 g | Fat 17 g | Saturated Fat 7 g | Cholesterol 88 mg | Sodium 724 mg

Remove 1 cup of the cooking liquid and place in a small bowl. Stir in the masa harina until smooth (this ensures no lumps). Return to the slow cooker and stir until well combined. Let it sit for 5 minutes to thicken.

Ladle the chili into eight bowls and serve with any toppings you desire. Serve immediately.

TO FREEZE: Let it cool and transfer to 8 freezer-safe containers. Freeze, covered, for up to 3 months. To reheat, transfer to the refrigerator overnight to thaw then reheat or reheat from frozen in 30-second intervals until heated through.

No Slow Cooker? No Problem!

To cook this in a Dutch oven, add an additional 1 cup water or broth and simmer, covered, on low heat until the meat is fork-tender, 2½ to 3 hours.

Perfect Pairings

I love serving this over a bed of fluffy rice with chopped avocado and other toppings, but you can also serve it with chips or corn bread.

INSTANT POT FRENCH DIP AU JUS

If I want to make a meal I know my whole family will love, this French dip is it. Tommy asked me to keep this on our dinner rotation, he loved it! Tender beef, caramelized onions, and melted cheese are all tucked into a toasted roll, and of course it is served "au jus," with an irresistible oniony beef broth for dipping because this sandwich has it all! Thanks to the Instant Pot, the beef becomes melt-in-your-mouth tender and cooks in half the time it would on the stove. This sandwich is great for weeknight dinners or game day, and if you're lucky, you might even have leftovers for the next day.

Cut the beef into 4 pieces and season with the salt. Press the sauté button on an electric pressure cooker. When hot, spray with oil and add the beef. Sear the pieces evenly on all sides until browned, 3 to 4 minutes. Remove the meat and set aside.

Add the olive oil and onions to the pot and cook, stirring often, until lightly caramelized, 12 to 14 minutes.

Press cancel. Add 2 cups water and stir to deglaze the bottom of the pot. Add the bouillon cube, soy sauce, soup mix, and garlic.

Return the meat to the pressure cooker. Seal and cook on high pressure for 1 hour, until the beef is fork-tender. Quick or natural release, then open when the pressure subsides. Remove the beef and keep warm. Skim the fat from the cooking liquid and discard. Shred the beef with two forks and return it to the cooking liquid until ready to serve.

When ready to serve, remove the meat and onions and place in a large bowl. Strain the liquid (the jus) through a fine-mesh sieve into another bowl and reserve for dipping.

(recipe continues)

SERVES 10

2¼ pounds trimmed chuck roast

½ teaspoon kosher salt

Olive oil spray

1 tablespoon extra-virgin olive oil

2 large sweet onions, cut into ¼-inch-thick slices

1 beef bouillon cube, such as Knorr or Maggi

2 tablespoons reduced-sodium soy sauce or gluten-free tamari

3 tablespoons Homemade Dry Onion Soup Mix (recipe follows), or 1 (1.25-ounce) envelope dry onion soup mix

1 garlic clove, minced

10 Portuguese rolls, or 30 ounces French or gluten-free bread, toasted and split

10 slices provolone, Swiss, mozzarella, or nondairy cheese

Per Serving (1 sandwich + ⅓ cup jus) | Calories 543 | **Protein 36 g** | Carbohydrate 54 g | Fiber 3 g | Sugars 6 g | Fat 20 g | Saturated Fat 9 g | Cholesterol 85 mg | Sodium 1,335 mg

Preheat the boiler. Divide the meat and onions evenly among the toasted rolls (about ½ cup each). Top each roll with a slice of cheese. Transfer to a sheet pan and place under the broiler for 2 to 3 minutes to melt the cheese.

Serve the sandwiches with ⅓ cup of the jus per person on the side for dipping.

TIP: Choose good-quality rolls or French bread for the best results. If using French bread, I like to scoop out some of the inside to make a longer sandwich, aiming for a total of about 3 ounces of bread. Gluten-free rolls work just as well, and if you're dairy-free, you can simply skip the cheese or use a nondairy cheese alternative.

TO FREEZE: Transfer leftover meat and broth to a freezer-safe container. Freeze, covered, for up to 3 months. To reheat, transfer to the refrigerator to thaw or reheat from frozen in 30-second intervals until heated through.

No Instant Pot? No Problem!

To cook the beef in a Dutch oven, sauté the beef and onions as directed. Deglaze the pan as directed, adding the bouillon cube, soy sauce, soup mix, and garlic. Return the beef to the pot and bring to a boil. Reduce the heat to low, cover, and cook until the meat is fork-tender, 2½ to 3 hours.

HOMEMADE DRY ONION SOUP MIX

Use this mix in any recipe that calls for a packet of dry onion soup mix. One packet of store-bought is about 1¼ ounces or 3 tablespoons of this mix.

In a small bowl, combine the dried onion, bouillon granules, onion powder, garlic powder, pepper, paprika, and parsley. Store the mixture in an airtight container for up to 6 months.

TIP: If you want it lower in sodium, use a low-sodium beef bouillon.

Per Serving (1 tablespoon) | Calories 16 | **Protein 0 g** | Carbohydrate 2 g | Fiber 0 g | Sugars 0 g | Fat 0 g | Saturated Fat 0 g | Cholesterol 0 mg | Sodium 588 mg

Perfect Pairings
I serve this with a big green salad full of seasonal produce to balance out this meal.

MAKES 7½ TABLESPOONS

¼ cup minced dried onion

2 tablespoons beef bouillon granules, or 2 crushed beef bouillon cubes

½ teaspoon onion powder

½ teaspoon garlic powder

¼ teaspoon freshly ground black pepper

¼ teaspoon sweet paprika

¼ teaspoon dried parsley flakes

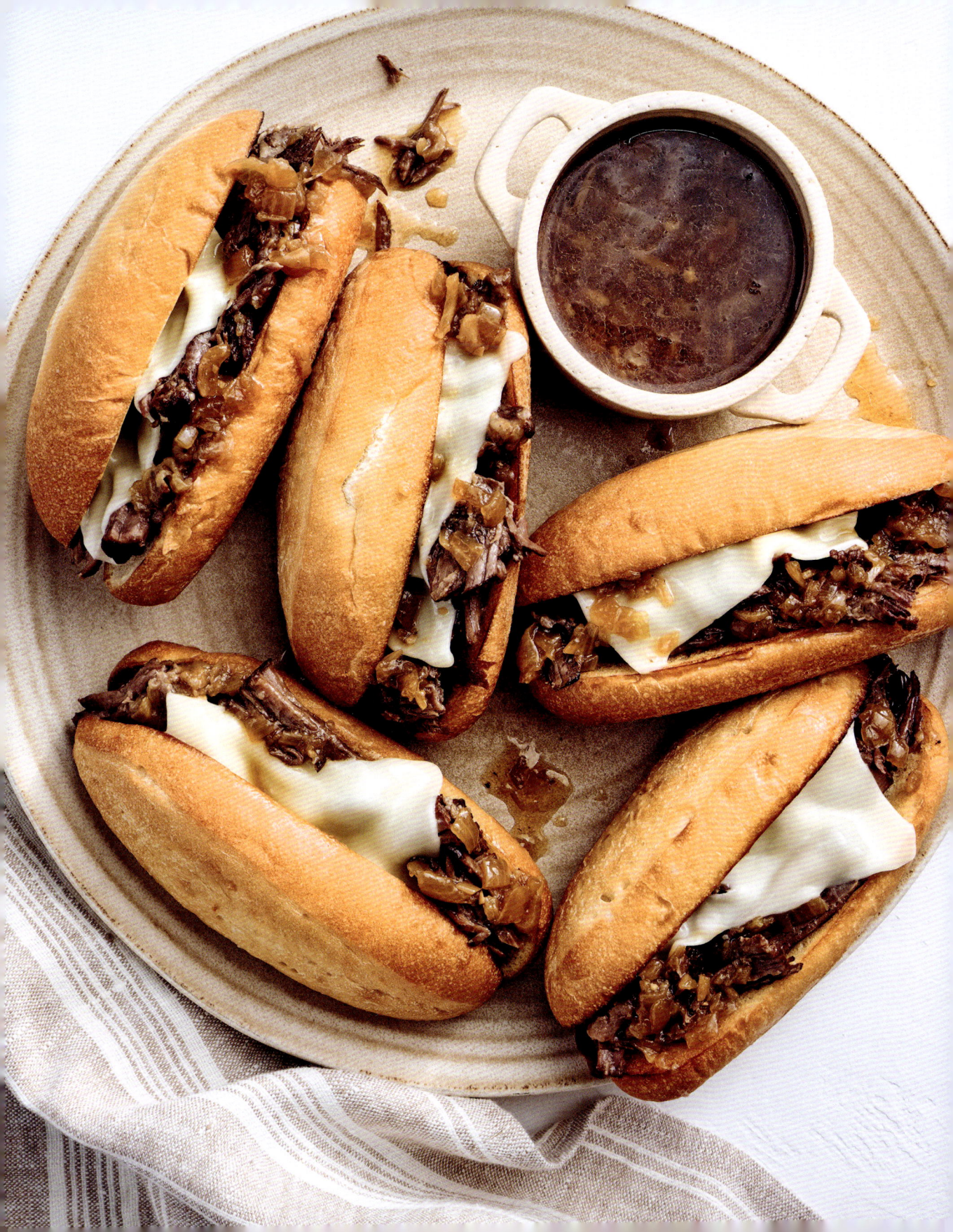

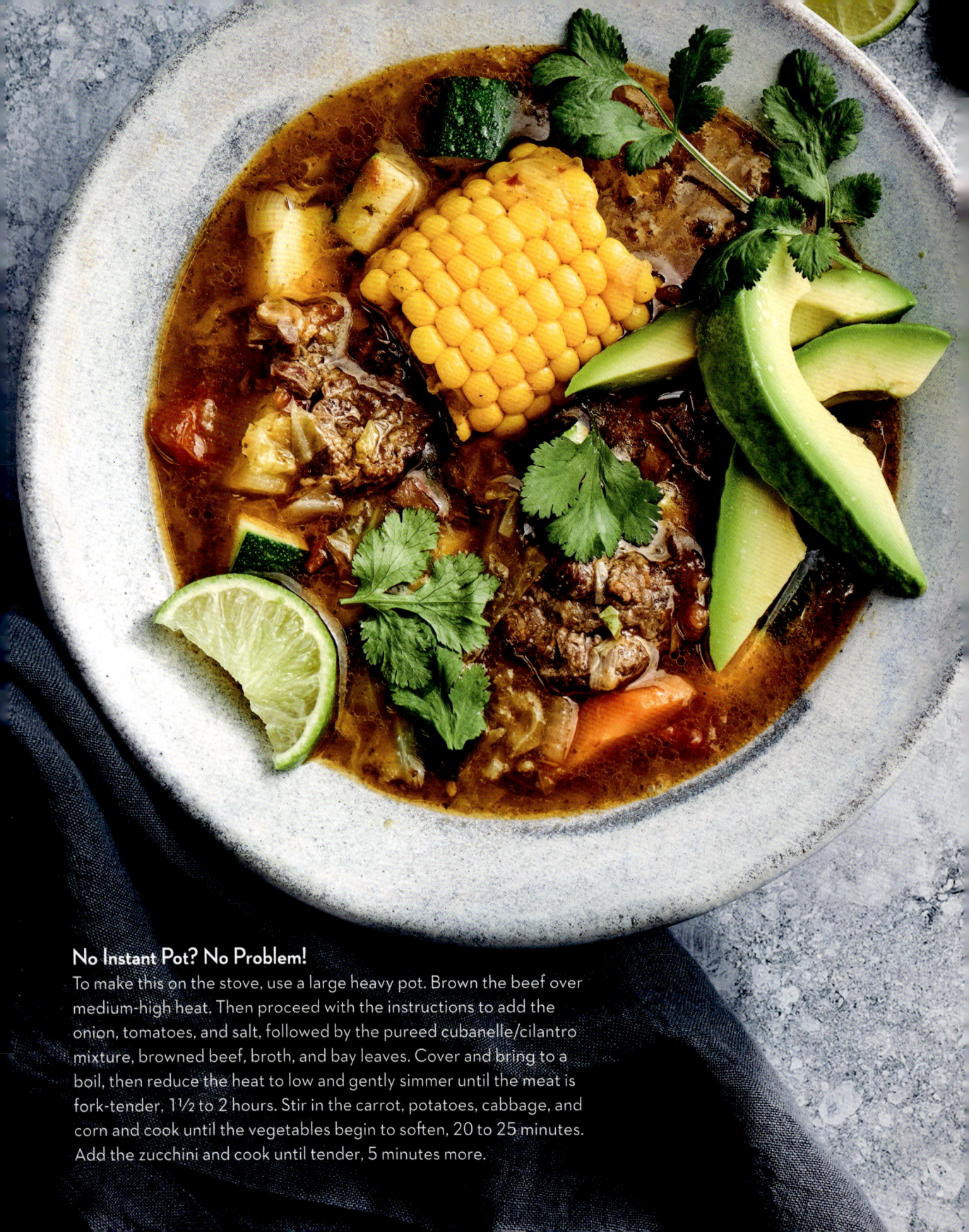

No Instant Pot? No Problem!

To make this on the stove, use a large heavy pot. Brown the beef over medium-high heat. Then proceed with the instructions to add the onion, tomatoes, and salt, followed by the pureed cubanelle/cilantro mixture, browned beef, broth, and bay leaves. Cover and bring to a boil, then reduce the heat to low and gently simmer until the meat is fork-tender, 1½ to 2 hours. Stir in the carrot, potatoes, cabbage, and corn and cook until the vegetables begin to soften, 20 to 25 minutes. Add the zucchini and cook until tender, 5 minutes more.

INSTANT POT CALDO DE RES

Mexican Beef Soup

When the weather turns cold and I'm craving a hearty, comforting soup that warms me to the bone, I love caldo de res. This Mexican beef soup is packed with tons of vegetables like cabbage, potatoes, zucchini, and corn, along with tender chunks of beef, and it's as nourishing as it is delicious.

In a blender, combine the cubanelle pepper, cilantro, beef bouillon base, 2 cups water, the garlic, and ¾ teaspoon of the salt and blend until smooth. Set aside.

Press sauté on the electric pressure cooker and heat until very hot. Spray with oil and add the beef. Cooked until browned on all sides, 4 to 5 minutes per side. Transfer to a plate and set aside.

Add the onion, tomatoes, and remaining ¼ teaspoon salt to the pot and sauté, stirring, until softened, 4 to 5 minutes.

Pour the pureed cubanelle/cilantro mixture into the pot and add the seared beef, bone broth, and bay leaves. Seal and cook on high pressure for 45 minutes. Natural release, then open when the pressure subsides.

Stir in the carrot, potatoes, cabbage, and corn. Seal and cook on high pressure for 10 minutes. Quick release, then open when the pressure subsides. The potatoes and carrot should be tender; if not, press sauté and simmer for a few more minutes.

Add the zucchini and press sauté. Partially cover and cook until the zucchini is tender, about 5 minutes. Season with salt to taste (since all brands of broth and bouillon vary in sodium levels).

Ladle the soup into large bowls. Garnish with the cilantro, squeeze lime juice over top, and serve with avocado.

TO STORE: Refrigerate for up to 4 days. To freeze, let the soup cool and freeze in freezer-safe containers for up to 6 months. In either case, prepare the cilantro, limes, and avocado just before serving.

Per Serving (1¾ cups soup + 1 piece corn + 2 ounces avocado) | Calories 354 | **Protein 40 g** | Carbohydrate 26 g | Fiber 7.5 g | Sugars 7 g | Fat 11 g | Saturated Fat 2.5 g | Cholesterol 44 mg | Sodium 816 mg

SERVES 6

1 cubanelle pepper, stemmed and seeded

1 cup loosely packed fresh cilantro, plus more for garnish

1 tablespoon Better than Bouillon Beef Base

3 garlic cloves, peeled

1 teaspoon kosher salt, plus more to taste

Olive oil spray

1½ pounds trimmed bone-in beef shanks, or 1¼ pounds trimmed beef chuck, cut into 1-inch cubes

1 small onion, chopped

2 Roma tomatoes, diced

4 cups beef bone broth*

3 bay leaves

1 medium carrot, cut into ¼-inch pieces

1 medium yellow potato (6 ounces), peeled and cut into 1-inch cubes

1 small green cabbage, cored and roughly chopped

2 ears corn, husked and cut into thirds

1 medium zucchini, cut into ½-inch cubes (about 1½ cups)

FOR SERVING

2 limes, cut into wedges

8 ounces avocado (2 small Hass), cut into wedges

*Read the label to be sure this product is gluten-free.

SPICED YOGURT-MARINATED LAMB CHOPS

Yogurt makes a great marinade for meats like lamb because the lactic acid in the yogurt tenderizes the meat and keeps it moist during cooking. I love the flavors of Indian cuisine, so here I've seasoned the marinade with warm, bold Indian spices like curry powder and garam masala. The lamb chops stay juicy after grilling, and the cilantro topping adds the perfect fresh contrast to the richness of the dish.

MARINATE THE LAMB: Season the lamb chops with the salt and black pepper to taste. In a large bowl, stir together the yogurt, garlic, ginger, lemon juice, curry powder, garam masala, and turmeric. Add the lamb chops and spread the spiced yogurt mixture over them to coat. Cover and marinate at room temperature for least 30 minutes or in the refrigerator as long as overnight.

MAKE THE CILANTRO TOPPING: When ready to cook, in a medium bowl, combine the cilantro, red onion, lime juice, jalapeño, and salt.

Preheat a grill or grill pan to medium heat. Remove most of the marinade from the lamb chops with the back of a spoon and discard. Oil the grill or grill pan and add the chops. Cook until a thermometer inserted in the side of each chop registers 145°F for medium-rare, about 5 minutes per side, or longer to your preferred doneness.

Place 2 chops on each of four plates and top with the cilantro mixture. Spoon ¾ cup rice and 1 sliced cucumber alongside.

SERVES 4

LAMB

8 lamb loin chops (about 3½ ounces each)

¾ teaspoon kosher salt

Freshly ground black pepper

¼ cup whole-milk plain yogurt (not Greek)

3 garlic cloves, minced

1 teaspoon grated fresh ginger or ginger paste

2 tablespoons fresh lemon juice

1 teaspoon curry powder

1 teaspoon garam masala

½ teaspoon ground turmeric

Olive oil spray

CILANTRO TOPPING

⅓ cup roughly chopped fresh cilantro

¼ small red onion, thinly sliced

2 tablespoons fresh lime juice

1 small jalapeño pepper, sliced into rounds, including seeds

¼ teaspoon kosher salt, or more to taste

FOR SERVING

3 cups cooked basmati rice

4 Persian (mini) cucumbers, sliced

Per Serving (2 chops + ¼ cup topping + ¾ cup rice + 1 sliced cucumber) | Calories 447 | **Protein 45 g** | Carbohydrate 39 g | Fiber 1.5 g | Sugars 2 g | Fat 11 g | Saturated Fat 4.5 g | Cholesterol 129 mg | Sodium 419 mg

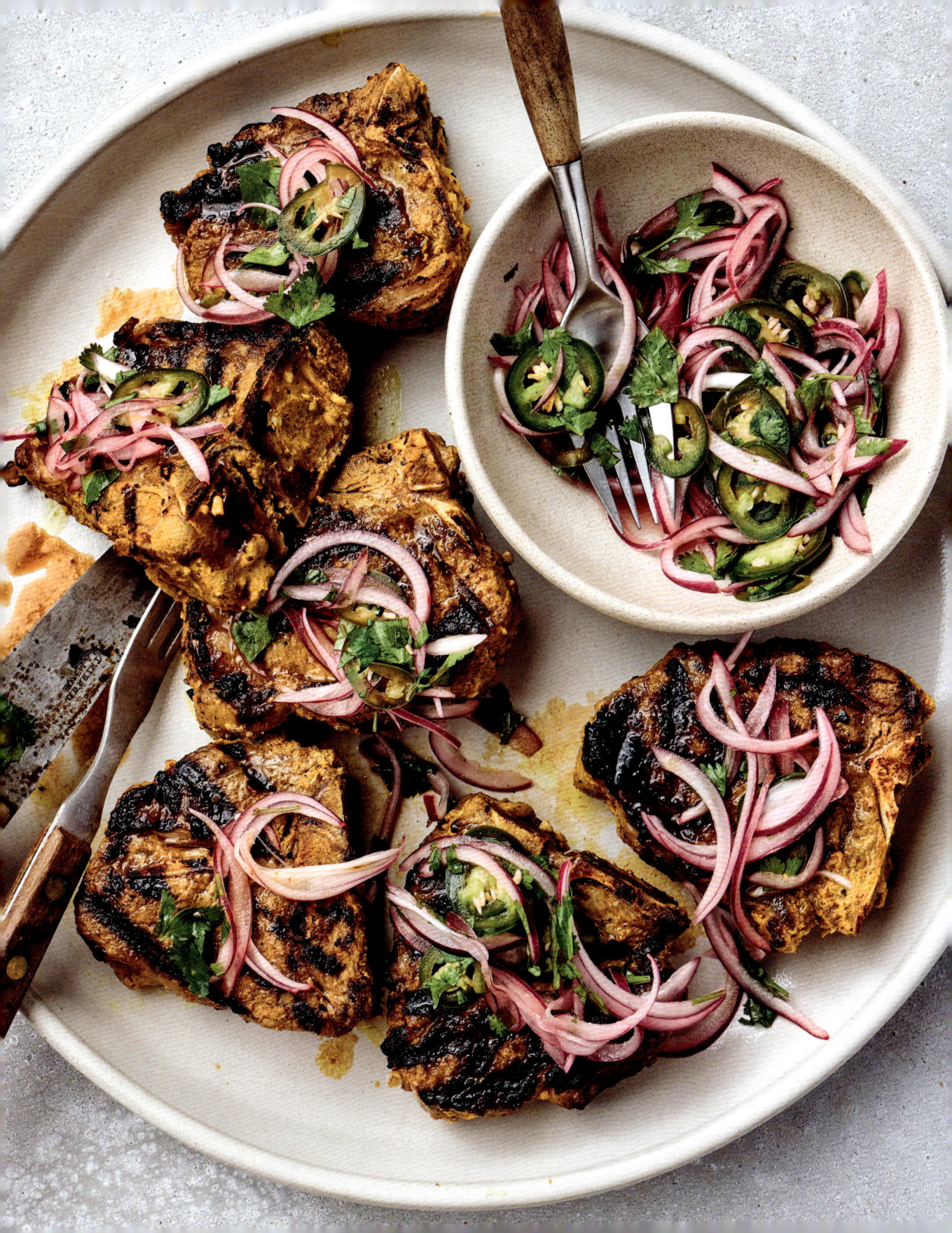

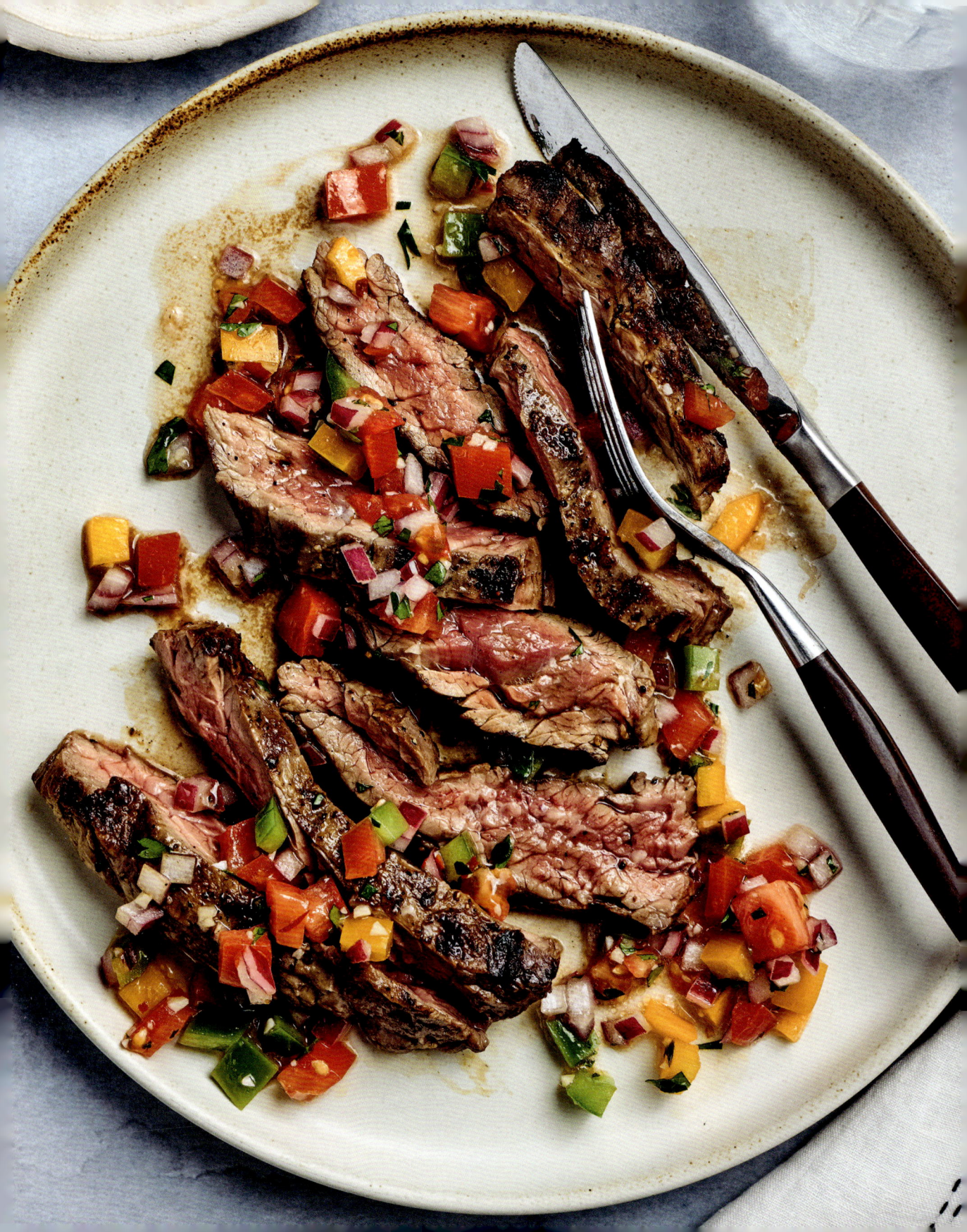

CHURRASCO with Salsa Criolla

I *love* churrasco—it's the South American name for grilled beef, and it's one of my favorite ways to enjoy steak. Growing up with Argentine relatives, we spent many a summer night firing up the grill to cook the classic meats, including skirt steak, chorizo, and morcilla. They were all served alongside chimichurri and salsa criolla—a bright, flavorful side made of tomatoes, peppers, and red onion that perfectly complements the richness of the meat. I always have the ingredients for salsa criolla in my garden, and it's so easy to whip up. The longer the salsa marinates, the better, and you can even prepare it a day ahead.

MAKE THE SALSA CRIOLLA: In a small bowl, combine the onion, salt, garlic, and vinegar and let sit for 5 minutes to mellow out the onion.

Add the tomato and its juices, the bell pepper, olive oil, pepper flakes, and parsley and mix to combine. Set aside until ready to use. It's ideal to make it 3 hours ahead if time permits; if making ahead, refrigerate until ready to use.

GRILL THE STEAKS: Season the steaks with the salt and black pepper to taste and let them rest on the counter for 10 to 20 minutes before grilling.

While they rest, preheat a grill to high heat.

When the grill is hot, place the steaks on the grill and sear until nicely charred on one side, 2 to 3 minutes. Flip the steaks over and continue to grill until the internal temperature reads 135°F for medium-rare, about 2 minutes, or longer to your desired doneness. Be careful not to overcook or the steak will be tough.

Remove the steaks from the grill and let them rest for 5 to 7 minutes. Serve topped with the salsa criolla or on the side.

Per Serving (1 piece of steak + ⅓ cup salsa) | Calories 279 | **Protein 31 g** | Carbohydrate 3 g | Fiber 1 g | Sugars 2 g | Fat 16 g | Saturated Fat 5 g | Cholesterol 91 mg | Sodium 517 mg

SERVES 4

SALSA CRIOLLA

¼ medium red onion, finely diced

½ teaspoon kosher salt

1 garlic clove, minced

1 tablespoon red wine vinegar

1 medium vine tomato, diced

½ cup diced bell pepper (I use a mix of green and yellow)

1 tablespoon extra-virgin olive oil

⅛ teaspoon crushed red pepper flakes

1 tablespoon chopped fresh parsley

STEAK

1¼ pounds skirt steak, trimmed of fat and cut into 4 pieces

1 teaspoon kosher salt, plus more to taste

Freshly ground black pepper

Perfect Pairings
A simple mixed salad with lettuce, tomatoes, and onions, dressed with olive oil and vinegar, is a fresh, easy option. Alternatively, grill some vegetables like bell peppers, onions, eggplant, and zucchini alongside the meat for a delicious side. For a starchy accompaniment, consider rice, potatoes, or crusty bread.

INSTANT POT UZBEK PLOV

My husband, Tommy, who grew up in Queens, New York, introduced me to Uzbek cuisine by bringing me home samsa, a flaky, lamb-filled pastry, from his favorite Uzbek restaurant. But the real surprise came when he accidentally received the delicious rice dish plov (also known as osh or pilaf) in one of his orders. As a rice lover, I was so obsessed with this dish that I just had to re-create it at home, and now it's on regular rotation in our household! While it's traditionally made with lamb, I found that beef chuck works just as well. Using my Instant Pot makes the dish ready quicker, and I love that it's a one-pot meal—hearty, flavorful, and perfect for busy nights.

In a large bowl, season the meat with 1 teaspoon of the salt, the ground cumin, and black pepper. Press the sauté button on an electric pressure cooker and spray with oil. Sear the meat until browned on all sides, 4 to 5 minutes. Set the meat aside.

Add the onions to the pot and cook until soft and golden brown, 5 to 8 minutes. Return the meat to the pot. Add 1 cup water, the bone broth, remaining 1½ teaspoons salt, the cumin seeds, and carrots and stir to combine. Seal and cook on high pressure for 35 minutes, until the meat is tender. Natural release, then open when the pressure subsides.

Stir in the rice and chickpeas and place the garlic bulb on top, cut side down.

Cover and cook on high pressure for 4 minutes. Let the pressure release naturally for 8 minutes, then quick release. Open when the pressure subsides. Discard the garlic and fluff the rice with a fork. If the rice isn't cooked enough, cover the pot and keep it closed for 5 more minutes to let it finish steaming. Serve immediately.

SERVES 6

1⅓ pounds trimmed boneless leg of lamb or beef chuck, cut into 1-inch pieces

2½ teaspoons kosher salt

1 teaspoon ground cumin

¼ teaspoon freshly ground black pepper

Olive oil spray

2 medium yellow onions, diced

1 cup low-sodium beef bone broth*

½ teaspoon cumin seeds or coriander seeds

5 medium carrots, peeled and julienned

2 cups uncooked basmati rice

1 cup canned chickpeas, rinsed and drained

1 garlic bulb, halved horizontally

*Read the label to be sure this product is gluten-free.

Perfect Pairings
A fresh, crisp salad made with tomatoes, cucumbers, onions, and a light vinaigrette is traditionally served on the side.

Per Serving (1⅔ cups) | Calories 467 | **Protein 31 g** | Carbohydrate 71 g | Fiber 5 g | Sugars 9 g | Fat 6 g | Saturated Fat 1.5 g | Cholesterol 65 mg | Sodium 676 mg

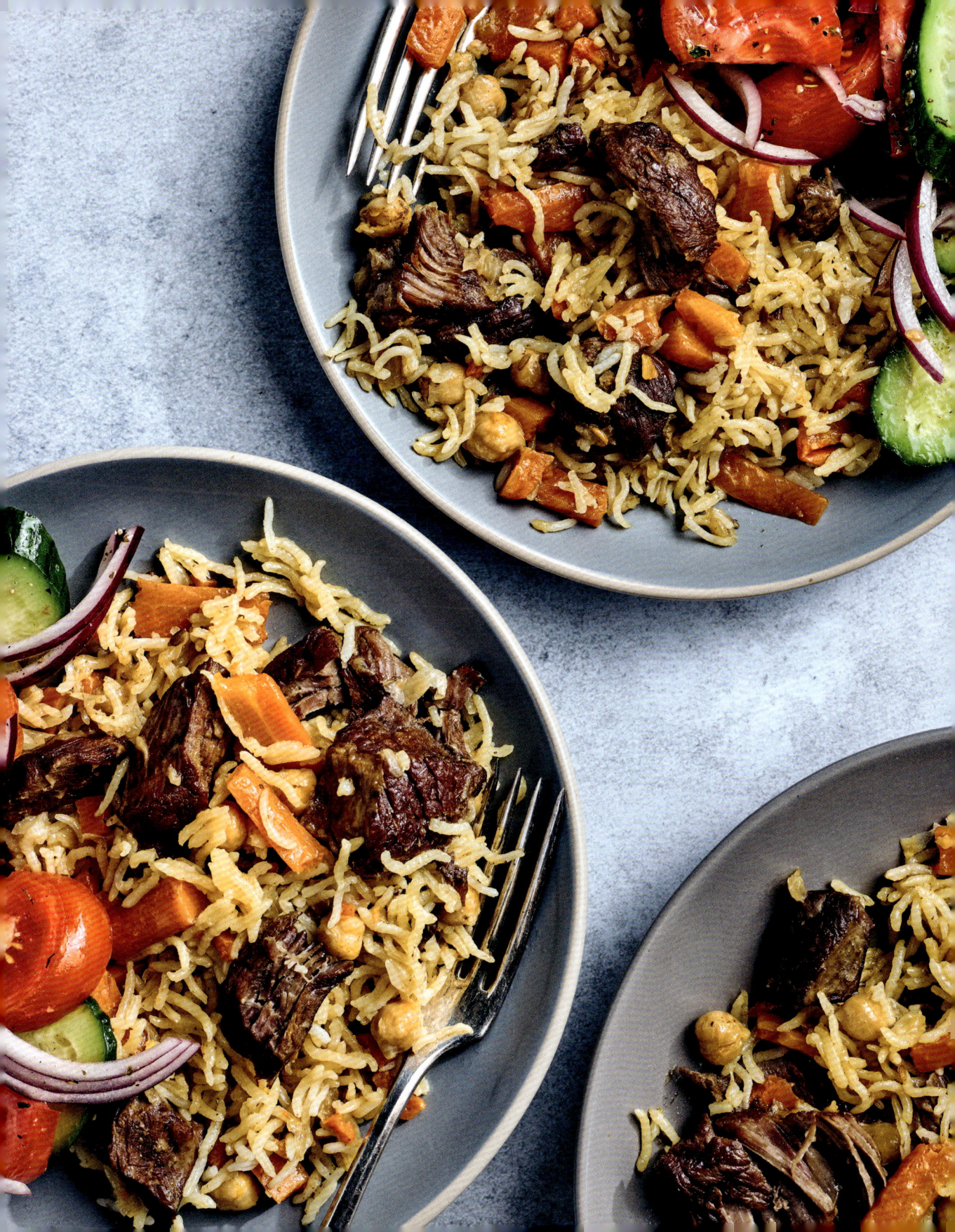

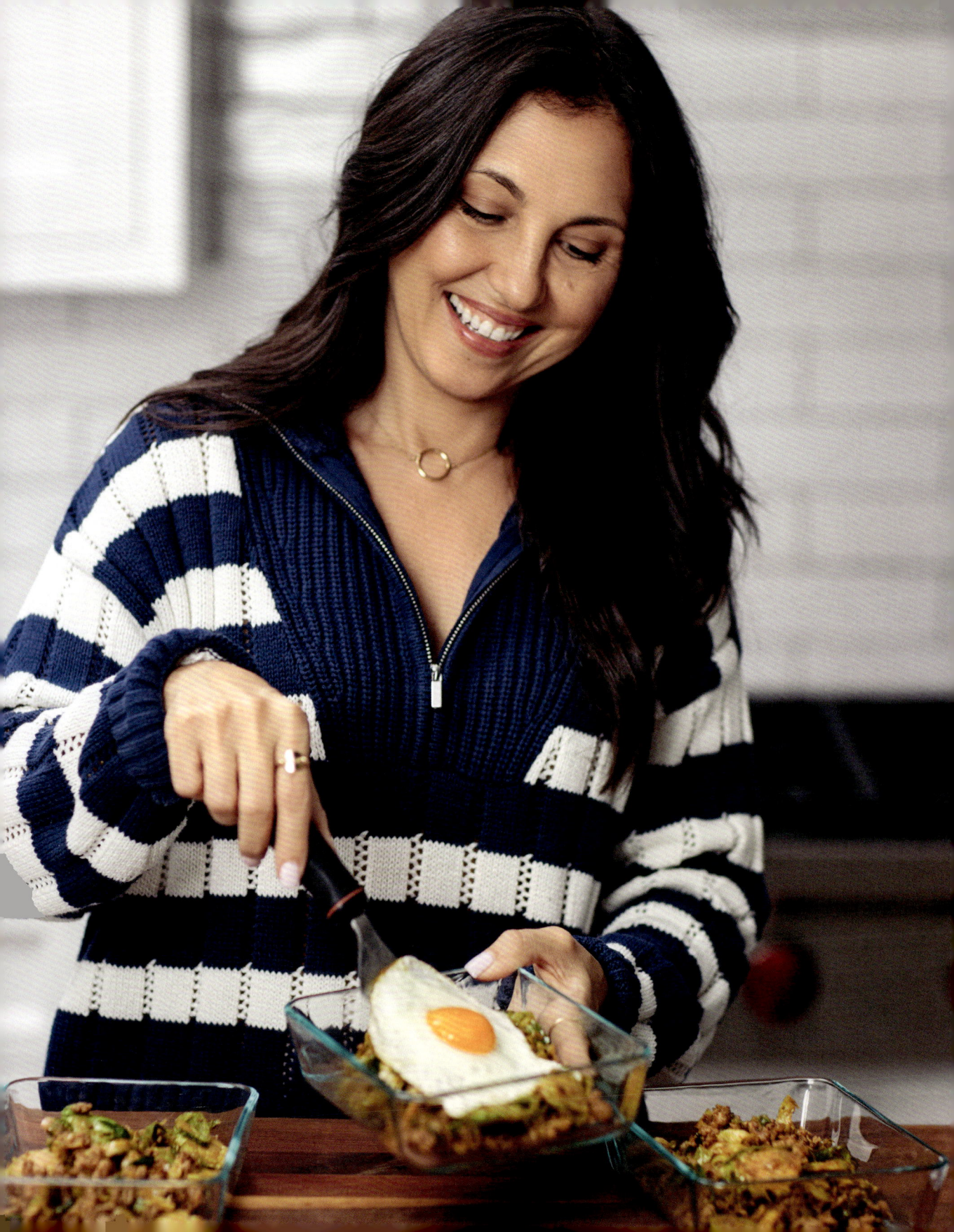

SPICY PORK BRUSSELS BOWLS

These delicious, protein-packed bowls are a fan favorite on Skinnytaste and in my house! They're a low-carb and easy-to-make dish with shredded Brussels sprouts, smoky ground pork, and a runny egg on top. I season the pork with a blend of smoky spices, but you can also change up the spices or sub out the ground pork for veggie crumbles, ground chicken, or ground turkey. If you want to meal prep this, divide it into four bowls and refrigerate up to 5 days.

In a small bowl, combine the ancho powder, smoked paprika, salt, cayenne, black pepper, oregano, and cumin.

Heat a large cast-iron or heavy nonstick skillet over medium heat and spray with oil. Add the pork and cook the meat, breaking it up in small pieces, about 5 minutes.

Add the spice mixture, garlic, and vinegar and cook until browned and no longer pink in the middle, 8 to 10 minutes. If dry, add 2 to 3 tablespoons water, as needed. Transfer to a plate and set aside.

Add the Brussels sprouts and onion to the skillet and cook over high heat, stirring occasionally, until the Brussels start to brown and are crisp-tender, 6 to 7 minutes. Return the pork to the skillet and mix everything together to warm through, 1 to 2 minutes.

Heat a nonstick skillet over medium heat and spray with oil. Add the eggs, cover, and cook until the whites are just set and the yolks are still runny, 2 to 3 minutes.

To serve, divide the Brussels pork mixture among four serving bowls or plates and top each with an egg.

SERVES 4

2 teaspoons ancho chile powder

1 teaspoon smoked paprika

1 teaspoon kosher salt

¼ teaspoon cayenne pepper

¼ teaspoon freshly ground black pepper

¼ teaspoon dried oregano

¼ teaspoon ground cumin

Olive oil spray

1 pound ground pork (90% lean), ground meat of choice, or plant-based ground "meat"

3 garlic cloves, minced

2 tablespoons red wine vinegar

6 cups shredded Brussels sprouts

¼ cup chopped onion

4 large eggs

Per Serving (1½ cups + 1 egg) | Calories 336 | **Protein 35 g** | Carbohydrate 15 g | Fiber 6 g | Sugars 4 g | Fat 17 g | Saturated Fat 5 g | Cholesterol 257 mg | Sodium 491 mg

CARNE BISTEC A CABALLO
Colombian Thin-Cut Steaks with Fried Egg

Bistec a caballo is a traditional Colombian dish that was a staple in my house growing up. The dish consists of thinly cut cut steaks served in a flavorful tomato and onion sauce and topped with a sunny-side-up egg. For me, it's the runny egg on top of the steak that truly makes the dish—I just love how the yolk creates a velvety sauce in every bite. (A caballo means "on horseback," referring to the egg served on top.) These thin steaks cook incredibly fast, needing less than a minute per side in a hot pan, so make sure everything is prepped and ready to go before you start cooking.

Season both sides of the steak slices with 1 teaspoon of the salt and the garlic powder.

Heat a large cast-iron or enamel skillet over high heat until very hot. Spray the skillet with oil. Working in batches to avoid overcrowding, add a few slices of steak at a time and cook until browned on both sides, 30 to 60 seconds per side. Set the meat aside on a plate.

Reduce the heat to medium-low and add the olive oil, onion, and ¼ teaspoon of the salt. Cook, stirring, until the onions are soft and browned, 2 to 3 minutes. Add the tomatoes and season with the remaining ¼ teaspoon salt, the cumin, and black pepper to taste. Add ½ cup water and simmer for a few minutes, until the tomatoes get saucy, adding more water if needed.

Return the meat to the skillet along with their juices and combine well with the sauce. Remove from the heat and keep covered to stay warm.

Heat a large nonstick skillet over medium-high heat. Spray with oil and add the eggs. Reduce the heat to medium-low, cover, and cook until the whites are set and the yolks are still runny, or to your desired doneness, 3 to 4 minutes. Divide the meat and tomato sauce among 4 serving plates and top each with a fried egg. Serve immediately.

SERVES 4

1¼ pounds sirloin tip steak, very thinly sliced

1½ teaspoons kosher salt

½ teaspoon garlic powder

Olive oil spray

1 tablespoon extra-virgin olive oil

1 medium onion, halved and thinly sliced into semicircles

2 large or 3 medium vine tomatoes, halved and thinly sliced into semicircles

½ teaspoon ground cumin

Freshly ground black pepper

4 large eggs

Perfect Pairings
I always love this with cooked white rice, but my mom also served it with roasted potatoes or oven fries. A simple salad of lettuce and avocado on the side pairs really well with this, too.

Per Serving (4 ounces steak + sauce + 1 egg) | Calories 333 | **Protein 38 g** | Carbohydrate 7 g | Fiber 1.5 g | Sugars 4 g | Fat 16 g | Saturated Fat 4.5 g | Cholesterol 273 mg | Sodium 574 mg

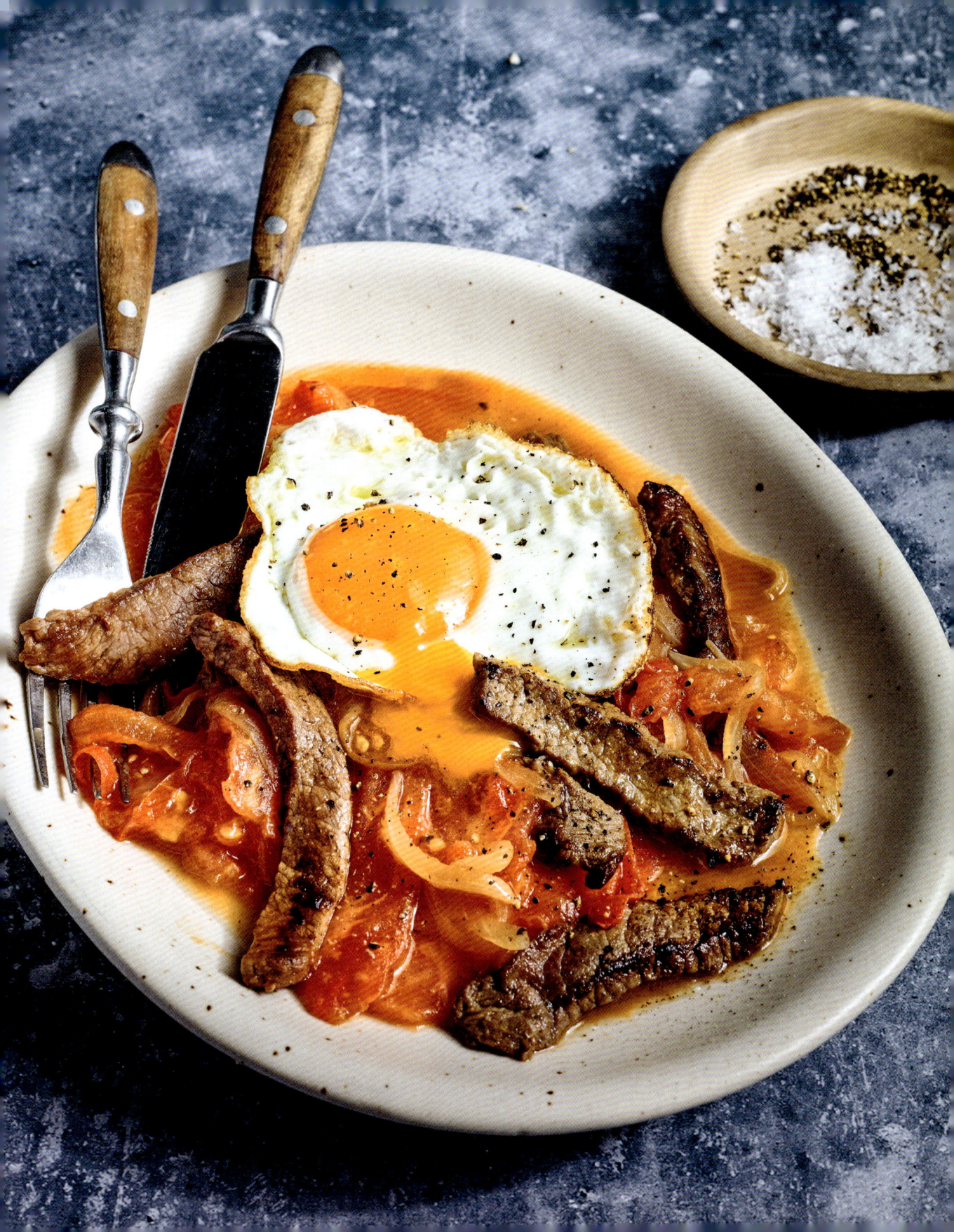

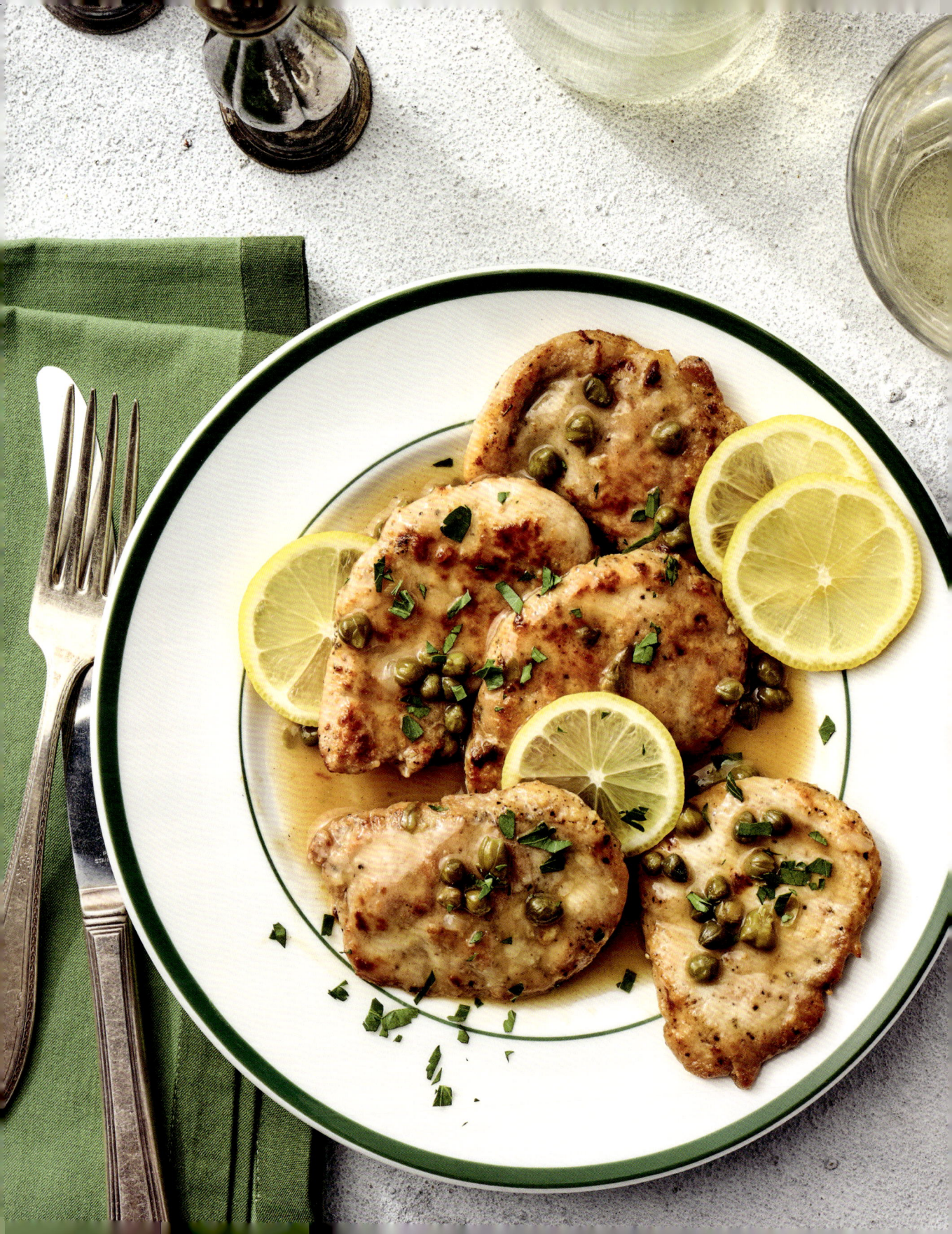

PORK TENDERLOIN PICCATA

If you're looking for a dish that's elegant yet quick enough to make any night of the week, this dish is a winner. It's a family favorite. My daughter Madison absolutely loves the tangy combination of capers and lemon, and I love how tender the pork turns out, even when using lean pork tenderloin. The light, flavorful sauce perfectly complements the delicate medallions of pork, and best of all, it comes together in just 30 minutes.

Trim and remove any silver skin from the pork tenderloin. Cut the pork across the tenderloin into 12 medallions ¾ inch thick. Place the medallions between wax paper and pound to a ¼-inch thickness. Season both sides of the pork with the salt and pepper to taste.

Place the flour on a shallow plate. Dredge the pork in the flour and shake off any excess.

Heat a 12-inch nonstick skillet over medium-high heat and add the oil. Working in batches if needed, sear the pork until golden brown on both sides and just cooked through in the center, about 1 minute per side (they will finish cooking in the sauce later). Remove and set aside on a plate.

Reduce the heat to medium and melt 1 tablespoon of the butter. Add the white wine to deglaze the pan, scraping up any browned bits. Add the lemon juice, reserved lemon halves, bone broth, and black pepper to taste. Simmer until the sauce is slightly reduced, 3 to 4 minutes.

Discard the lemon halves and add the remaining ½ tablespoon butter. Return the pork medallions and accumulated juices to the skillet, spooning the sauce over them. Add the capers and simmer until the pork is cooked through (the internal temperature should register 145°F), 3 to 4 minutes.

To serve, sprinkle with parsley and garnish with lemon slices.

SERVES 4

1½ pounds pork tenderloin

½ teaspoon kosher salt

Freshly ground black pepper

¼ cup all-purpose flour or gluten-free flour

2 tablespoons extra-virgin olive oil

1½ tablespoons unsalted butter or nondairy butter

⅓ cup low-calorie dry white wine (I like Kim Crawford Illuminate 70-calorie Sauvignon Blanc)

Juice of 1 large lemon, lemon halves reserved

¾ cup chicken bone broth*

2 tablespoon capers, drained

Chopped fresh parsley, for garnish

1 lemon, thinly sliced

*Read the label to be sure this product is gluten-free.

Perfect Pairings

Serve over pasta or rice, or with crusty bread to soak up the delicious sauce. Roasted vegetables and a simple salad on the side would be great, too.

Per Serving (3 slices pork + sauce) | Calories 327 | **Protein 38 g** | Carbohydrate 6 g | Fiber 0 g | Sugars 1 g | Fat 15 g | Saturated Fat 5 g | Cholesterol 122 mg | Sodium 395 mg

SAVOR
THE SEA

Living on the coast, I'm lucky to have access to fresh fish and seafood all the time, and not surprisingly, it's a staple in our home. I eat seafood at least twice a week, if not more, and I'm constantly inspired by the incredible variety of dishes you can create with it.

This chapter features some of my absolute favorite seafood recipes, each bursting with flavor and packed with protein. For a sushi craving, the Spicy Salmon Sushi Bake (page 244) is the perfect at-home solution. My husband, Tommy, can't get enough of the Air Fryer Blackened Mahimahi Sandwiches (page 240), inspired by our many trips to the Sunshine State. My daughter Madison loves the Sheet Pan Tajín Salmon Tacos (page 224) so much, I almost named them after her! And when I'm in the mood for something lighter and low-carb, the Chili Crisp Shrimp Lettuce Wraps with Pickled Veggies (page 223) are my go-to.

This chapter has something for everyone, from bold, spicy flavors to lighter, refreshing options—recipes that will help you incorporate more fish and seafood into your weekly high-protein meals.

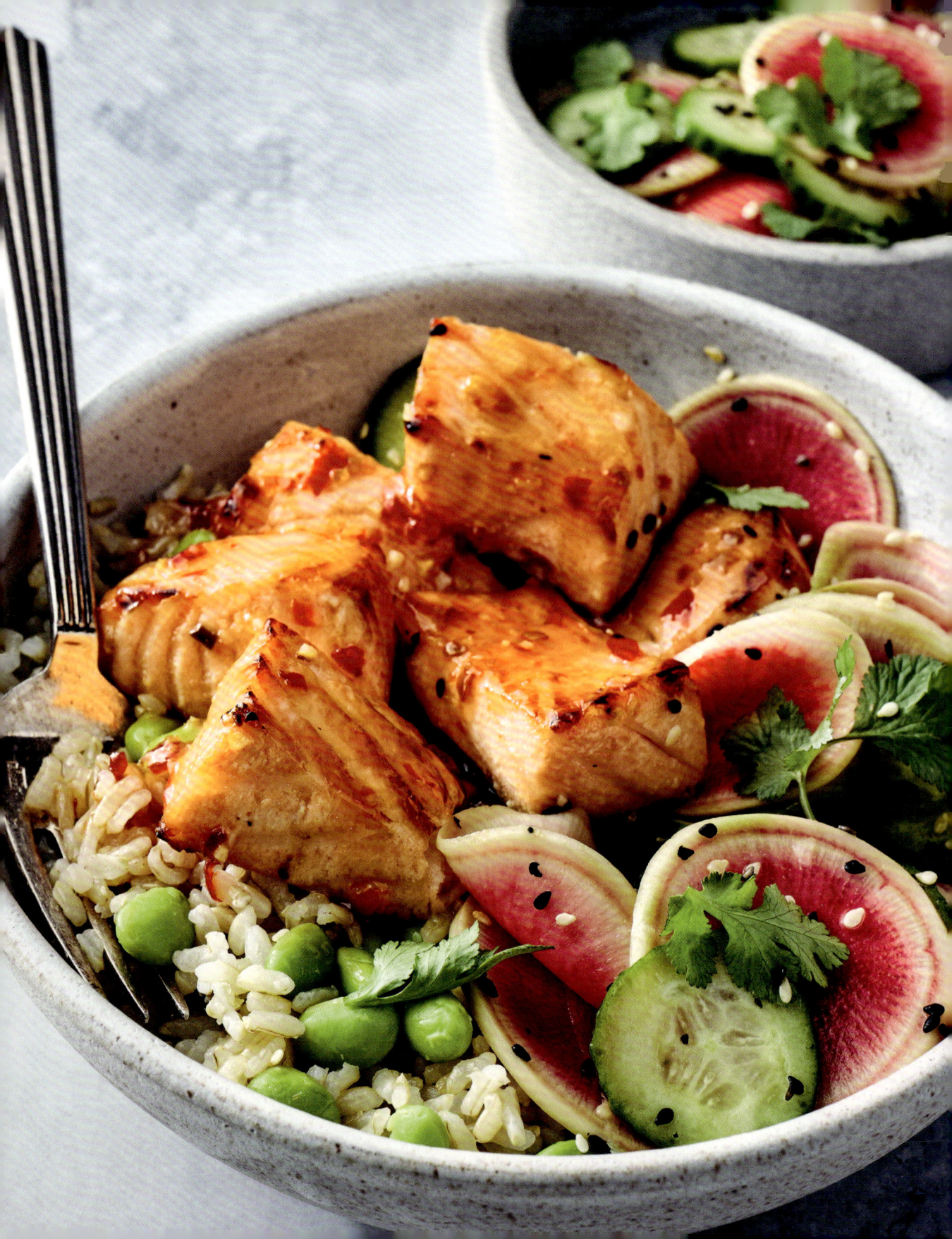

SWEET & SPICY SALMON BOWLS

with Edamame Rice

I eat salmon at least twice a week, and not just because it's my favorite fish, but also because it's packed with omega-3 fatty acids! These healthy fats are critically important for heart health, brain function, and reducing inflammation. My husband, Tommy, is not the biggest fan of salmon, so I usually make this bowl for myself for lunch. It comes together really fast, and the edamame rice adds even more protein. You can easily double this recipe to serve four or halve it for just one serving.

Preheat the oven to 425°F. Line a baking sheet with parchment paper.

In a medium bowl, combine the radish, cucumber, vinegar, 1 teaspoon of the sesame oil, the sesame seeds, and ¼ teaspoon of the salt. Let the shaved veggie salad marinate while everything else cooks.

In a large bowl, toss the salmon with the chili sauce, garlic, sambal, and ¼ teaspoon of the salt. Let marinate while the oven is preheating.

Transfer the salmon to the prepared baking sheet and bake until golden and cooked through, about 10 minutes. (Alternatively, to cook in an air fryer, cook for 5 to 6 minutes at 400°F.)

Meanwhile, in a medium skillet, combine the remaining ½ teaspoon sesame oil and the ginger over medium heat and cook for about 30 seconds. Add the rice, edamame, and remaining ¼ teaspoon salt and stir to heat through, 2 to 3 minutes. Set aside.

Right before serving, gently mix the cilantro into the shaved veggie salad. Build your bowls with edamame rice at the bottom, chili-garlic salmon on one side, and shaved veggie salad on the other. If desired, sprinkle the salmon with sesame seeds and serve with extra sweet chili sauce or sambal.

TIP: Any radish will work, but watermelon radish is my favorite for this!

SERVES 2

¼ cup thinly sliced watermelon radish

1 cup sliced Persian (mini) cucumbers

1 tablespoon seasoned rice vinegar

1½ teaspoons toasted sesame oil

1 teaspoon black and white sesame seeds or furikake, plus more (optional) for serving

¾ teaspoon kosher salt

2 skinless salmon fillets (4 ounces each), cut into bite-size pieces

2 tablespoons Thai sweet chili sauce, plus more (optional) for serving

2 garlic cloves, minced

1½ teaspoons sambal oelek, plus more (optional) for serving

1 teaspoon grated fresh ginger

1 cup cooked brown rice

½ cup shelled edamame, thawed if frozen

¼ cup fresh cilantro leaves

Per Serving (1 bowl) | Calories 407 | **Protein 31 g** | Carbohydrate 41 g | Fiber 6.5 g | Sugars 12 g | Fat 13 g | Saturated Fat 1.5 g | Cholesterol 62 mg | Sodium 1,020 mg

SEARED COD with Roasted Cherry Tomato Sauce

I love how the juices from the tomatoes mix with the cod to create such a light and flavorful sauce for the couscous. After testing this dish a few times, I realized that searing the cod before baking it results in a seriously tasty fish dish, but using thick fillets is key to keep the fish from overcooking.

Preheat the oven to 400°F.

In a 12 × 9-inch baking dish, combine the tomatoes, white wine, bay leaves, 1 tablespoon of the olive oil, the garlic, ¼ teaspoon of the salt, and black pepper to taste. Toss to combine.

Bake, undisturbed, until the tomatoes have started to collapse and release their juices and you see a few charred spots, 30 to 35 minutes.

Meanwhile, in a small bowl, stir together ½ teaspoon of the salt, ¼ teaspoon black pepper, the paprika, and cayenne. Pat the cod dry and season generously with the spice mixture.

Cook the couscous according to the package directions.

When the tomatoes are ready, remove them from the oven (but keep the oven on).

In a nonstick medium skillet, heat the remaining 1 tablespoon oil over medium heat until shimmering. Add the cod and cook on each side until golden and starting to crisp, about 2 minutes per side. Flip the cod carefully to keep the fillets intact. The cod will still be uncooked in the center.

Carefully nestle the cod fillets in the baking dish with the tomatoes and return to the oven. Bake until the fish flakes easily with a fork, another 5 to 6 minutes. Season with the remaining ⅛ teaspoon salt and top with the parsley.

Spoon the tomatoes and juices over the fish and serve with the couscous.

SERVES 4

1 pint cherry tomatoes

½ cup low-calorie dry white wine (I like Kim Crawford Illuminate 70-calorie Sauvignon Blanc)

2 bay leaves

2 tablespoons extra-virgin olive oil

2 garlic cloves, minced

¾ teaspoon plus ⅛ teaspoon kosher salt

Freshly ground black pepper

½ teaspoon sweet paprika

⅛ teaspoon cayenne pepper, or to taste

1⅓ cups uncooked pearl couscous (see Tip for gluten-free options)

4 thick skinless cod fillets (6 ounces each) or other firm white fish, such as striped bass, thawed if frozen

1 tablespoon finely chopped fresh parsley

TIP: To make this gluten-free, swap out the pearl couscous for quinoa or roasted vegetables.

Per Serving (1 fillet + ½ cup sauce + ⅔ cup cooked couscous) | Calories 398 | Protein 33 g | Carbohydrate 43 g | Fiber 4 g | Sugars 2 g | Fat 8 g | Saturated Fat 1 g | Cholesterol 80 mg | Sodium 770 mg

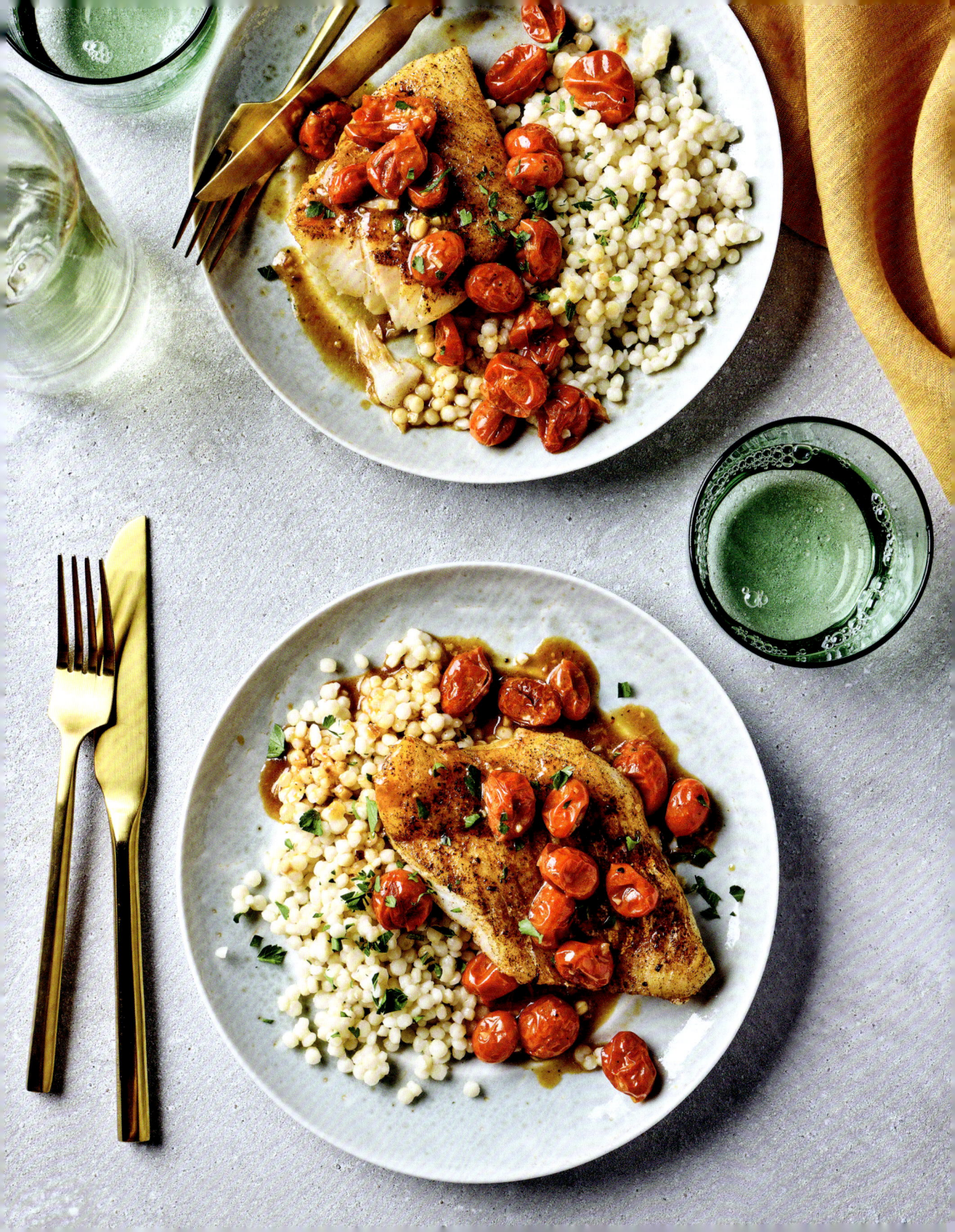

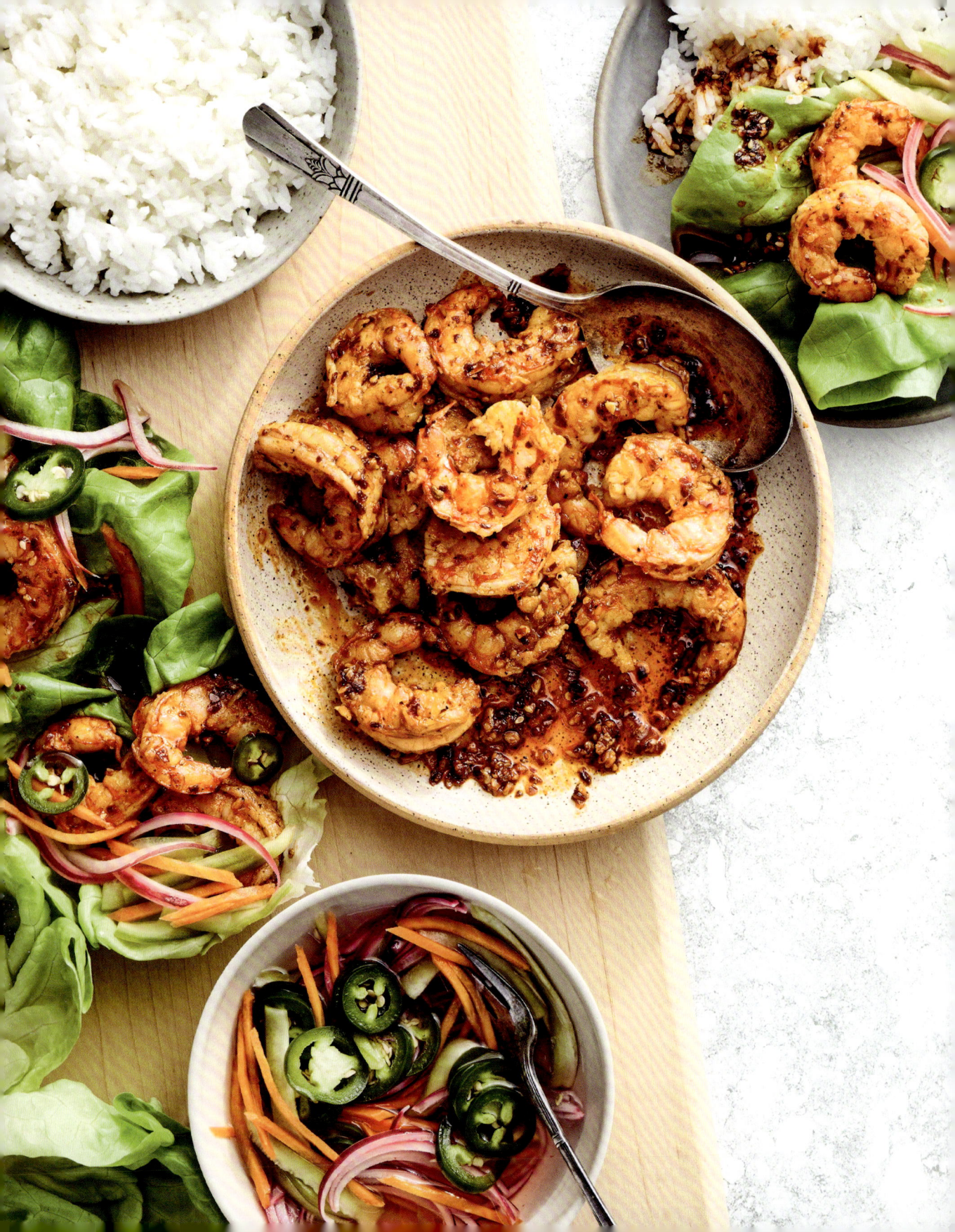

CHILI CRISP SHRIMP LETTUCE WRAPS
with Pickled Veggies

Eating this dinner with your hands is so fun and laid back—I set everything on the table and let everyone create their own wrap. Chili crisp oil is a delicious spicy condiment that's widely available from many brands, such as Mr Bing Mild Chili Crisp, Fly By Jing, and S&B Crunchy Garlic with Chili Oil, to name a few. If you want to turn this into a rice bowl, skip the lettuce and serve over rice.

MAKE THE QUICK-PICKLED VEGGIES: Arrange the carrots, cucumber, onion, and jalapeño (if using) in a 1-pint glass jar.

In a small saucepan, combine the vinegar, ¼ cup water, and the salt. Heat over medium heat, stirring until the salt dissolves, 1 to 2 minutes. Let it cool for a few minutes, then pour the liquid over the veggies. Let it continue to cool to room temperature, then refrigerate until ready to eat.

MAKE THE CHILI CRISP SHRIMP: Heat a large nonstick skillet over medium heat. Season the shrimp with the salt and pepper. When the skillet is hot, spray it with oil, then add the shrimp and sauté until fully cooked, 2 to 3 minutes on each side. Remove from the heat and stir in the chili crisp.

Drain and discard the liquid from the pickled vegetables.

TO ASSEMBLE: Set out the lettuce leaves, rice, shrimp, and the pickled vegetables for people to assemble their own wraps.

TIP: If your lettuce leaves are on the smaller side, cut the shrimp in smaller pieces so the wraps are easier to eat.

SERVES 4

QUICK-PICKLED VEGGIES

½ cup matchstick-cut carrots, pre-cut

½ seedless cucumber, peeled and cut into matchsticks

¼ red onion, thinly sliced

1 jalapeño (optional), thinly sliced into rings

½ cup seasoned rice vinegar

1 teaspoon kosher salt

CHILI CRISP SHRIMP

50 peeled and deveined large shrimp (see Tip), about 1½ pounds

¼ teaspoon kosher salt

¼ teaspoon freshly ground black pepper

Olive oil spray

5 tablespoons chili crisp

ASSEMBLY

20 large lettuce leaves, such as butter lettuce, Bibb, Boston, or Little Gem (about 2 heads)

3 cups cooked white or brown rice

Per Serving (5 lettuce wraps) | Calories 447 | **Protein 40 g** | Carbohydrate 41 g | Fiber 4 g | Sugars 2 g | Fat 11 g | Saturated Fat 2.5 g | Cholesterol 251 mg | Sodium 487 mg

SHEET PAN TAJÍN SALMON TACOS

My daughter Madison loves these salmon tacos so much that I usually make them for her a few times a month. They're super easy to prepare because I don't take the skin off the salmon before I cook it. Instead, I roast the salmon on a sheet pan skin side down, and once baked, the fish comes right off the skin and right onto the tortillas. My husband is not a fan of salmon, so I usually swap his salmon for another protein, like chicken.

Preheat the oven to 425°F. Line a sheet pan with foil and spray with oil.

In a small bowl, combine the red onion, juice from 1½ limes, and a large pinch of kosher salt. Toss to combine and let the mixture pickle while you prepare the other ingredients, stirring occasionally.

In a small bowl, combine the mashed avocado, juice of the remaining lime half, and ¼ teaspoon kosher salt.

Place the salmon on the sheet pan skin side down, spray the flesh with olive oil, and season with the Tajín.

Bake until the fish is cooked through in the center, 12 to 14 minutes, depending on the thickness. (Alternatively, to cook in an air fryer, preheat the air fryer to 400°F. Use air fryer parchment for easy cleanup, then air-fry the salmon skin side down for 6 to 9 minutes, depending on the thickness of the fish.) With a spatula, break each fillet into 3 pieces, leaving the skin behind.

Meanwhile, lightly char the tortillas over a flame or in a hot skillet, 30 seconds on each side, and keep warm.

To serve, place some of the cabbage on the bottom of each tortilla, top with the salmon, then the avocado, and finish with the pickled red onions. Serve with lime wedges.

SERVES 4

Olive oil spray

½ medium red onion, thinly sliced

2 limes, halved

Kosher salt

5 ounces avocado (about 1 medium Hass), mashed with a fork

4 salmon fillets (6 ounces each)

1 tablespoon Tajín (Mexican chile-lime seasoning salt)

12 corn tortillas

2 cups shredded red cabbage

8 lime wedges, for serving

Per Serving (3 tacos) | Calories 490 | **Protein 39 g** | Carbohydrate 42 g | Fiber 8 g | Sugars 3 g | Fat 19 g | Saturated Fat 3 g | Cholesterol 94 mg | Sodium 760 mg

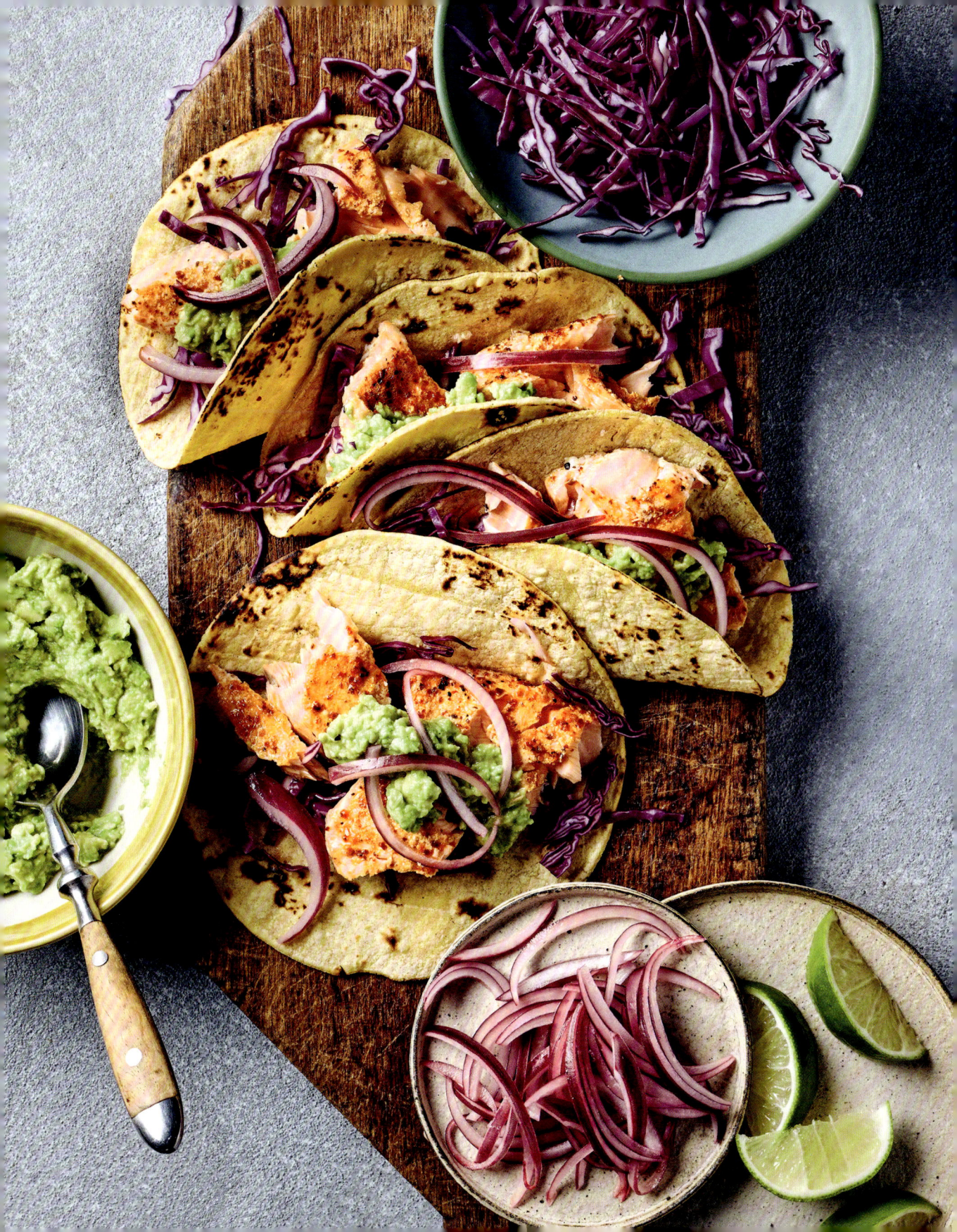

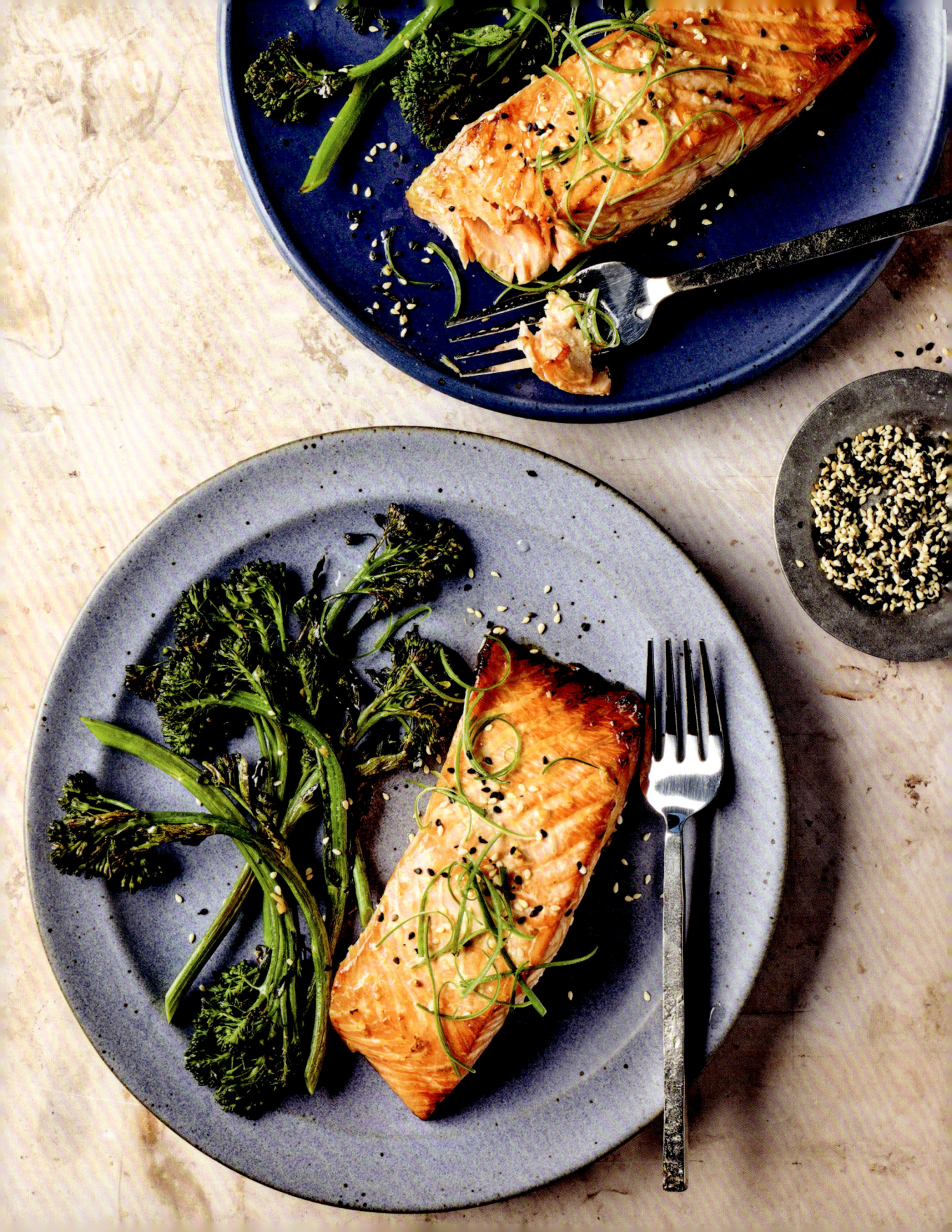

SHEET PAN MISO-SOY STEELHEAD TROUT

with Charred Broccolini

This seriously tastes like a fancy restaurant dish, but it's actually so easy to make at home! If you have only 20 minutes to marinate the fish, it will work fine, but 1 or 2 hours would be ideal. Steelhead trout looks very similar to salmon, only it's milder and less fatty, and it doesn't have as much of that "fishy" flavor that some people shy away from. The broccolini comes out perfectly charred, and if you want to serve this with a grain, it's great with some hot sticky white rice.

In a shallow bowl large enough to hold the fish, whisk together the soy sauce, mirin, miso, garlic, and ginger. Add the fish to the bowl and coat it in the marinade. Cover and let it marinate for 20 minutes, or ideally 1 to 2 hours in the fridge.

When ready to cook, adjust an oven rack in the center and another 6 inches from the broiler and preheat the oven to 425°F. Spray a large sheet pan with oil.

Place the fish on the sheet pan skin side down. Reserve 1 tablespoon of the marinade (discard the rest). In a bowl, mix the broccolini with the reserved 1 tablespoon marinade and the sesame oil and toss well. Place on the sheet pan around the fish.

Bake on the center rack until the fish is cooked through, 10 to 12 minutes, depending on the thickness of the fish. Switch the oven to broil, move the pan to the higher rack, and broil until the fish is golden brown, 2 to 3 minutes (be careful not to let it burn).

Divide the vegetables and fish between two plates and sprinkle with sesame seeds and scallions. Serve immediately.

TIP: I buy my steelhead trout from the food market Aldi's, but you can easily swap it for salmon, Arctic char, or Chilean sea bass in this recipe.

SERVES 2

¼ cup reduced-sodium soy sauce or gluten-free tamari

¼ cup mirin (Japanese sweet rice wine)

2 tablespoons white miso* (I like Miso Master Organic)

2 garlic cloves, minced

1½ teaspoons grated fresh ginger

Olive oil spray

2 steelhead trout, Arctic char, or salmon fillets (6 ounces each)

1 bunch broccolini

1 teaspoon toasted sesame oil

½ teaspoon black and white sesame seeds

1 scallion, sliced

*Read the label to be sure this product is gluten-free.

Per Serving (1 fillet + ½ bunch broccolini) | Calories 334 | **Protein 37 g** | Carbohydrate 11 g | Fiber 3.5 g | Sugars 5 g | Fat 15 g | Saturated Fat 2.5 g | Cholesterol 99 mg | Sodium 328 mg

SALMON & POTATO LEEK SOUP

On a cold night, I love warming up with this creamy and cozy salmon soup—it's filling, takes less than 30 minutes to prepare, and is made all in one pot. Filled with chunks of fresh salmon, hearty potatoes, leeks, carrots, sour cream, and dill, this buttery soup is the ultimate comfort food. It's inspired by the Finnish soup lohikeitto, which is very similar to an American chowder, but without the corn and bacon. While salmon is traditional in this soup, other fish like steelhead trout or Arctic char can also be used.

Heat a large heavy pot or Dutch oven over medium heat and add the butter. When melted, add the leeks and cook, stirring occasionally, until soft and translucent, 2 to 3 minutes.

Add the carrots, potatoes, stock, ½ cup water, bay leaf, salt, pepper to taste, and the dill and bring to a boil. Reduce the heat to medium-low, cover, and simmer until the potatoes and carrots are cooked and soft, 15 to 18 minutes.

In a small bowl, combine the sour cream with 1 cup of the hot stock from the pot and mix well until smooth and no lumps appear. Add the sour cream mixture along with the fish to the soup and gently stir to combine. Cook uncovered for 1 more minute, then remove from the heat. Cover with the lid and set aside for 4 to 5 minutes for the salmon to poach. Be careful not to overcook the salmon; you'll know it's done when the salmon flakes easily with a fork.

Discard the bay leaf and adjust the seasoning with more salt and pepper if needed. Divide the soup among four bowls. Garnish with more dill and serve immediately.

SERVES 4

1 tablespoon unsalted butter

2 large leeks, white and light-green parts only, chopped and rinsed well

3 medium carrots, peeled and chopped

¾ pound new potatoes, cut into ½-inch pieces

5 cups reduced sodium vegetable stock

1 bay leaf

½ teaspoon kosher salt, plus more to taste

Freshly ground black pepper

2 tablespoons chopped fresh dill, plus more for serving

⅓ cup sour cream

20 ounces skinless Atlantic salmon fillet, cut into ¾-inch cubes

Perfect Pairings
This soup is delicious and filling on its own, but if you want to serve this with a side dish, a green salad or crusty bread would be lovely.

Per Serving (2 generous cups) | Calories 391 | **Protein 31 g** | Carbohydrate 30 g | Fiber 4 g | Sugars 9 g | Fat 16 g | Saturated Fat 5.5 g | Cholesterol 94 mg | Sodium 792 mg

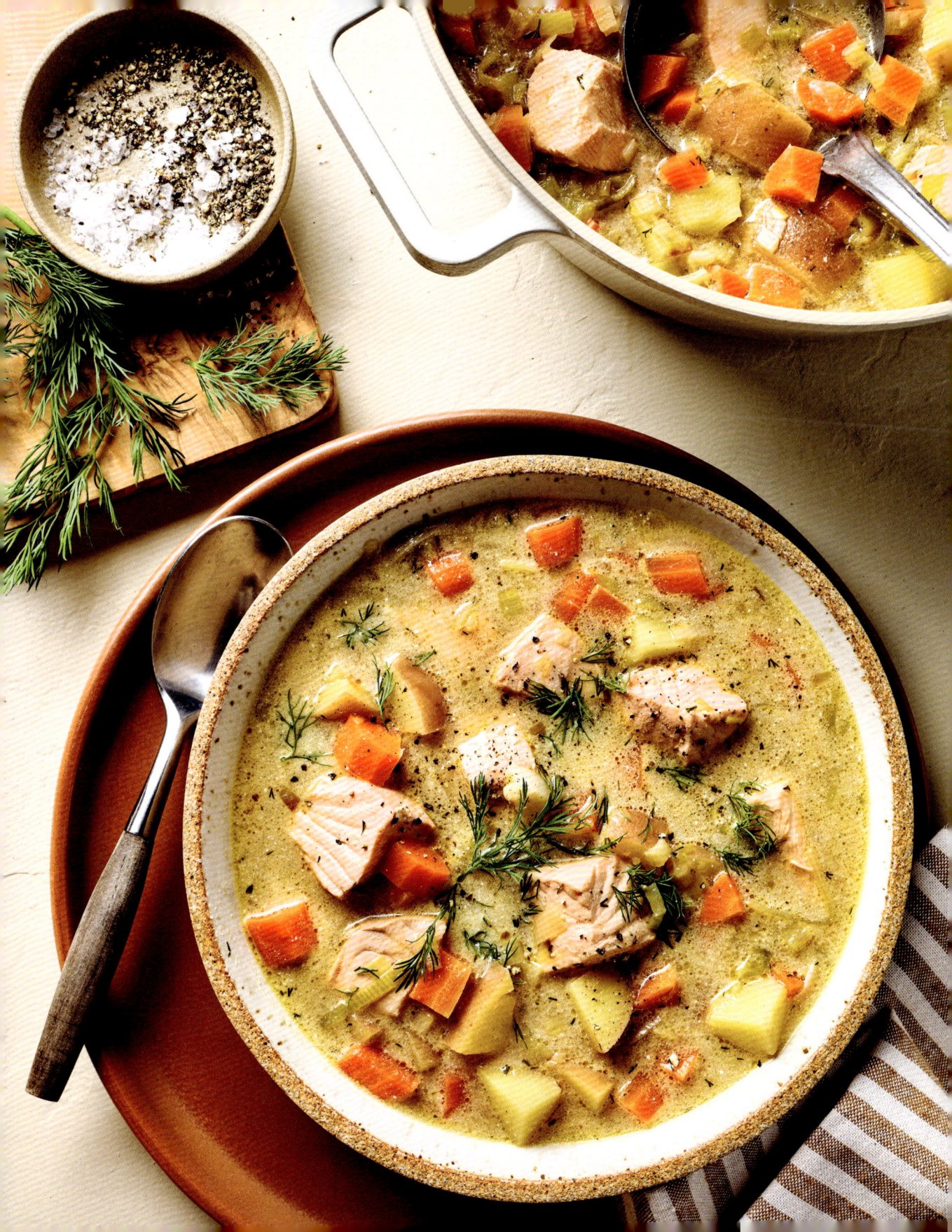

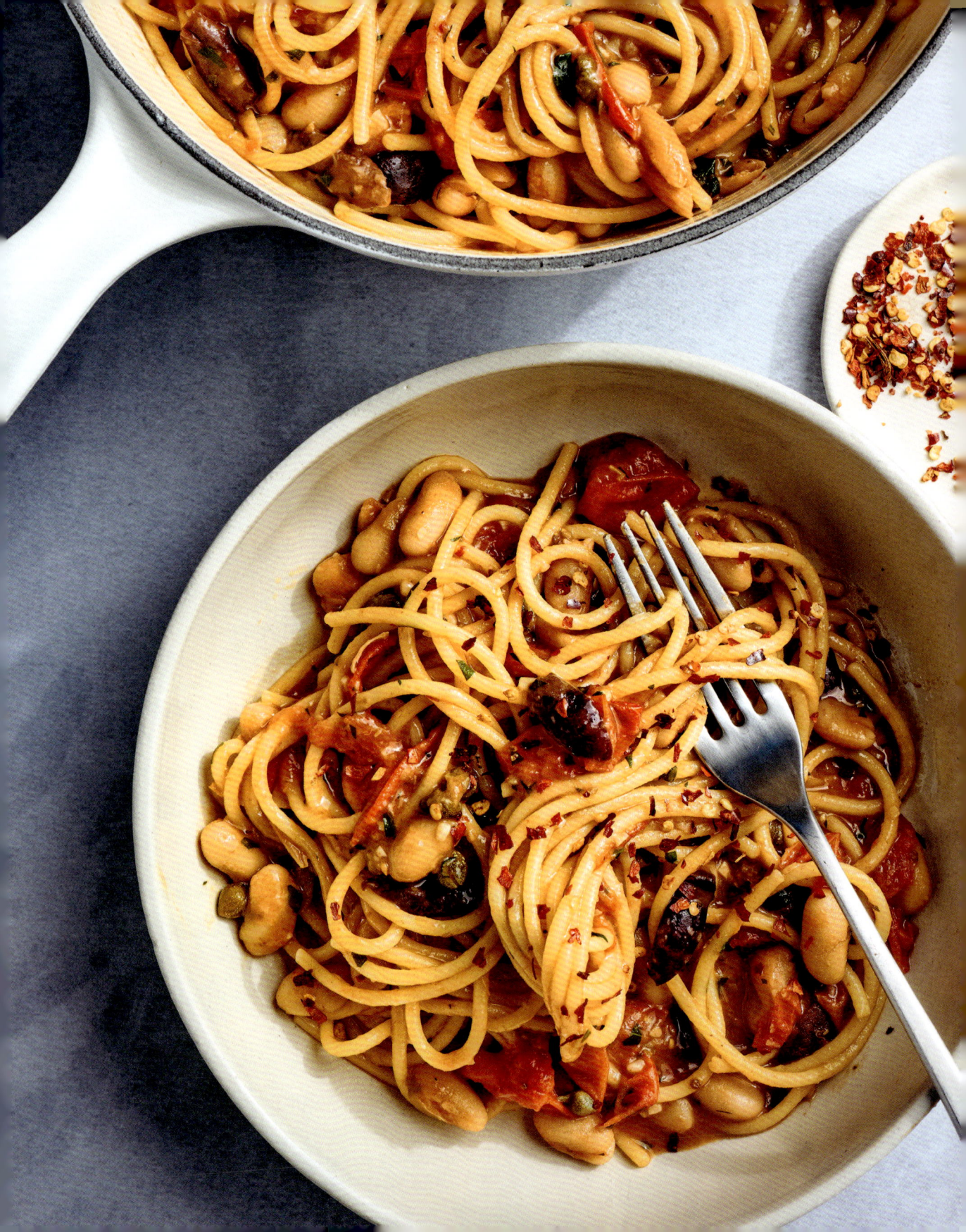

ONE-POT WHITE BEAN PASTA PUTTANESCA

This one-pot pasta dish gets its big, bold flavors from anchovies, kalamata olives, and capers—the trifecta for a winning puttanesca. It tastes incredibly rich and velvety, without any butter or cream. Don't be afraid of using anchovies; they truly make the dish, and trust me, they don't add a fishy flavor! Instead, they just melt away into the sauce leaving a mild and delicious saltiness. If you don't want to use fillets, you can use anchovy paste instead. This pasta dish is not only packed with flavor, it's got plenty of protein from the beans, bone broth, and protein pasta.

In a large deep skillet with high sides, heat the oil over medium heat. Add the garlic and cook, stirring, until fragrant, about 2 minutes. Stir in the tomato paste and continue to cook for 1 more minute. Add the anchovies, oregano, and 2 teaspoons of the capers and cook, stirring, until the anchovies break down, for 1 minute.

Stir in the broth, beans, and ½ cup water, scraping to release any caramelized bits from the bottom of the pan. Add the pasta, tomatoes, and pepper flakes, then increase the heat to medium-high and bring to a boil. Once boiling, cook, stirring occasionally, until the pasta starts to soften, about 6 minutes.

Stir in the olives and remaining 2 teaspoons capers, reduce the heat to medium, cover, and cook, stirring occasionally, until the pasta is al dente and the tomatoes have softened, 5 to 6 minutes. Remove from the heat and stir in the parsley.

Serve right away with more pepper flakes, if desired.

TIP: The pasta will continue to soak up liquid as it sits, so the dish is best eaten right away. You can add a little more broth if you have leftovers.

SERVES 4

1 tablespoon extra-virgin olive oil

4 garlic cloves, minced

2 teaspoons tomato paste

3 oil-packed anchovy fillets, finely chopped

2 teaspoons chopped fresh oregano, or 1 teaspoon dried

4 teaspoons capers

3 cups unsalted chicken bone broth*

1½ (15-ounce) cans small white beans,* rinsed and drained (2¼ cups)

8 ounces high-protein spaghetti (I like Barilla Protein+) or your favorite gluten-free option

1 pint grape tomatoes, halved

¼ teaspoon crushed red pepper flakes, plus more (optional) for serving

¼ cup sliced kalamata olives

¼ cup chopped fresh parsley

*Read the label to be sure this product is gluten-free.

Per Serving (1½ cups) | Calories 479 | **Protein 31 g** | Carbohydrate 78 g | Fiber 14 g | Sugars 5 g | Fat 7 g | Saturated Fat 1 g | Cholesterol 6 mg | Sodium 780 mg

SUMMER FARMERS' MARKET LOBSTER FRIED RICE

I've put a summery spin on my favorite Chinese takeout with some delicious lobster and fresh farmers' market veggies! Adding lobster to this fried rice loaded with summer corn, cherry tomatoes, and zucchini is delicious, but you can also just use shrimp. This can also be made with frozen corn if it's not in season, and you can swap the zucchini for asparagus or broccoli.

In a large skillet or wok, heat 1½ teaspoons of the sesame oil over medium heat. Add the lobster and cook until opaque and cooked through, 4 to 5 minutes. Remove from the pan and set aside.

Add another 1½ teaspoons sesame oil and the corn and cook until browned, 4 to 5 minutes. Add the zucchini and cook until just tender, 3 to 4 minutes. Add the garlic and the scallion whites and light greens and cook until aromatic, about 1 minute. Add the cherry tomatoes, cooked rice, and soy sauce and mix to combine. Cover to steam, 2 to 3 minutes.

Push all of the ingredients to one side of the pan and add the remaining 1 teaspoon sesame oil. Add the eggs and scramble. Once fully cooked, mix to combine with the rice.

Increase the heat to medium-high and crisp the rice for about 1 minute, then add the lobster meat and cook for 1 minute to heat through. Top with the scallion greens and serve.

SERVES 4

4 teaspoons toasted sesame oil

1 pound lobster meat, from 4 lobster tails (6 ounces each), chopped

1⅓ cups fresh corn kernels

1⅓ cups diced zucchini

2 garlic cloves, minced

3 scallions, chopped, white and green parts kept separate

1⅓ cups cherry tomatoes, quartered

3 cups cooked white or brown rice

2½ tablespoons reduced-sodium soy sauce or gluten-free tamari

3 large eggs, beaten

Per Serving (2 cups) | Calories 433 | **Protein 30 g** | Carbohydrate 55 g | Fiber 3 g | Sugars 5 g | Fat 10 g | Saturated Fat 2 g | Cholesterol 284 mg | Sodium 882 mg

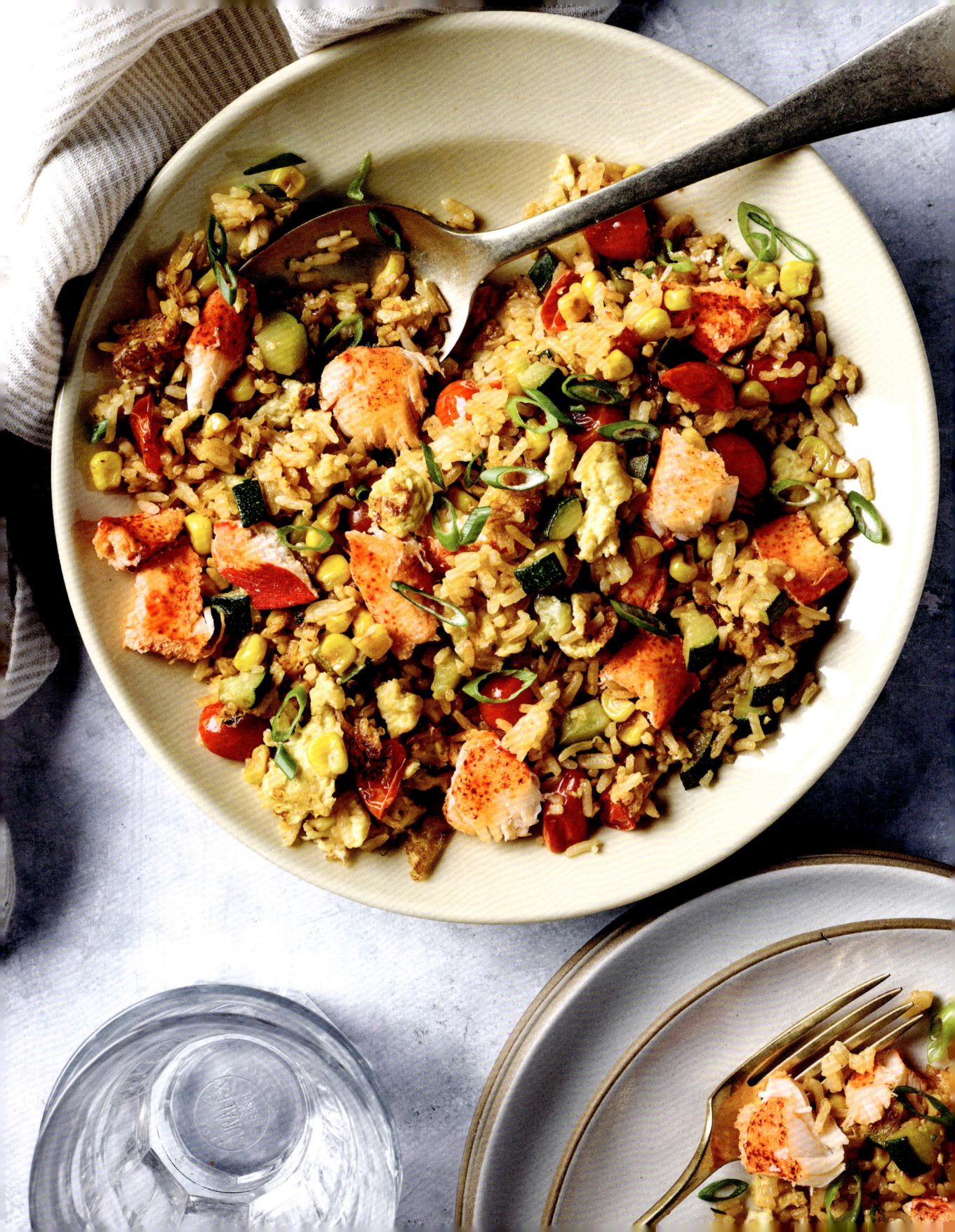

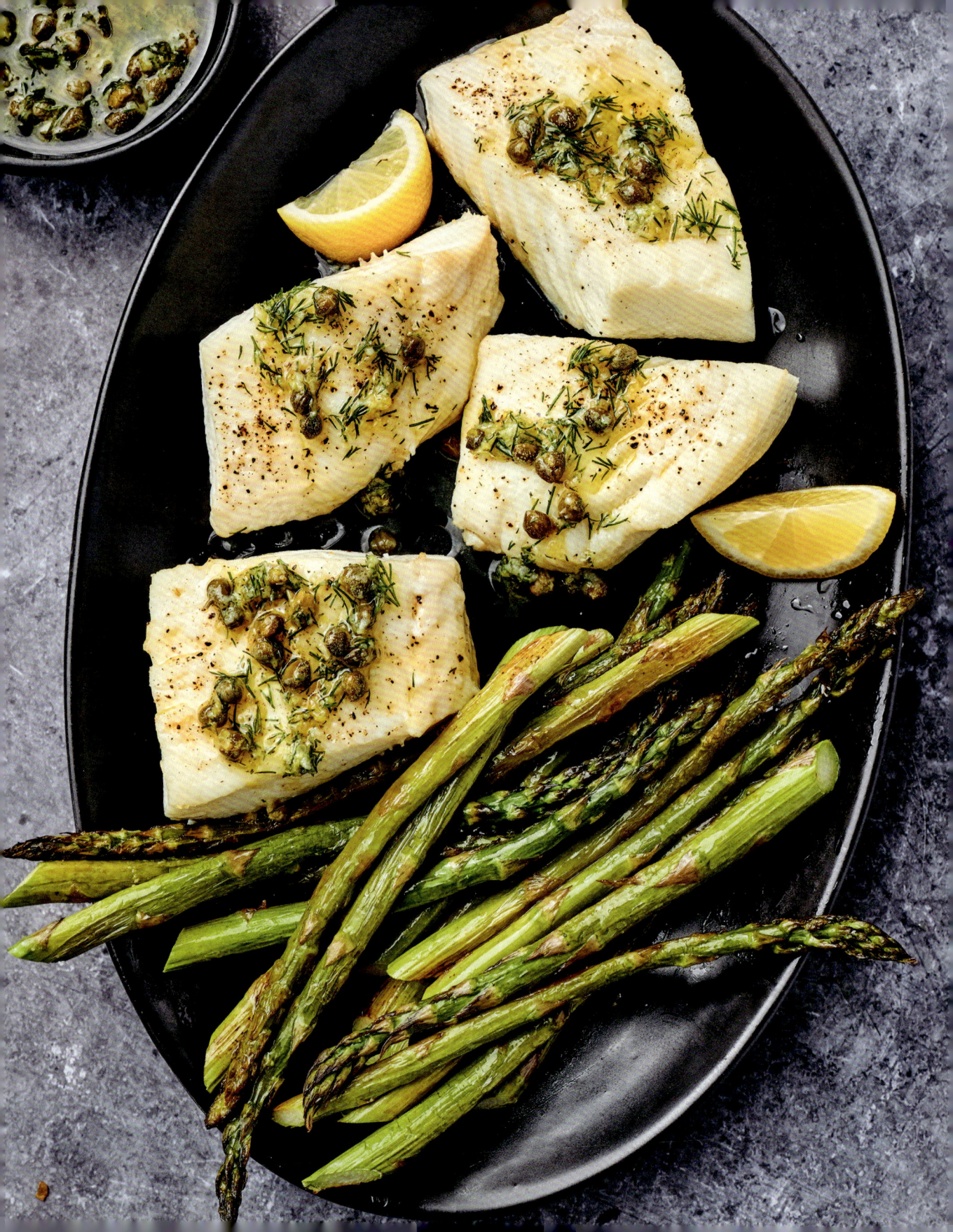

BROILED FISH
with Lemony-Dill Sauce

What I love about this dish is its simplicity and elegance, making it perfect for both a quick meal and a dinner party. Pairing white fish with lemons, dill, and capers creates a classic combination that's close to my heart. The lemony tang perfectly complements the flaky fish, but it's the capers that steal the show with their briny bite. Fresh dill has also become a favorite herb of mine—I even grow it in my garden.

Adjust an oven rack to 6 inches from the heating element and preheat the broiler to high.

In a small bowl, combine the olive oil, lemon zest, lemon juice, garlic, capers, caper brine, and dill.

Place the fish on a sheet pan (if desired, for easier cleanup, line it first with foil). Season the fish with the salt and black pepper to taste. Broil until opaque and cooked through, 5 to 8 minutes, depending on the thickness. (No need to flip.)

Transfer the fish to a platter or four plates and spoon the lemon-dill sauce over the fish.

SERVES 4

¼ cup extra-virgin olive oil

Grated zest of 1 lemon

1 tablespoon fresh lemon juice

2 garlic cloves, grated on a Microplane

2 tablespoons capers

1 teaspoon caper brine

⅓ cup loosely packed chopped fresh dill

4 white-fleshed fish fillets (6 ounces each), such as halibut, grouper, striped bass, or cod

¾ teaspoon kosher salt

Freshly ground black pepper

Perfect Pairings
I usually serve this with whatever vegetables are in season. Roasted asparagus, green beans, or zucchini are all great options.

Per Serving (1 fillet) | Calories 279 | **Protein 32 g** | Carbohydrate 1 g | Fiber 0 g | Sugars 0 g | Fat 16 g | Saturated Fat 2.5 g | Cholesterol 83 mg | Sodium 445 mg

CALABRIAN CHILI MUSSELS
with Garlic Toast

If you love quick and flavorful meals with minimal fuss, this dish is calling your name. Mussels are bathed in a spicy, tangy broth infused with the bold kick of Calabrian chili. It's a dish that feels like it came straight from a fancy restaurant, yet it's still light enough for a weeknight dinner. If you typically only eat mussels when dining out, you'll be surprised by how easy it is to make them at home! Don't forget the garlicky toast, it's perfect for dipping and soaking up every last drop of the rich, flavorful broth.

In a large pot, heat the olive oil over medium heat and add the anchovies. Cook, stirring, until the anchovies break down, about 1 minute. Add the Calabrian chili oil and minced garlic and let sizzle until fragrant, about 30 seconds.

Quickly add the wine, broth, and Calabrian chili peppers to the pan. Bring to a boil and cook for 3 to 4 minutes, then stir in the mussels and cover immediately. Shake the pot and cook for 1 minute. Stir the mussels, cover, and cook until the shells begin to open, 3 to 4 minutes.

Meanwhile, spray the baguette slices with oil and place under the broiler or toaster oven to toast until golden, 2 to 3 minutes. Rub the toasts with the halved garlic clove.

Stir the parsley into the mussels and divide among four bowls. Serve with the garlic toast.

SERVES 4

1 tablespoon extra-virgin olive oil

5 oil-packed anchovy fillets

1 tablespoon oil from a jar of Calabrian chili peppers

7 garlic cloves, 6 minced and 1 clove halved for rubbing toasts

¾ cup dry white wine

¾ cup no-salt-added vegetable broth*

¼ cup jarred Calabrian chili peppers, sliced

48 mussels (about 2¼ pounds), scrubbed and debearded

4 slices baguette (about 1 ounce each) or gluten-free bread

Olive oil spray

⅓ cup chopped fresh Italian parsley

*Read the label to be sure this product is gluten-free.

Perfect Pairings
Serve this with grilled asparagus or roasted vegetables, or opt for a simple arugula salad with lemon and shaved Parmesan cheese. For a sweeter option that cuts through the heat and richness of the dish, a shaved fennel and orange salad would be perfect.

Per Serving (12 mussels + broth + 1 ounce toast) | Calories 422 | **Protein 36 g** | Carbohydrate 29 g | Fiber 1 g | Sugars 1 g | Fat 14 g | Saturated Fat 2.5 g | Cholesterol 76 mg | Sodium 1,151 mg

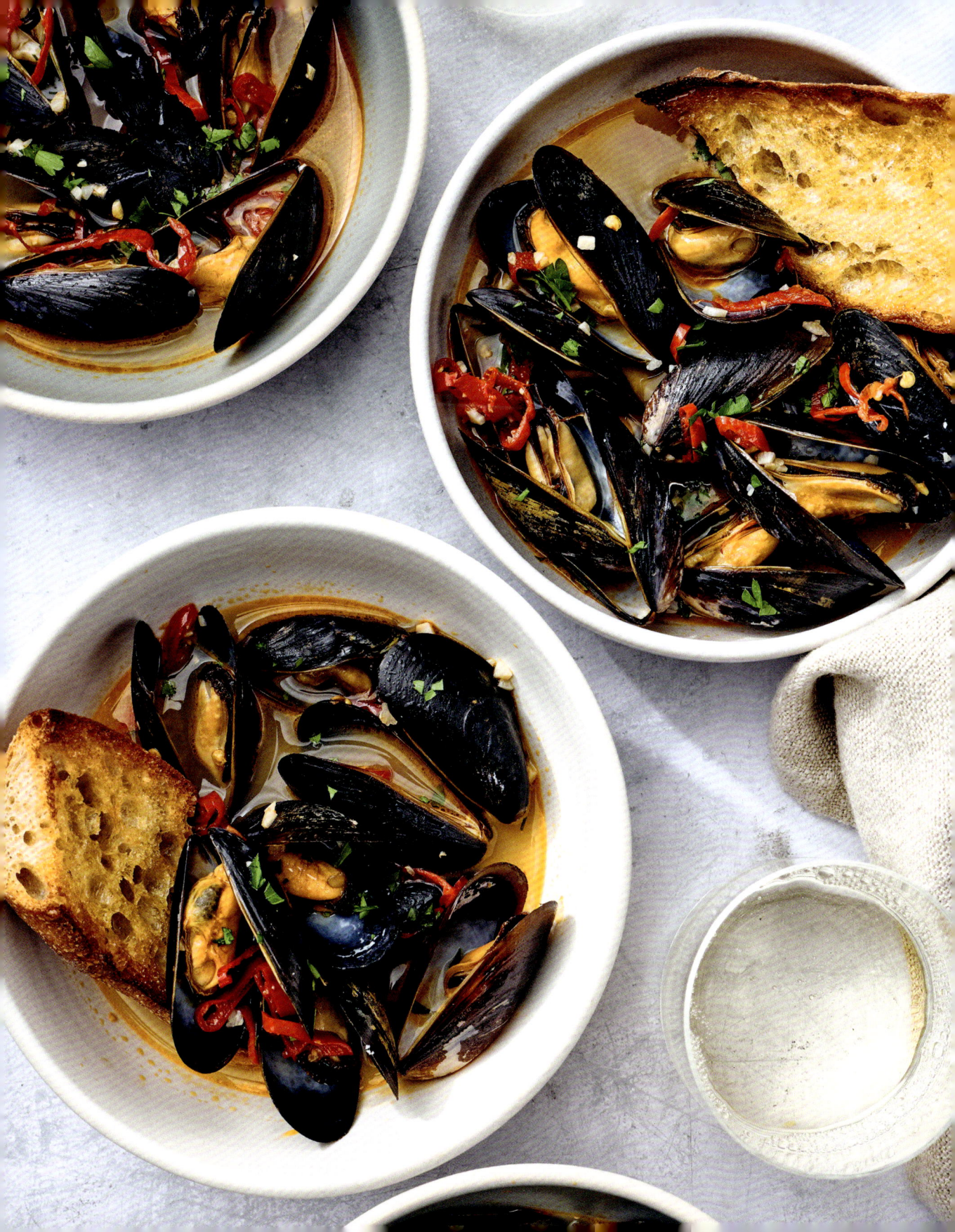

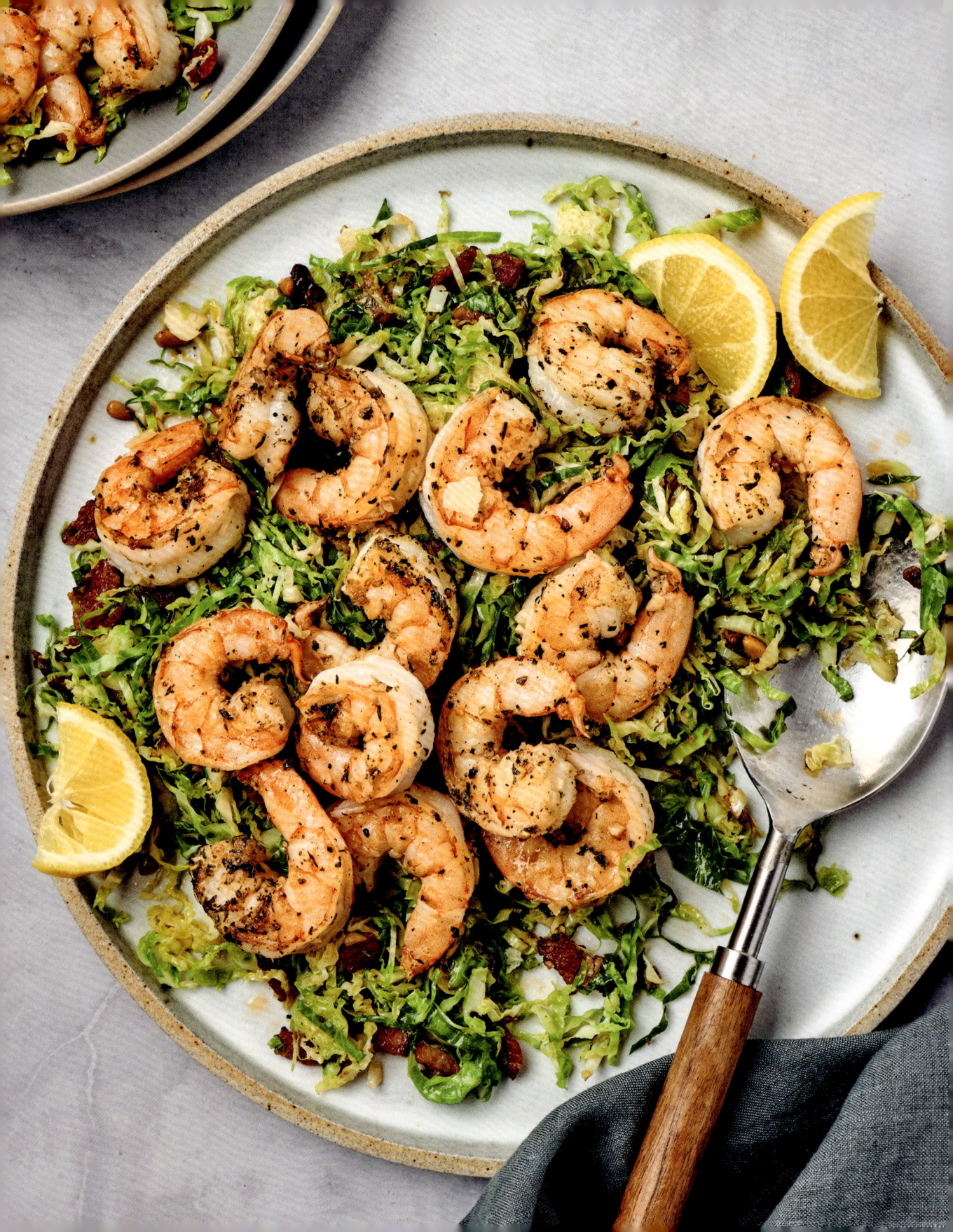

SAUTÉED SHRIMP

with Shredded Brussels & Bacon

I was never a big fan of Brussels sprouts until I tasted my friend Nicole's shredded Brussels recipe quickly sautéed in the skillet with bacon. Now it's my favorite way to prepare Brussels sprouts and I want to share it with you! Here they're sautéed with bacon and pine nuts, making a wonderful base for sautéed shrimp. The savory, smoky bacon enhances the earthy Brussels sprouts, while the pine nuts add a bit of nuttiness and crunch. This dish is not only packed with flavor but is also a light and low-carb meal. It's perfect for any shrimp lover looking for new ways to enjoy a quick and satisfying weeknight dinner.

In a large bowl, gently toss the shrimp with the olive oil. Add the Italian seasoning, half of the garlic, ¼ teaspoon of the salt, and pepper to taste and mix to evenly coat. Set aside to marinate for 5 minutes.

In a large dry skillet, toast the pine nuts over medium-low heat until fragrant and starting to brown, 3 to 5 minutes. Shake the skillet or stir occasionally with a wooden spoon to allow for even toasting. When toasted, remove the nuts from the skillet so they don't burn.

Spray the same pan lightly with olive oil and increase the heat to medium-high. Remove the marinated shrimp with a slotted spoon and add to the pan. Cook until the shrimp are opaque and cooked through, about 3 minutes, flipping halfway. Transfer the shrimp to a plate and cover with foil to keep warm and rest while you make the Brussels sprouts.

Wipe out the skillet, set over medium heat, add the bacon, and cook until just crisped. Add the remaining garlic and cook for about 20 seconds. Add the Brussels sprouts, remaining ¼ teaspoon salt, and pepper to taste. Sauté until the Brussels wilt slightly but still have a crisp bite, about 3 minutes. Stir in the pine nuts, then transfer the Brussels sprouts to a serving platter.

Top the Brussels sprouts with the cooked shrimp and serve with lemon wedges on the side.

Per Serving (about 4 ounces shrimp + generous ½ cup Brussels sprouts) | Calories 339 | **Protein 36 g** | Carbohydrate 12 g | Fiber 4.5 g | Sugars 3 g | Fat 16 g | Saturated Fat 4.5 g | Cholesterol 215 mg | Sodium 569 mg

SERVES 4

1¼ pounds peeled and deveined extra-large shrimp, tail-off

1 tablespoon extra-virgin olive oil

¾ teaspoon Italian seasoning

2 large garlic cloves, minced

½ teaspoon kosher salt

Freshly ground black pepper

2 tablespoons pine nuts

Olive oil spray

4 slices center-cut bacon, or 2 ounces pancetta, finely chopped

16 ounces shredded Brussels sprouts (about 6 cups)

½ lemon, cut into wedges

TIP: There are a few ways to get shredded Brussels—buy them preshredded, use a sharp knife and shave them thin, or use a food processor.

AIR FRYER BLACKENED MAHIMAHI SANDWICHES

SERVES 4

Every time I visit the Florida Keys, I indulge in blackened fish—mahimahi, grouper, you name it—paired with creamy Key lime tartar sauce. On my last trip, I had a blackened mahimahi sandwich that was so incredible because it was so fresh and perfectly seasoned. I re-created it as soon as I got home! I prefer to use the broiler or air fryer to cook all four sandwiches at once, though a cast-iron skillet works great, too. The original sandwich was served on a brioche bun, but a potato bun is just as delicious. Tommy loved this!

MAKE THE KEY LIME TARTAR SAUCE: In a small bowl, combine the sour cream, mayo, pickles, dill, pickle juice, lime juice, salt, and black pepper and refrigerate until ready to serve.

Cook the blackened fish: In a small bowl, combine the paprika, cayenne, garlic powder, thyme, oregano, salt, and black pepper and mix to blend. Spritz the fish on both sides with oil and coat all over with the spice mix.

Spray the air fryer basket with oil. Working in batches, place the fish in the basket in a single layer and cook at 400°F until the fish flakes easily with a fork, 6 to 7 minutes, depending on the thickness of the fish, flipping halfway.

TO SERVE: Spread the tartar sauce on both sides of the buns. Add the fish, lettuce, tomato, and red onion. Eat right away.

No Air Fryer? No Problem!

Place the fish on a sheet pan covered with foil and broil 6 inches from the heating element for about 5 minutes, or until cooked through in the center and browned (no need to flip). (Alternatively, cook in a hot cast-iron skillet on both sides until browned.)

Per Serving (1 sandwich) | Calories 454 | **Protein 40 g** | Carbohydrate 23 g | Fiber 3.5 g | Sugars 6 g | Fat 23 g | Saturated Fat 8 g | Cholesterol 92 mg | Sodium 759 mg

KEY LIME TARTAR SAUCE

¼ cup reduced-fat sour cream or nondairy sour cream

3 tablespoons light mayonnaise

⅓ cup finely chopped dill pickles

1 tablespoon chopped fresh dill

1 tablespoon dill pickle juice

1 teaspoon lime juice

⅛ teaspoon kosher salt

⅛ teaspoon black pepper

BLACKENED FISH

1 tablespoon sweet paprika

½ teaspoon cayenne pepper

1 teaspoon garlic powder

1 teaspoon dried thyme

1 teaspoon dried oregano

1 teaspoon kosher salt

⅛ teaspoon black pepper

4 pieces skinless mahimahi, grouper, red snapper, or sea bass fillets (6 ounces each)

Olive oil spray

FOR SERVING

4 potato buns, soft whole wheat burger buns, or gluten-free buns

4 Boston lettuce leaves

4 slices tomato

Sliced red onion

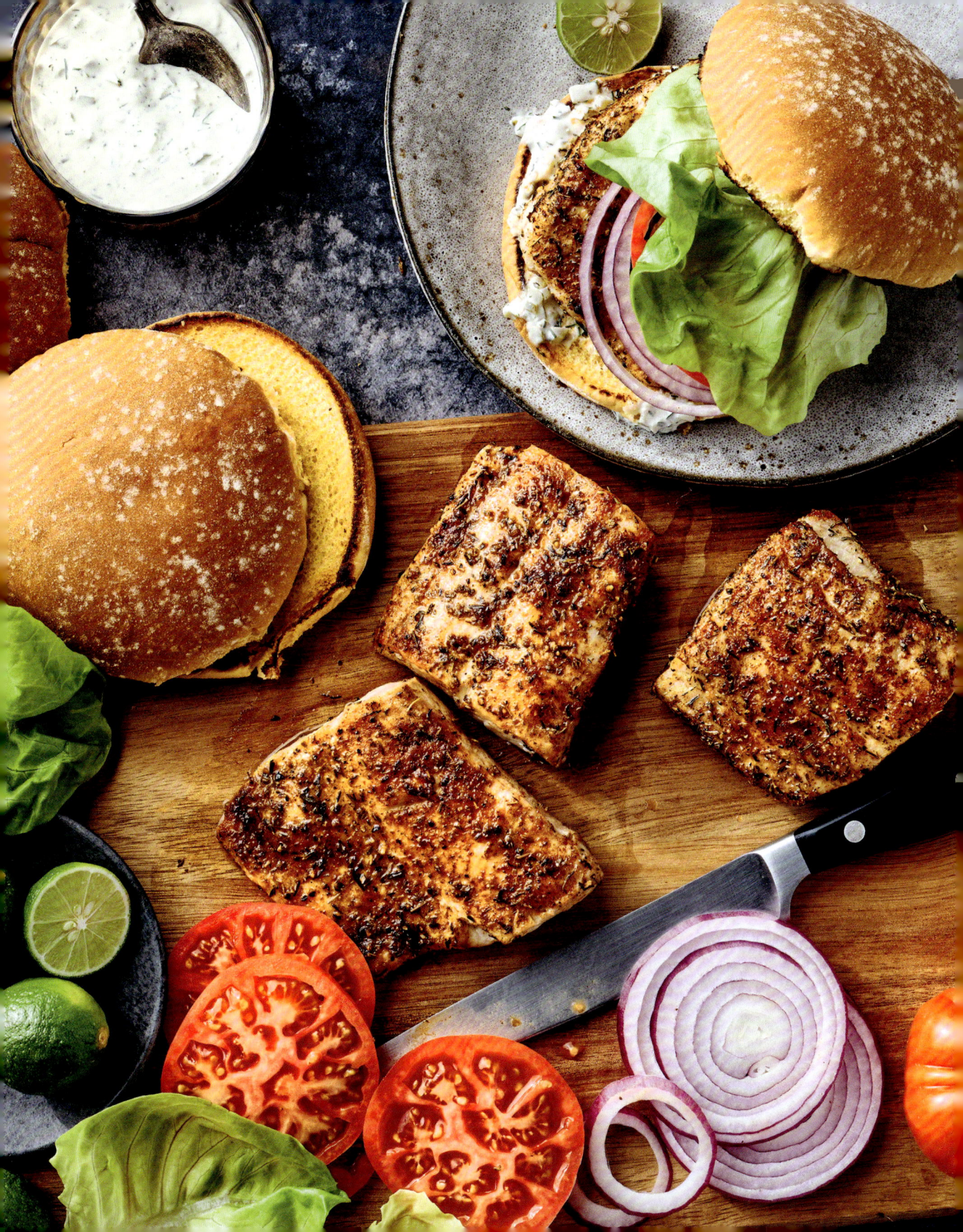

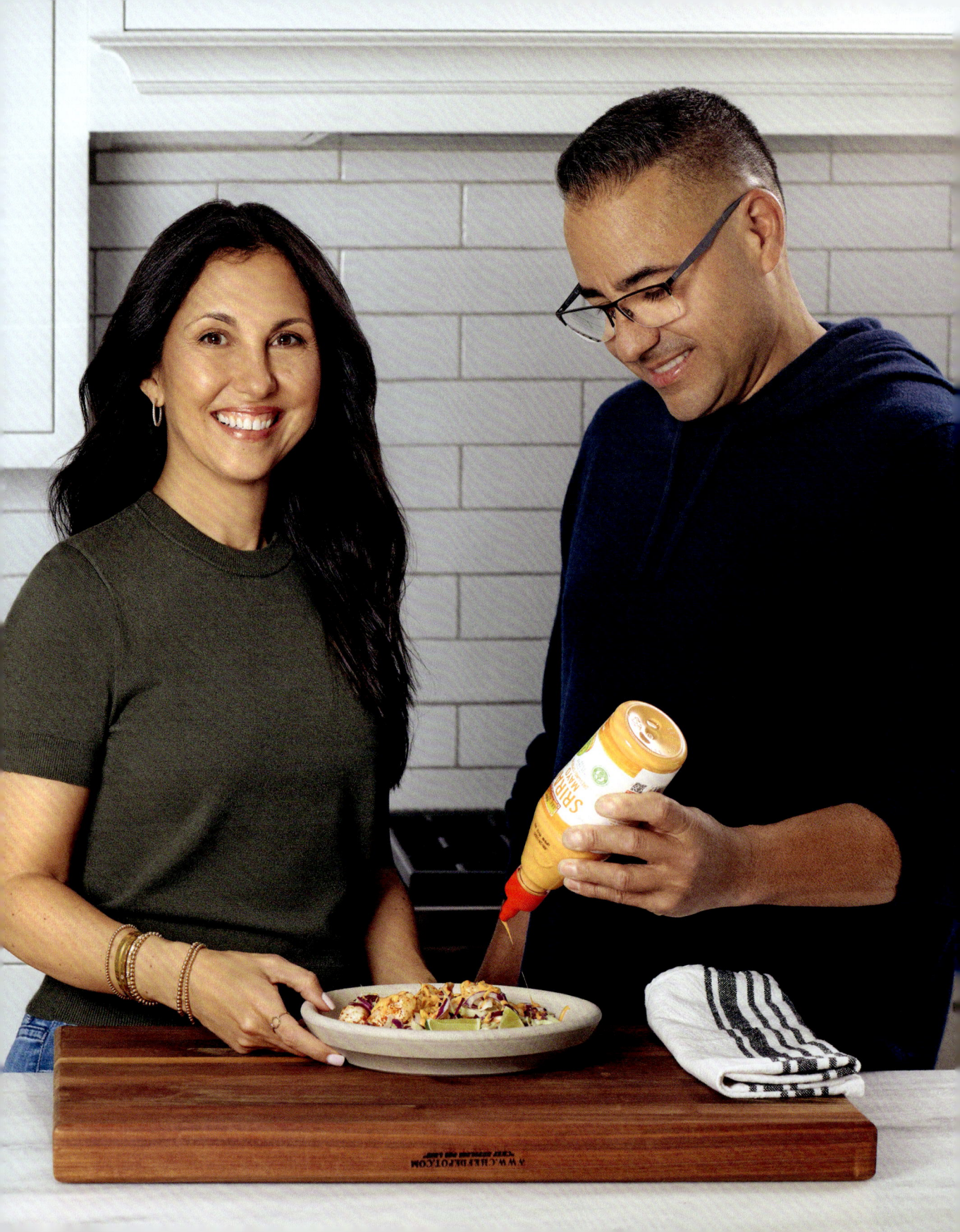

AIR FRYER FISH TACO BOWLS

If you want a high-protein, low-carb dish you can whip up in under 20 minutes, this is it! Sometimes the recipes I put the least amount of thought into turn out to be my most popular, and these fish bowls are the perfect example. I had some leftover fish with no plans on how I was going to use it, and since I always have cabbage in my refrigerator (because my daughter Madison loves cabbage slaw), I created these fish taco bowls and shared them with the world not expecting them to be so popular! They're super simple to prepare and can be made in the air fryer or a skillet.

Spritz the fish all over with oil and season with the Cajun seasoning. Cut 1 lime into wedges and halve the other.

In a small bowl, combine the mayo and Sriracha and squeeze in the juice of ½ lime. Add a little water until it's easy to drizzle. Set aside.

Air-fry the fish for 6 minutes at 400°F, shaking the basket halfway, until cooked through.

Meanwhile, combine the slaw with the olive oil, the juice of the remaining ½ lime, and the salt.

Divide the slaw among four bowls, then add the fish on the side and drizzle the spicy mayo over the fish. Serve with lime wedges and garnish with cilantro.

No Air Fryer? No Problem!
Heat a large skillet over high heat, spray with oil, and cook the fish for 5 to 6 minutes, flipping halfway, until cooked through.

SERVES 4

4 skinless white fish fillets, such as blackfish, mahimahi, or grouper (6 ounces each), cut into 1-inch pieces

Olive oil spray

2 to 3 teaspoons Cajun seasoning, to taste

2 limes

¼ cup mayonnaise

1 teaspoon Sriracha sauce or chipotle peppers in adobo sauce

5 cups coleslaw mix (red cabbage, green cabbage, and shredded carrots)

1½ teaspoons extra-virgin olive oil

½ teaspoon kosher salt

Chopped fresh cilantro, for garnish

Perfect Pairings
You can serve this with rice, quinoa, beans, avocado, or pickled red onions.

Per Serving (6 ounces fish + ¾ cup slaw) | Calories 418 | **Protein 32 g** | Carbohydrate 6 g | Fiber 2 g | Sugars 3 g | Fat 28 g | Saturated Fat 7 g | Cholesterol 95 mg | Sodium 558 mg

SPICY SALMON SUSHI BAKE

You've been asking for a lighter sushi bake, and I'm thrilled to finally deliver—it's good! I usually go for salmon or tuna when I order sushi, but since I prefer my tuna raw, salmon was the perfect choice here. This dish comes together in no time and it was an instant hit in my house. Even my aunt, who typically steers clear of raw sushi, couldn't get enough! This one's a keeper and will definitely be on my regular dinner rotation.

Preheat the oven to 425°F. Spray a 9 × 9-inch or an 8 × 8-inch baking dish with oil.

MAKE THE SPICY MAYO: In a small bowl, mix together mayo and Sriracha.

MAKE THE SALMON SUSHI BAKE: In a medium bowl, combine the vinegar and 1 teaspoon of the sesame oil. Add the rice and mix so that each grain is coated evenly.

In another medium bowl, combine the salmon, soy sauce, remaining 1 teaspoon sesame oil, 1 teaspoon of the Sriracha, and the scallion whites and mix together well until evenly combined.

Add a layer of seaweed to cover the bottom of the baking dish. Evenly spread the rice over the nori, then spread the salmon mixture on top.

Bake until the salmon is cooked and golden on top, 10 to 12 minutes.

Drizzle the top with the spicy mayo and the remaining 2 teaspoons Sriracha. Top with the avocado slices, spacing them out evenly. Sprinkle with the scallion greens and sesame seeds.

TO SERVE: Cut in 4 pieces and serve with more soy sauce on the side, if desired.

SERVES 4

Olive oil spray

SPICY MAYO

¼ cup Kewpie mayonnaise

2 tablespoons Sriracha sauce

SALMON SUSHI BAKE

1 tablespoon seasoned rice vinegar

2 teaspoons toasted sesame oil

2 cups cooked sticky white or brown rice (I like using frozen)

20 ounces skinless salmon fillet, finely chopped into small pieces

1½ tablespoons reduced-sodium soy sauce or gluten-free tamari, plus more (optional) for serving

3 teaspoons Sriracha sauce

¼ cup thinly sliced scallions, white and green parts kept separate

2 packs toasted nori seaweed snack sheets (12 sheets total)

3 ounces avocado (about 1 small Hass), thinly sliced and halved

1 teaspoon black and white sesame seeds

Per Serving (1 slice) | Calories 509 | **Protein 33 g** | Carbohydrate 27 g | Fiber 4 g | Sugars 4 g | Fat 28 g | Saturated Fat 3.5 g | Cholesterol 103 mg | Sodium 855 mg

Perfect Pairings
Serve this with cucumber sticks.

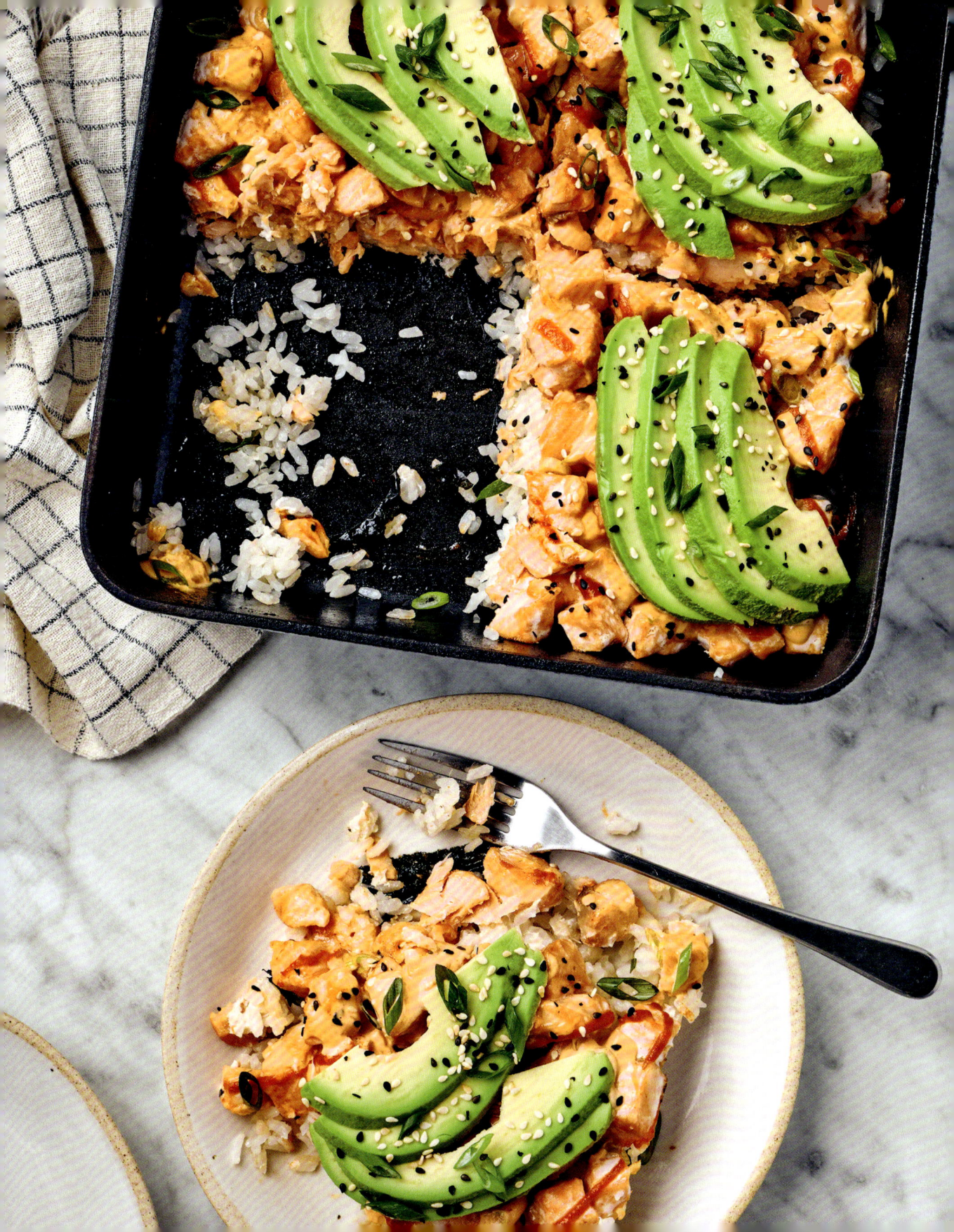

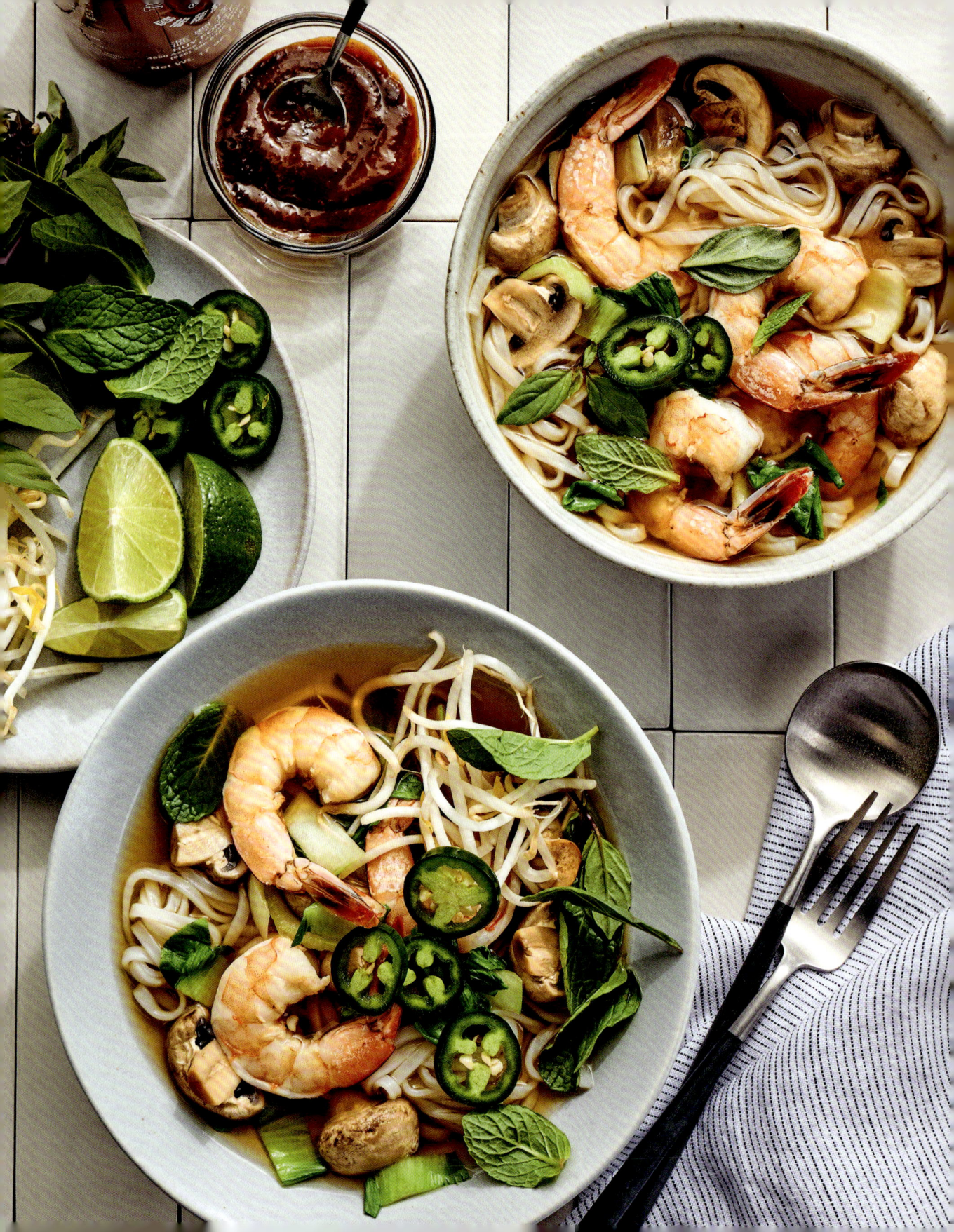

PHO THE LOVE OF SHRIMP

My family loves Vietnamese pho, and this quick pho-inspired soup makes smart use of kitchen scraps to create a shortcut stock that delivers deep, rich flavor with zero waste. You'll be amazed at the complexity achieved in under 30 minutes of simmering. It's a fan favorite on my Skinnytaste website, and while shrimp pho may not be as iconic as its beef or chicken counterparts, it's a lighter, equally satisfying take on the classic that still captures the essential pho experience. I swapped bok choy for cauliflower florets on my website, but feel free to use any veggies you have on hand.

If you're using frozen shrimp, thaw it completely and drain as much water as possible, using a paper towel to pat it dry. If you're using unfrozen, shell-on shrimp, peel and reserve the shells for the stock.

In a medium saucepan, combine the broth, fish sauce, soy sauce, cinnamon stick, star anise, fresh ginger, and shrimp shells (if applicable) and bring to a simmer over high heat.

Meanwhile, chop the leafy tops from the bunch of cilantro. Add all the stems to the saucepan. Chop ½ cup of the leaves for garnish and set aside.

Cook the broth until very fragrant, 20 to 25 minutes. Use a slotted spoon to remove and discard the solids. Keep at a gentle simmer.

Just before the broth is ready, fill a wide skillet with water and bring to a boil over high heat. Remove from the heat and add the rice noodles. Let the noodles soak for 3 to 5 minutes, or according to the package directions. Drain and set aside.

Add the mushrooms and bok choy to the broth and cook until the bok choy is tender but still crisp, 4 to 5 minutes. Add the shrimp and cook until firm, opaque, and pink, 1 to 2 minutes.

To serve, divide the rice noodles among four bowls. Using a slotted spoon, distribute the shrimp and veggies, about 1¼ cups per bowl. Ladle 1 cup broth over the top and garnish with the reserved chopped cilantro and any favorite toppings you desire. Serve immediately.

Per Serving (1 bowl) | Calories 321 | **Protein 31 g** | Carbohydrate 41 g | Fiber 2.5 g | Sugars 4 g | Fat 3 g | Saturated Fat 1 g | Cholesterol 169 mg | Sodium 1,420 mg

SERVES 4

1 pound large shrimp

6 cups chicken broth*

2 teaspoons fish sauce*

1 tablespoon reduced-sodium soy sauce

1 cinnamon stick

1 star anise pod

1-inch piece fresh ginger, sliced

1 bunch fresh cilantro

6 ounces thin rice noodles

8 ounces white mushrooms, halved

3 cups chopped baby bok choy (from 1 small head)

FOR SERVING (OPTIONAL)

Thinly sliced jalapeño, lime wedges, mung bean sprouts, fresh mint, Thai basil, sliced scallions, Sriracha sauce

*Read the label to be sure this product is gluten-free.

Acknowledgments

Creating a book is a collective effort, and I'm endlessly grateful for the incredible support I've received every step of the way—from the initial concept, to testing, to photography and design. This journey wouldn't have been possible without my Skinnytaste community, and without my amazing team and family by my side.

To the dedicated Skinnytaste readers and fans—you're the heart of this book. Seeing your love for my recipes in your kitchens and hearing about your health journeys fill me with so much happiness. Your enthusiasm for my high-protein recipes sparked the idea for this book, and I'm thrilled to bring it to life!

To my husband and two daughters, thank you for your unwavering support and for always being my eager taste testers, no matter the dish or the hour.

A special shout-out to my dear friend Heather K. Jones for being my partner and dietitian on this eighth cookbook. Your energy, positivity, and vision make the entire process a joy. And to Danielle Hazard for your attention to every little detail, and to the rest of Heather's team, Alexandra Beane and Jackie Price.

To my aunt Ligia Caldas, your help in the kitchen and the time we've spent together testing recipes mean the world to me—I truly couldn't do this without you. And to Camila Caldas, Nina Caldas, Katia Toninni, DyAnne Iandoli, Monica Stevens Le, and Erin Alvarez, whose invaluable contributions helped bring this book to life.

To my fierce agent, Janis Donnaud—your guidance and dedication are unparalleled, and I'm truly grateful for your support.

To the incredible team at Clarkson Potter—Jenn Sit, Elaine Hennig, Stephanie Huntwork, Jan Derevjanik, Mia Johnson, Patricia Shaw, Kim Tyner, Stephanie Davis, and Jina Stanfill—working with you all is a dream.

To the talented Eva Kolenko and her team, thank you for capturing such stunning photos. Thank you also to Victoria Janashvili for the lifestyle images.

Mom, Ivan, and the rest of my family—your love and support have been my foundation since day one, and I'm forever grateful.

And finally, to all my girlfriends, near and far—thank you for riding alongside me on this wild, wonderful adventure. Your encouragement means the world to me!

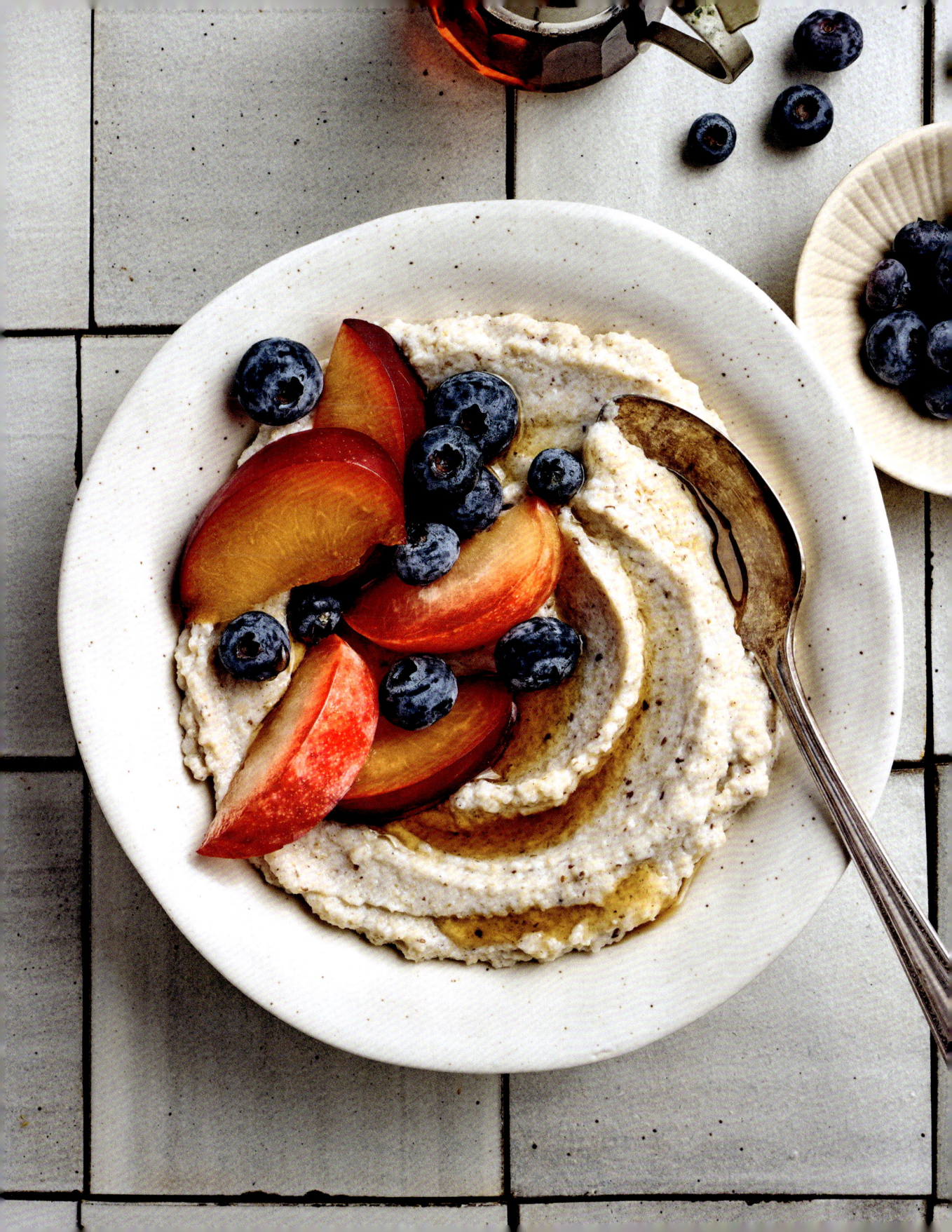

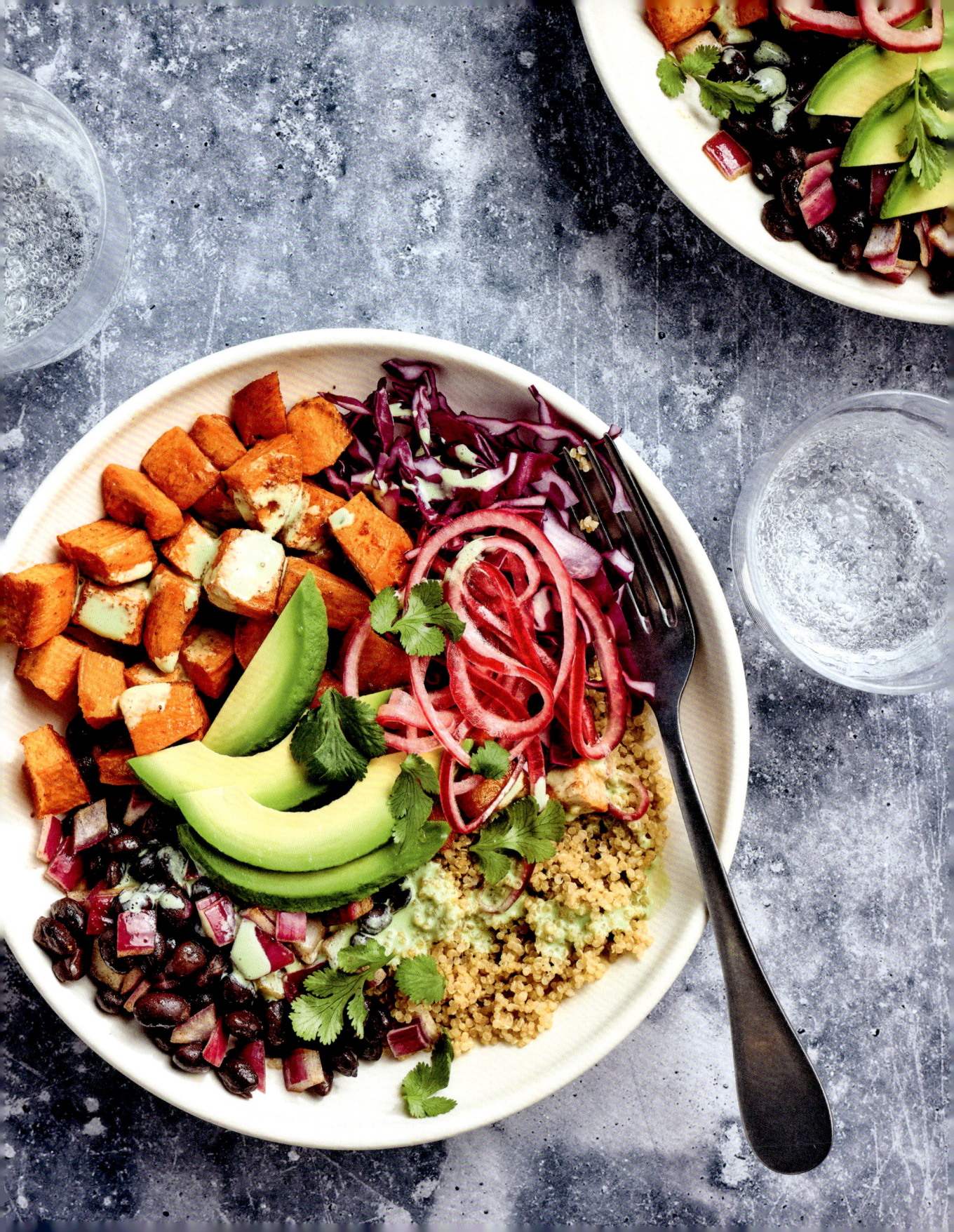

Index

CLARKSON POTTER/PUBLISHERS
An imprint of the Crown Publishing Group
A division of Penguin Random House LLC
1745 Broadway
New York, NY 10019
clarksonpotter.com
penguinrandomhouse.com

Library of Congress Cataloging-in-Publication Data
is available upon request.

ISBN 979-8-217-03394-2
Deluxe edition ISBN 979-8-217-03527-4
B&N Black Friday edition ISBN 979-8-217-03528-1
Ebook ISBN 979-8-217-03395-9

Editor: Jennifer Sit
Editorial assistant: Elaine Hennig
Designer: Jan Derevjanik
Design manager: Mia Johnson
Production designer: Christina Self
Production editor: Patricia Shaw
Production: Kim Tyner
Compositors: Merri Ann Morrell and Hannah Hunt
Food stylist: Emily Caneer | Food stylist assistant: Carrie Beyer
Lifestyle food stylist: Ksenia Radkevich
Prop stylist: Genesis Vallejo
Copy editor: Kate Slate
Proofreaders: Robin Slutzky, Mark McCauslin, Sigi Nacson, and Nicole Ramirez
Indexer: Elizabeth T. Parson
Publicist: Jina Stanfill
Marketer: Stephanie Davis

Manufactured in China

10 9 8 7 6 5 4 3 2 1

First Edition

The authorized representative in the EU for product safety and compliance is Penguin Random House Ireland, Morrison Chambers, 32 Nassau Street, Dublin D02 YH68, Ireland, https://eu-contact.penguin.ie.